BATTLE STATION SICK BAY

BATTLE STATION
Sick Bay

Navy Medicine in World War II

Jan K. Herman

Naval Institute Press
Annapolis, Maryland

© 1997 by Jan K. Herman

All rights reserved. No part of this book may be reproduced without written permission from the publisher.

Library of Congress Cataloging-in-Publication Data

Herman, Jan K.
    Battle station sick bay: Navy medicine in World War II / Jan K. Herman
      p. cm.
    Includes bibliographical references and index.
    ISBN 1-55750-361-3 (acid-free paper)
      1. World War, 1939–1945—Medical care—United States. 2. United States. Navy—Medical care. 3. Medicine, Naval—United States—History—20th century. 4. World War, 1939–1945—Personal narratives, American.   I. Title.
D807.U6H47 1997
940.54'7573—dc21   96-44536

Printed in the United States of America on acid-free paper ∞

04 03 02 01 00 99 98 97   9 8 7 6 5 4 3 2
First printing

Unless noted otherwise, all photos are from the Bureau of Medicine and Surgery Archives and are used by permission.

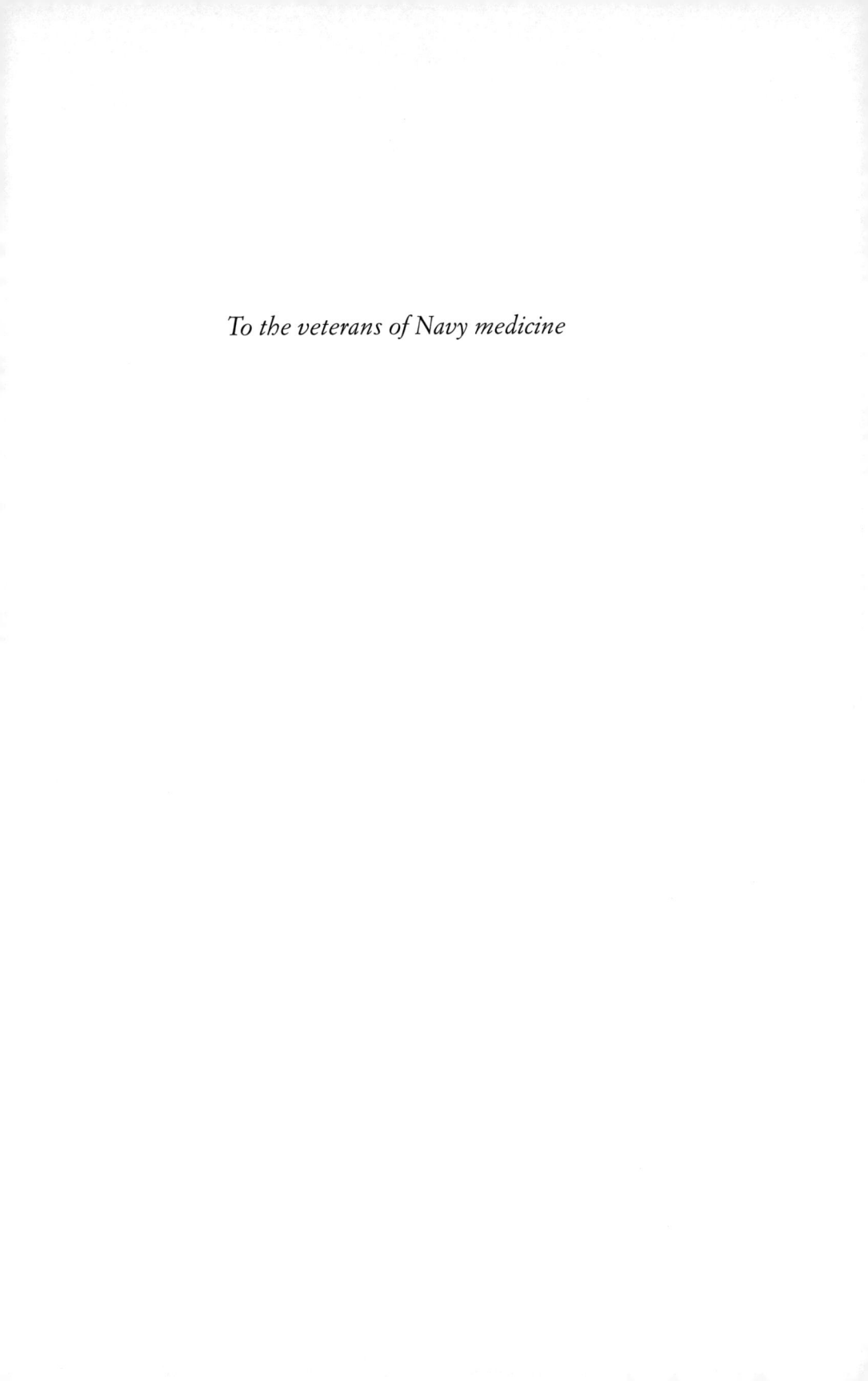

To the veterans of Navy medicine

CONTENTS

	Foreword	ix
	Preface	xi
	Introduction	1
ONE	Pearl Harbor	19
TWO	The Navy's War	35
THREE	Guests of the Emperor	61
FOUR	Island Warfare	83
FIVE	Submarine Surgeons	119
SIX	With the Surface Fleet	129
SEVEN	Mercy Ships	158
EIGHT	The Rice Paddy Navy	181
NINE	D-Day	189
TEN	Uncommon Duty	208
ELEVEN	Ecstatic to Be Free	224
TWELVE	Peace	238
	Glossary	251
	Bibliography	255
	Index	259

FOREWORD

Much of the history of Navy medicine in World War II resides in libraries and archives, embedded in official reports and documents seldom seen by anyone but scholars. Until now a significant portion of that untold history also lay hidden, buried in the memories of the veterans who, over fifty years ago, helped decide the contest between fascism and freedom.

The story of Navy medicine in World War II has not been told like this before. For the first time, an aging generation of physicians, nurses, and corpsmen tells the way it was, matter-of-factly, with pride and pathos but not without humor. These are recollections of men and women tested at Pearl Harbor, Corregidor, Guadalcanal, Peleliu, Normandy, Iwo Jima, and Okinawa. Some were aboard vessels under kamikaze attack, others languished in POW camps scattered throughout Japan and the Philippines.

The author shows us how oral history brings passion and color to a period that often appears as a one-dimensional chronicle of battles lost and won, punctuated by the dueling egos of generals and admirals. In this compilation, we appreciate as never before the single-minded purpose with which the ordinary men and women of Navy medicine dedicated themselves to their healing art, often under unimaginable circumstances. In the mirror of their sacrifices, we may ask ourselves: How does my generation measure up to theirs? What would I have done in their place?

Battle Station Sick Bay is a compelling book not because it evokes such self-examination but because it gives voice to the uncelebrated players in the most pivotal drama of our century.

Vice Adm. Harold M. Koenig, MC, USN
Surgeon General of the Navy

PREFACE

Pass the scuttlebutt with any World War II enlisted veteran of the Navy Medical Department and you will likely hear the heroic tale of how one of their own removed a shipmate's appendix while his patient and their submarine withstood an avalanche of Japanese depth charges.

When I first heard this story back in 1985, the theme sounded vaguely familiar. As a youngster and a fan of the 1950s TV series *The Silent Service,* I had seen such an episode. And hadn't a similar scenario appeared in the Hollywood film *Destination Tokyo?*

Not long thereafter, while thumbing through an old anthology, I discovered a story entitled "Doc Lipes Commandeers a Submarine's Wardroom." That was it! I now knew I had to find Doc Lipes and learn what had really happened nearly a half century earlier.

After a short search, I contacted Wheeler B. Lipes, then president of Memorial Medical Center in Corpus Christi, Texas, and conducted my first oral-history interview. Ten years and 130 oral histories later, that first talk with Doc Lipes would represent the birth of the Navy Medical Department's oral-history project.

I soon realized that the men and women of my parents' generation were already in their sixties, seventies, and eighties. The timing seemed right, with the fiftieth anniversary of the war rapidly approaching. Along with the articles, books, celebrations, reunions, and national attention that would focus on the significance of their contributions, many veterans might be willing to share memories.

And share them they did, often with unbounded enthusiasm. More than a few admitted that World War II was the pinnacle event in their lives. Nothing since 1945 had offered the same sense of purpose, adventure, and camaraderie born of shared danger and adversity. To others, though, World War II was not the zenith but a brief interlude, a stop along the way. They had gone on to other major adventures after the great crusade.

Nevertheless, many saw the interviews as their last opportunity to set the record straight, and a few wished to leave children and grandchildren a detailed record of their service. The sessions were very emotional. More than one confided that this was the first time in fifty years they had talked of their experiences. Neither wives nor children had heard any of it. After offering "I have nothing really important to contribute," they revealed significant episodes and events never before discussed.

Why had they remained silent for so many years? One physician offered an explanation. "When we got back from the war we tried to pick up where we left off. We married, raised families, threw ourselves into our work, and never found the time to contemplate what we'd been through. Now we're retired, the kids are gone, and we have plenty of time on our hands to think about what it all means."

As an oral historian, I became privy to long-dormant emotions—pride at having served, grief over losing beloved comrades, guilt at having survived. Some ex-POWs expressed the still-simmering hatred for their captors. And humor, the soldier's and sailor's timeless survival tool, wove its way through many accounts.

I gradually recognized that the project had become a two-way street. As interviewer, I earned a privilege many historians only dream of. If the discussions were a catharsis for the veterans, for me they were gripping testimony. It was thrilling to hear Dr. Henry Heimlich describe firsthand how a failed chest surgery performed on a wounded Chinese soldier was the first step to developing the lifesaving maneuver that made his name a household word; there was drama, even fifty years later, in Dr. Howard Bruenn's story of how he struggled to revive the fatally stricken FDR at Warm Springs, Georgia. Corpsman Stanley Dabrowski took me to

World War II Iwo Jima, where, under fire, he treated his first sucking chest wound; at that same loathsome little island, nurse Kathryn Van Wagner performed the un-nurselike act of lobbing a mortar round at the Japanese "to see what it was like." I tried to imagine how Dr. Ferdinand Berley must have felt when, after three years as a POW, he heard the radio voice of the emperor telling his nation that the war was over.

There were many accounts I had never read in any book, revelations filtered through a veteran's eyes about such highly charged events as Hiroshima and Nagasaki. Dr. Murray Glusman, a former POW, related how he and his fellow prisoners regarded the atomic bomb. Reduced to eating rice sweepings from warehouse floors and watery soup flavored with weeds, Glusman calculated that he and his comrades would not survive beyond October 1945. To them and the pitiful survivors of other camps, the atomic bombs meant salvation. With the nation again debating the significance and morality of our use of the bomb, here was a point of view worth contemplating.

Collecting these stories during the last decade has been fascinating. Not all interviews were face-to-face meetings; out of necessity, many began with an introductory telephone call and ended, many calls later, with a set of reminiscences successfully recorded, a new friendship in hand, and promises of a visit in the not-too-distant future. Because an individual's home can offer additional insight into a personality, I preferred meeting the men and women of Navy medicine on their own turf. Several interviews come to mind:

It was a brooding, overcast February day when I visited Dr. Howard Bruenn in his New York apartment overlooking the New Jersey Palisades across the Hudson. He was retired after spending a long, distinguished career on the staff of the Columbia Presbyterian Medical Center. Our discussions centered on what he referred to as the most exciting year of his life—March 1944 to April 1945. As Franklin Delano Roosevelt's cardiologist, Bruenn's job was to keep the gravely ill commander in chief alive while he prosecuted the war, oversaw domestic policy, ran for a fourth term, and negotiated the future of Europe with Winston Churchill and Joseph Stalin.

Even after a half century, Bruenn's recollections were clear and his loyalty unwavering for a revered leader he confessed was not of his political party. When we took a break for light refreshment, the old man showed me mementos in his study. One was a Soviet ruble note from

Yalta with three autographs across its face—Winston Churchill, Joseph Stalin, and Franklin D. Roosevelt.

On a bright summer day several years later in New Britain, Connecticut, I interviewed Stanley Dabrowski in his modest home close to the house he grew up in. Flowers and fruit trees were in full bloom in his manicured yard, which looked more like a park, and he was justifiably proud of his handiwork.

He told me that at age eighteen he became a corpsman: "the Navy had nice clean sheets and berths, three square meals a day, beautiful big battleships, carriers, destroyers . . ." It all had a familiar ring. It was the account of many young men just out of high school who joined the Navy to stay out of foxholes. Dabrowski ended up serving with the Marines at Iwo Jima.

He escorted me to his den, which had the aura of a shrine. Everywhere were souvenirs of the man's service—dog tag, heavy steel helmet, a miniature of the Marine Corps memorial, and the most celebrated photograph of World War II, the flag raising at Iwo Jima, inscribed to Dabrowski and autographed by Joe Rosenthal, the man who took that immortal image.

I met others, such as Henry Heimlich, at their workplaces. At the Heimlich Institute in Cincinnati, the noted physician supports a variety of medical projects and now promotes his maneuver for resuscitating drowning victims. "What's it like to have your name in the dictionary?" I asked him.

"What can I say?" he responded. "Did you know a six-year-old boy saved his four-year-old brother just last week using the maneuver? It was on the national news." Nothing needed to be added.

When we spoke of his World War II service as a young Navy doctor on "prolonged extra-hazardous overseas duty in China," his eyes lit up. Even with the brilliant accomplishments of the last fifty years, those adventures as a jaygee were still the most exciting of his life.

It had just begun snowing in the former coal-mining town of Exeter, Pennsylvania, as I neared the end of a session with retired Navy nurse Ann Bernatitus. "You had better take my shovel with you," she ordered, pointing out that an additional eight inches were expected that evening. I complied, realizing that an argument with this feisty survivor of Bataan and Corregidor would be fruitless. Of the twelve Navy nurses stationed in the Philippines at the beginning of the war, Bernatitus was the only one who escaped capture. I had been so enthralled by her saga that the impending blizzard had seemed trivial.

As you read the first-person accounts that follow, I think you will find, as I did, that very little qualifies as trivial.

On the contrary, many of the stories put new perspective on historical events many of us have taken for granted.

This book is based on the recollections of World War II veterans—personal testimony derived from interviews, or accounts found in letters and other documents in the Bureau of Medicine and Surgery archives. Some stories have previously appeared in the *Hospital Corps Quarterly,* a rare journal seldom seen outside the military medical community. Others have been published in *Navy Medicine,* the Navy Medical Department's bimonthly journal. With the exception of the interviews with Cecil Coggins by Katherine Herbig and with Grace Lally by Irene Matthews, I conducted all of the interviews between 1984 and 1996. *Battle Station Sick Bay* is the story of the most cataclysmic event of the twentieth century as told by the men and women of the Navy Medical Department who were there.

I am grateful not only to the veterans who spent long hours dictating their recollections into a microphone, but also to two others whose efforts and support helped make this book possible: my aide and colleague, David R. Klubes, separated the wheat from the chaff; my wife, De, for many months read drafts, suggested refinements, and put up with the exchange of family evenings and weekends for what became known as The Night Shift.

BATTLE STATION SICK BAY

Introduction

When Japanese bombs fell on Pearl Harbor, 7 December 1941, Navy medicine was already 166 years old. The physicians, dentists, nurses, and corpsmen who treated the badly burned and wounded survivors of that tragedy could trace their heritage back to the very birth of the Navy in 1775.

During the first year of the Revolution, the Continental Congress authorized both a Navy and Marine Corps. It also provided for surgeons and surgeons' mates and for the setting apart of spaces aboard naval vessels for treating the sick and injured. These spaces became known as sick berths and later sick bays. Because Congress made no allowance for a central organization to run navy medical matters, ships' captains selected and hired surgeons and surgeons' mates to care for the crew and accompanying marines. Navy medical personnel ever since have provided medical care to the Marine Corps.

Joseph Harrison of the *Alfred* and Henry Tillinghast of the *Providence* share the distinction of being the first surgeons to serve in the Continental Navy. Assisting these two pioneers and their fellow surgeons and surgeons' mates were the so-called Loblolly Boys, named for the thick porridge fed to the sick aboard ship. Trained to feed, wash, and shave the sick and wounded, these men also had the dubious honor of providing containers for amputated limbs, hot tar for cauterizing the stumps, and sand to spread on the decks to absorb any blood that might be shed during combat and surgical procedures. Loblolly Boys were the predecessors of the modern corpsmen.

After independence, the Continental Navy went out of business and the new nation remained without a navy until 1794, when Congress authorized six new ships to be built. These vessels were the nucleus for the new navy. Each was to have a surgeon and, for the larger ships, two additional surgeon's mates.

The new Department of the Navy was born in 1798. The Board of Navy Commissioners, which had the responsibility for conducting the navy's business, was cumbersome and inefficient. Because no central organization existed for medical personnel, the task of providing medical care suffered accordingly. Even though a congressional act provided for the establishment of naval hospitals in 1810, it took another twenty years to build the first permanent naval hospital.

On 31 August 1842, Congress passed a naval appropriations bill that replaced the Board of Commissioners with five bureaus controlling specific navy functions such as navigation and ordnance. The Bureau of Medicine and Surgery (BuMed) became the central administrative headquarters for the Navy Medical Department, and those names became interchangeable. BuMed's job was to oversee the construction of naval hospitals, procure medical supplies, hire competent physicians, and develop medical standards for the practice of Navy medicine.

The outbreak of the Civil War in April 1861 saw a tremendous expansion in the Navy's size. As President Abraham Lincoln called for a blockade of southern ports, the Medical Department's heavy responsibilities to the fleet proceeded apace.

Surgeons and surgeons' mates practiced their healing art aboard sailing ships and ironclads and, for the first time, aboard the first navy hospital ship. This vessel was the *Red Rover,* a captured Confederate sidewheeler that had been reconfigured as a hospital for the care of the sick and wounded. Among the *Red Rover*'s medical staff of about thirty were four Sisters of the Order of the Holy Cross, the first women to serve on a U.S. Navy ship. Assisted by several lay nurses' aides, these women were the predecessors of today's Navy Nurse Corps.

Due in part to a growing sentiment for providing better medical care for naval personnel, in 1871 Congress passed an appropriations act establishing the Medical Corps. Navy physicians had finally achieved full recognition as naval officers.

Meanwhile, by the mid-nineteenth century, the Loblolly Boys of the Revolutionary War began functioning as male nurses. After the outbreak of the Civil War, ships with a complement of under two hundred were allowed one male nurse, two nurses for larger ships. Navy Regulations in 1876 dropped the nurse title and adopted *bayman,* which was in common use by that time.

About the mid-1840s, the designation surgeon's steward appeared. These men ranked next after the master-at-arms, who was the senior petty officer on the ship. In 1866 steward's mates became known as apothecaries, revealing their primary task of distributing drugs. Nevertheless, baymen were still responsible for the everyday care of the sick and wounded.

In 1898, the same year the United States fought the Spanish-American War, Congress passed legislation establishing the Hospital Corps. The first group of corpsmen numbered but twenty-five pharmacists with the rank, pay, and privileges of warrant officers.

Although nurses made their debut aboard the *Red Rover* during the Civil War, it was 1898 before the first trained nurses cared for war casualties at the Norfolk Naval Hospital. These civilian women, although working for the Navy, were neither enrolled nor enlisted as naval personnel. Following the creation of the Army Nurse Corps in 1902 by congressional act, BuMed campaigned for a similar corps for the navy. That struggle finally paid off in 1908 with the establishment of the Nurse Corps. The first group of nurses to report for duty have since been known as the Sacred Twenty.

As with the Nurse Corps, there long had been the need for a professional Dental Corps. Since Revolutionary War days, naval personnel had had to rely on civilian dentists or ships' surgeons for dental treatment. In 1912 Congress finally authorized the Dental Corps, and the following year thirty dentists began their duties.

The United States' entry into World War I marked the most dramatic expansion of the Medical Department since the Civil War. Thirty-eight physicians, 5 dentists, and 348 corpsmen served with the Marine Brigade in France, distinguishing themselves in nearly all campaigns on the western front until the Armistice. Seventeen corpsmen were killed in action.

Two who returned home received the Medal of Honor. Two physicians and a dentist, Lt. (jg) Weeden Osborne, also were awarded the nation's highest honor, the latter following his death at the front.

The rapid expansion of the Navy and its Medical Department during the war quickly reversed itself in the 1920s. The Depression and renewed isolationism resulted in lean years for the Navy. Military budgets shrank under the Hoover administration and manpower dwindled. With reduced operations, warships either remained in port or were taken out of service. Nevertheless, Navy medicine prepared for future conflicts by developing base hospitals that could be moved and assembled on short notice; devising new systems to examine recruits; studying the latest advances in field sanitation; maintaining and training an adequate reserve for war of physicians, dentists, nurses, and corpsmen; and supporting the Marine Corps. BuMed also concerned itself with the new technology advanced by the recent war. It developed defense against chemical warfare, protection of submariners, and training of flight surgeons and undersea medical officers for the Navy's growing aviation and submarine communities.

The fleet continued to conduct periodic but abbreviated exercises, and a fully equipped, modern hospital ship usually took part. Until the USS *Solace* joined the Pacific Fleet in the summer of 1941, the Navy's sole hospital ship, the USS *Relief,* took turns in both the Atlantic and Pacific.

Despite reductions in military expenditures and the nation's isolationist tilt, the United States still had a modest foreign policy to maintain. Repeated interventions in the 1930s saw the Marines operating in the jungles of Central America, with Navy medical support as always.

Because the United States had traditional concerns in the Far East, American gunboats of the Yangtze Patrol cruised Chinese rivers safeguarding American missionaries and commercial interests. The Yangtze Patrol's blue-water parent organization, the Asiatic Fleet, maintained a token U.S naval presence in far Pacific waters. However, by the mid-1930s its obsolescent ships were no match for a superior Japanese fleet.

In 1931 Japan seized Manchuria and six years later invaded China proper. As the Japanese became more aggressive, relations with the United States soured. The Rape of Nanking, as it was known, and the continued brutalization of the Chinese revolted Americans. The *Panay* incident in December 1937 (in which Japanese planes sank the American gunboat) and U.S. sanctions directed toward thwarting Japanese expansionism presaged the inevitability of war between the two nations.

Meanwhile the European situation deteriorated, as Adolf Hitler consolidated his power and Germany rearmed. Benito Mussolini's ruthless invasion of Ethiopia and Japan's Chinese adventures demonstrated the League of Nations's failure as a peacekeeper and doomed it to an early death.

Thoroughly traumatized after losing a whole generation of young men in the trenches of World War I, France and Britain embraced the hazardous policy of appeasement. In Europe and Asia, fascism and imperialism marched unopposed. And the clock was ticking.

Superimposed over all was the Great Depression. Many young American men and women of limited means and with dim prospects saw a military career as a way up. The Army and Navy offered security, an education, and a future. And those with a college degree could compete for a position in the elite officer corps of either service. Qualified women might join the Army or Navy Nurse Corps. If one further aspired to a specialized profession in medicine and exotic locales in which to practice, a career as a military doctor was attractive indeed.

On the eve of World War II three young men took the oath of allegiance. One was an enlisted sailor, the other two commissioned officer-physicians. All three would sample the adventure promised in recruiting posters. After Pearl Harbor, all would taste combat firsthand.

BATTLESHIP SAILOR

Wheeler Lipes joined the Navy at age sixteen during the worst years of the Great Depression. He went through basic training in Norfolk, Virginia, and was assigned to Hospital Corps school at San Diego for further training. During the month-and-a-half trip to the West Coast, he served as a crewman aboard the ammunition ship USS *Nitro* (AE-2). Lipes soon learned what chores were expected of a common sailor. Later, as a corpsman assigned to a battleship, he experienced the rigorous discipline of the prewar Navy.

On the *Nitro* I was up scrubbing those decks at four o'clock in the morning using holystones, sand, and saltwater. There's a way you have to use a handle from a scrubber to make a holystone go back and forth on that wood. Then you bleached the deck until it became white with the salt and the sun. What a job!

Once I got to Hospital Corps school in San Diego we learned anatomy, physiology, pharmacy, general administration, clerical things, laboratory, X ray, nursing, a broad spectrum of those things which you would need in health care.

Those of us in that school recognized the value of getting an education. In those days, people had no jobs and usually no homes. But I thought the Depression was a time of prosperity, especially in the Navy. It [the Navy] gave us security, an education, and a future, which the country didn't really have at the time.

However, the rigidity of the Navy was evident. The only change that had been made since John Adams's time was that they had done away with keelhauling and flogging.

A friend of mine, a third-class pharmacist's mate, was three minutes late for muster at eight o'clock in the morning, and they gave him a bad-conduct discharge. When the war broke out, he came back into the Navy as a second class. He went with the Marines and had all sorts of commendations for valor.

But this was the extreme. So was my getting a thirty-day restriction. I had set a rack of six thermometers on the foot of the bed. The patient moved his foot and they flipped off on the floor and broke. I had to waste the executive officer's time to appear before a mast to talk about my terrible offense of breaking those thermometers.[1]

When I left Hospital Corps school in 1937, they sent me to the receiving ship at the destroyer base in San Diego. There I had to await transfer to the USS *Texas* [BB-35]. We lay to in Coronado Roads waiting for the *Texas* to show up. We finally went aboard and went through the Panama Canal and on into Norfolk.

I worked in the pharmacy on the *Texas* with fourteen or fifteen other pharmacist's mates. We had assignments in the sick bay itself—nursing care, making beds. In the pharmacy, you were triturating, pounding

---

1. A mast was a hearing for a minor offense before one's commanding officer that could result in non-judicial punishment.

capsules, doing whatever. We also participated in the various drills for which the medical department has to be ready.

The pharmacy was a long, narrow room, had a little counter, and behind that, under the porthole, a long leather bench. Sometimes I used to sleep on that bench rather than down in a hole someplace. But usually I slept in a hammock.

Your hammock had to be wrapped around your seabag. The hammock was brought around the seabag, tied up, and secured, so that you picked up the seabag and hammock all as one unit. It was an ingenious invention. There were bins on the outboard section where you stowed your seabags.

When they put out the signal you hooked your hammocks up. The berthing area extended a good long distance. I guess there must have been twenty people. When you were sick, it was a struggle getting in and out of that hammock. But you slept well, because it didn't matter what the ship did. Hammocks were practical.

It was hot below decks and there was no air-conditioning. Under way at sea, I used to take a blanket and go up under the number-one turret. Under that forward turret, you looked right up at solid steel, maybe fourteen or eighteen inches from your face. But there was always wind under there and it was cool. You always found a lot of people sleeping under the turrets.

If you look back in the history of sailing ships, we were doing the same things on the *Texas* that Lord Nelson and his crew did. With the hammocks stowed, the gun deck became the mess deck. There were long baronial-type tables with legs that folded. When we weren't eating, you'd fold the legs and up went the tables, fastened into the ceiling on some hooks.

With that table in the overhead the area was empty, like a big room with portholes along the side and those bin arrangements for the hammocks and seabags. That big open area was then ready to receive casualties or whatever was necessary to do when engagements were being fought.

At chow time, whoever the mess cook was would go to the galley and get a stack of interlocking tureens. They would stack, and they had a frame around them that snapped at the top so things didn't get spilled. He would take that rack, put the food in, and come back and serve it at the table on the mess deck.

Those of us in the medical department did a little better than most people because we would eat many of our meals in the sick bay. When we'd get food for the patients, we got enough for us. The food was excellent. I used to look forward to a meal that was fairly standard in the Navy, especially in naval hospitals—a New England boiled dinner. They'd have potatoes, cabbage, and carrots, and it was just excellent.

One of the things I remember was that terrible dog watch—twelve to two. You'd come off the bridge as a lookout when your watch was over. If you went by the galley at that time of morning, they were cooking navy beans and making fresh bread. I don't think you could avoid going by and getting some. You would get a big soup bowl full of beans and big slab of bread. It was a good reward for a wet, cold night up on that bridge.

The battleship navy was a rugged, rigid navy. One time we were in the Canal Zone tied up at the pier in Balboa. Liberty began on the hour, exactly on the hour. If you missed that group to go ashore, you had to wait until the next full hour—ten o'clock, eleven o'clock, twelve o'clock.

I had on a pair of bell-bottom trousers, which you weren't supposed to wear on liberty. We were lined up for inspection. The officer of the deck came down and inspected everybody, giving us left face and right face. And then it was over the gangway and under the pier. Well, I got to the left-face part all right, but when I made the right face and put my foot up to take that first step to go over the gangway, they took me out of ranks because of those bell-bottom trousers. I had to wait for the next cycle. They sent a coxswain with me back down to my locker. He took my bell-bottom trousers and a huge pair of canvas scissors and cut them up in little pieces.

ON THE ASIATIC STATION

Lt. (jg) Ferdinand Berley joined the Navy as a line officer fresh out of college in 1934, but his true ambition was to become a navy physician. Times were bad and the few Navy medical officers on active duty were kept busy caring for young men at Civilian Conservation Corps (CCC) camps scattered around the country.

In 1937, the year Berley graduated from Northwestern Medical School, the Navy had only twenty openings for new physicians. Young Dr. Berley took the examination and secured one of them.

After a surgical internship at the San Diego Naval Hospital, he volunteered for duty with the Asiatic Fleet. First as a destroyer-division medical officer and then a physician assigned to the 4th Marines, Berley saw the Orient as quite a contrast from what he'd left behind.

China of the late 1930s was a nation of extremes—grinding poverty and indecent wealth. As its largest port, Shanghai was certainly the most westernized of cities, a condition brought about by years of foreign presence. This was evident in its architecture and by the number of Americans, Russians, Germans, French, and British who resided in specially designated sections of the city and traveled its beggar-filled streets in coolie-drawn rickshaws.

Shanghai was divided into foreign enclaves, each immune from Chinese law and enjoying the protection of its own troops and gunboats. In the squalid Chinese quarter where the so-called Green Gang ruled, opium dens and houses of prostitution flourished amidst crime and the open exploitation of Chinese citizens.

Adding to the misery was the harvest of Japanese imperialism. Bodies of victims slain by the invaders floated down Soochow Creek and choked Shanghai's canals; destitute refugees clogged its streets and regularly froze to death during the cold winter nights.

I arrived in Manila in September of 1939 and was assigned as medical officer of Destroyer Division 58. At that time there was a medical officer for four destroyers which constituted a division. A squadron was made up of three divisions. The four ships in DesDiv 58 were the *Parrott* [DD-218], the *Bulmer* [DD-222], the *Edsall* [DD-219], and the *Stewart* [DD-224]. My quarters were on the *Parrott*.

As the medical officer, I was responsible for the health of crews and staffs. When we were together, I would hold sick call once a week or whenever necessary. Each of the destroyers had a chief or first-class pharmacist's mate, and they were darned good. In fact, they were as good as any doctors.

One of the problems we had in those days was treating syphilitics. Part of the treatment consisted of intravenous drugs. I had written several letters requesting permission for some of my pharmacist's mates to give the drugs because many times we would be separated for several weeks at a time. I might not see one of my ships for two weeks and that might interrupt the treatment. We used salvarsan, which we gave intravenously, and intramuscular bismuth preparation. I never did get permission.

In February of 1940 the *Parrott* was ordered to south China for a month's duty at Swatow and Amoy. When we arrived in Amoy, liberty was not allowed in Amoy proper but on a small island which lay across the bay from Amoy called Kulangsu. It was a beautiful island with a shrine at the very highest point that could be seen for miles around, just like a Chinese painting.

The medical officer of the *Asheville* and his corpsman conducted me and my corpsman on a tour of the bars around Kulangsu and on his recommendation only one passed, a bar operated by a former mess boy named Sam. I made an agreement with Sam to set up a prophylactic station on the second floor, and each afternoon upon coming ashore, I would inspect the new prostitutes who came to work there.

A Japanese destroyer was also in the harbor—the *Harukaze,* a beautiful ship compared to the old four-stackers that comprised the destroyers of the Asiatic Fleet. On the 2,600th anniversary of the founding of the Japanese Empire the skipper of the *Parrott,* Butch Parker, sent an ensign to the *Harukaze* to see whether they were going to dress ship [display their flags]. If they were, Parker would dress ship to return the honor. They told the ensign that they were not going to, but he returned with an invitation from the captain to come aboard, which we did. They had chairs set up for us amidships and put on an exhibition of bayonet and sword exercises. Afterward, we were invited to their wardroom and served cheese and scotch.

Two weeks later we sailed for Swatow and, lo and behold, there was the *Harukaze* at anchor. They must have known of our plans well ahead of time. They invited us aboard and we were treated to a luncheon by the captain in charge of the port, a very gracious host. The luncheon was complete with refreshments and geisha girls.

In those days the destroyers spent the hot months—June, July, and August—in Tsingtao and Chefoo, with a stop off in Shanghai on the return to the Philippines. The wives would follow to Tsingtao and

Chefoo and there they would live. They had their own rickshaw boys outfitted with uniforms, and amahs, Chinese servants who acted as cooks and babysitters. Life on the Asiatic station was pretty plush.

Living in Shanghai as a bachelor was most interesting. The European powers were at war, so the Americans had the run of the city. There were two parts to Shanghai, the international settlement and the French. On the outskirts of the settlements was an international police force and guards with barricades to inspect cars coming in. Something was going on nearly every day. The newspapers were always reporting a bombing or a kidnapping.

The Japanese were on the opposite side of Soochow Creek. They had their sentries on one side of the bridge and the Marines on the international side. There were no sampans along the bank on the Japanese side. All the sampans were on the international side. People lived and died on those sampans; they were truly boat people.

The Japanese were not allowed to come into the international settlements unless they had permission, and we were not allowed in their section unless we had their permission. And they were constantly creating incidents.

On the outskirts of the international settlement were several nightclubs, several of which were placed out of bounds because of the incidents that might occur there. The Japanese controlled many of them.

I was assigned to the urology ward at the regimental hospital, on a street named Gordon Loo. I knew nothing about urology except what I'd learned at medical school. I would have the duty about every third day overnight; the normal hours ran from eight o'clock to four. Our Marine driver would pick me up and take me to the hospital. I'd have lunch there and then he'd take me back to my quarters. In the winter we counted as many as eight bodies along the way, lying on the street near the curb. This was very common.

About two or three months before I left Shanghai, we began taking conditioning hikes because the Marines at that time had gotten absolutely spoiled. Once a week in the morning we marched through the streets of Shanghai and always saw women coming out to empty their toilets—potties—in the honey cart that came by. Our hike took us down along the Whangpoo River. The stench was terrific in the area where they unloaded the honey carts onto barges to be used for fertilizer. And a little farther down were barges loaded with coffins. The Chinese believed that their bodies should be returned to their place of birth. These coffins may have been on those barges for a year or more waiting to be taken where they supposed to go. We always had to hold our noses when we went by.

One time we saw a cart loaded with rice sacks just ahead of us as we proceeded up the street. All of a sudden, out of nowhere, a bunch of people appeared and swarmed all over the cart climbing over the top of one another. They had pockets in their aprons, and within three minutes those sacks were completely empty. It was just like a pack of rats. The coolies who were carting that stuff—there were about five of them—stood around completely dazed.

While in Shanghai, I was given temporary duty on board the *Isabel* [PY-10], a river gunboat. The *Isabel* was the flagship of the Asiatic Fleet. We cruised all the way up the Yangtze to a place called Wuhu where I met a woman doctor who was the chief of surgery there at the hospital. She and I spent the time discussing medicine. The next morning she invited me to assist her in operations. She had so many cases, it was unbelievable.

I saw things there I had never seen before. Of course, in those days, in general surgery you did everything—brain surgery, orthopedics, everything. And she did all of that. We used cotton for sutures. I had been used to using catgut and silk, but never cotton. After World War II, cotton became very commonly used for sutures. We used paper for sponges and wore two pairs of gloves. Because they didn't have equipment to sterilize with, the instruments were boiled, put in a Lysol solution, and then rinsed off with sterile water.

This was in December of 1940. After Col. Sam Howard, our new commanding officer, came and took over the 4th Marines, he allowed bachelor officers to live in the French section if they wished. Prior to that, we could only live in the international section. There were three Marine officers down the hall from me and we got together and got ourselves a penthouse in the French quarter. We had the furniture made, had a number-one boy, a cook, and a coolie. All the coolie did was sit off in the kitchen and open the door for us; we never carried a key. We lived like kings.

MR. ROOSEVELT'S WAR

On 1 September 1939 Hitler unleashed his mechanized divisions and Stukas on Poland, igniting World War II. Most American citizens may have sympathized with the European democracies, but a Congress strongly influenced by persistent and highly vocal isolationist sentiment was determined to keep the war on the other side of the Atlantic. President Roosevelt argued that the best way to do this, short of intervention, was to aid Britain and France.

At first, the threat of German U-boats operating in contiguous waters such as the Caribbean gave the president the pretext to order the Navy to track all belligerent ships, with an emphasis on U-boats and other vessels flying the German flag. Their positions were then broadcast on frequencies monitored by the British. Roosevelt's distaste for Hitler and his sympathy for the Allies was slowly but surely maneuvering the United States into outright hostilities.

> Dr. Lewis L. Haynes, still a very junior officer assigned to the outpatient dispensary at the U.S. Naval Base Norfolk, Virginia, got an unexpected opportunity to participate in Mr. Roosevelt's war. It was December 1939.

I was ordered to depart at once to Destroyer Division 62, as the doctor had become ill and they were sailing the next day. I dashed home, packed, and went to sea. The division had four destroyers, the *Overton* [DD-239], the *Bainbridge* [DD-246], the *Sturtevant* [DD-240], and the *Reuben James* [DD-245].

We first went to Key West, Florida, for "neutrality patrol." This was in January or February 1940. We went out on patrol for seven days, came into port for three or four days, and then went back on patrol for seven days. Our orders were to follow any ship belonging to nations that were at war in Europe and broadcast our position every fifteen minutes. This meant German ships coming out of Brazil and other South American ports. The British knew where all their ships were and when we were broadcasting they knew we weren't following a British man-of-war but a German ship. We felt like Judas's goats and were not happy with this assignment. One German ship sent us a message: "Are you here to protect me." Our skipper replied, "No. We're here only in the interests of American neutrality." We set up pools on the destroyer as to the time the British destroyers would show up to catch the German vessel. And when they arrived, the Germans scuttled the *Odenwald* and got into lifeboats. The British took them on board and we resumed our patrol.

I recall friendliness toward the British and resentment toward the Germans, but I don't recall any great hostility. The hostility came after the invasion of France in June 1940 and the stories began coming out. Suddenly we realized that sooner or later, we were going to war with Germany.

Shortly after Germany defeated France, we received orders to join a newly formed fleet. It seems that some of the French fleet sympathetic to the Vichy government, an aircraft carrier, a cruiser, and some destroyers, had just crossed the Atlantic and were now in Martinique. President Roosevelt was very upset that these armed combatants were now in the Caribbean. Invoking the Monroe Doctrine, he asked them to disarm but they would not. So our orders were to prepare for the invasion of Martinique.

We had transports with Marines and the most antiquated landing equipment you've ever seen. There were old-fashioned landing craft—pre-Higgins boats. We left Guantanamo Bay every day to practice-fire our guns at Culebra Island, an island off the Puerto Rican coast. And the Marines made practice landings.

When we arrived, the Vichy French backed down, took their planes off the carrier, off-loaded ammunition, and allowed the United States to put observers ashore. The ships remained in the harbor until the end of the war. We returned to Guantanamo Bay, the invasion fleet dispersed, and we went back to our neutrality patrol. For a time we even patrolled out of Panama and covered the whole Caribbean.

At first we only had five officers aboard the *Bainbridge*. The commanding officer, Edward Patrick Crehan, qualified me as an officer of the deck. When I came aboard, he told me I would have other duties besides being a medical officer. So I was also the supply officer and the wardroom mess treasurer. I also qualified as officer of the deck under way, because we didn't have enough officers to fill the rotation. Until we got more people aboard, I took my turn and stood the four-to-eight watch every morning and the four-to-eight watch every night on the bridge.

When we had general quarters, I would be relieved; the old man would come up and take over the bridge. He did like to kick the doctor around. But I learned to be quite the seaman after a while. I could keep position on the convoy and had other skills. But I was very pleased when we got more officers aboard and I was relieved of that duty.

Those old four-piper destroyers were World War I vintage and very rugged ships to live on. They were 315 feet long and 31 feet wide. The midships were all engines and they could go like hell. The officers and deck crew lived forward and the engineers aft. Nevertheless, they were in pretty fair shape. We didn't have any breakdowns and I think the fifty we gave to the British did pretty well.[2]

In March of '41 we were ordered from the Caribbean to Argentia, Newfoundland. We went up there without any cold-weather clothing. After the first round-trip convoy we took up a collection aboard ship, went ashore in St. John's, and bought foul-weather clothing. We bought all the sheepskin coats we could find. We called them hot coats because when the men changed watch, they simply gave the coats to the next man. If someone said to me, "You can have four years in the Pacific under wartime conditions or six months in the Atlantic," I'd take the four years in the Pacific.

At Argentia we were stationed alongside a tender. We would get orders to proceed and pick up a convoy coming out of Halifax. We then relieved the Canadian corvette escorting that convoy and took it across to what was called Mid-Ocean Meeting Point. That was right off the tip of Ireland, about two hundred miles north, halfway to Murmansk. There we turned the convoy over to the British. Then we proceeded to Reykjavik, Iceland, and pulled up to the *Hecla,* a British destroyer tender, to refuel and provision. The American destroyers had good food and the British had good liquor, so when we were nested together we freely went back and forth.

---

2. In 1940 President Roosevelt signed the Lend Lease agreement with Britain. In exchange for bases in Newfoundland, Bermuda, and the Caribbean, the United States sent Britain World War I–era destroyers to help combat the German U-boat menace. Although the performance of these "four-stackers" was uneven due to age, their presence in the North Atlantic boosted British morale immeasurably when Britain stood alone against the Nazis.

After we fueled and provisioned, we would patrol the Denmark Straits for five or six days. Then we would come back in to refuel and reprovision again. Following this routine, we then picked up a convoy of mostly empty ships coming out of Britain at the same spot north of Ireland, and took it across until we got off Newfoundland. Then we'd turn the convoy over to the Canadians going into Halifax. Then it was back into Argentia again.

Our orders were to consider any German submarine or plane that came within fifty miles of us as hostile and we were to retaliate. Every time we picked up a sonar contact on a submarine, we made a run on it. One time when we were escorting a convoy off the tip of Greenland, we received a dispatch that the *Bismarck* and the *Prinz Eugen* were going out to raid in the Atlantic. The German goal was to destroy the cryolite mines at Ivigtut, Greenland. We were ordered to proceed northward to Ivigtut alone, and if we sighted anything we were to broadcast immediately. We went to general quarters every time an iceberg showed up on our not-very-good radar screen, and there were many in the ice cap.

As division medical officer, I rode either the *Reuben James,* the *Overton,* or the *Bainbridge.* I had a corpsman on each destroyer. I rode the *Reuben James* on one convoy to Iceland, and coming back we got into a hurricane, the most terrible storm I've ever seen in my life. The convoy got all broken up and all we did was fight to survive. The *James* had terrible damage. One time we fell off a huge wave and the inclinometer read 54 degrees to port. We landed flat on our side. The gyro binnacle in the forward living compartment tore from the deck and we had to tie it down. The old man, Tex Edwards, told us officers he didn't think we were going to make it.

We also had a lot of injuries. Our sick bay was nothing more than a small closet. If I wanted to examine a patient, I took him out of sick bay and laid him down in one of the crewman's bunks. Sometimes it was very rough up forward. Men would complain of seasickness, and even I had my big bucket right alongside of me. A crewman would say, "Doc, I'm seasick." And I'd reply, "I am too. Go on back to work." We didn't have the medications we do now. If I had a man who was sick with pneumonia or had come down with something, I would have to treat him in his own bunk.

During that hurricane, one of the engineers came up from the engine room and put his hand over the knife edge of the hatch just as a wave knocked the hatch down and smashed all his fingers. The only place a doctor had to do surgery on those old four-pipers was the wardroom mess table. I had two men hold him down to keep him from sliding off as the ship rolled and pitched. Other men held the instruments and trays. Two men had to hold me while I amputated two of his fingers and sewed them up. Then the man went to the engineering quarters back aft. When I had to change his dressings, I had to take the traveling lizard and run between waves.

The traveling lizard was a cable running from the forward deck house to the afterdeck house. Loops that ran along the cable came down so you put your hand through. You stood in the shelter of the bridge, watched for the roll of the waves, and ran like hell holding on to the loop, which slid the length of the cable. If a wave came along, you put your other hand up there and held on like hell.

Anyway, the *Reuben James* was so badly damaged that when we put into Argentia the ship was ordered back to Boston for repairs. I didn't go back with her. I was transferred to the USS *Roe* [DD-418].

The *Bainbridge, Sturtevant, Overton,* and *Roe* took the next convoy. Jack Daub, who was a very good friend of mine on the *Bainbridge,* was coming up the gangway of the *Reuben James* to report on board as I was going down. He was going to be executive officer relieving Sam Dealey, who went on to become a famous submariner out in the Pacific. Anyway, that was the last time I saw Jack Daub.

We went out with the convoy and as we were returning, the *Reuben James,* now fully repaired, was coming out with her convoy. She was torpedoed and sunk on October 31st, 1941, at 5:30 in the morning off Cape Fairwell, Greenland, by a German submarine and all officers were killed. I lost a lot of friends.

I was on the destroyers for nineteen months. We had gone north in March of '41 and this was October of the same year. We had been on convoy duty all that time. During Roosevelt's private war, I made six round trips in the North Atlantic.

ONE

Pearl Harbor

Pearl Harbor. Sneak attack. Treachery. Date of infamy. The single tragic, galvanizing event that plunged the United States into World War II. In the years since Japanese planes swarmed out of a balmy Sunday morning sky and nearly obliterated the Pacific Fleet, it seems that everything that could be said about 7 December 1941 has been said—and debated. Almost before the smoke had cleared, the search for answers began, and it continued even after final victory. A congressional investigation seeking the truth heaped up over forty volumes of testimony, shortened careers, and ensured by its quarrelsome deliberations that the controversy would live on.

What cannot be disputed is that Pearl Harbor was one of the greatest setbacks in U.S. military history. For the Navy, 7 December 1941 represents its greatest disaster. In less than three hours the pride of the Pacific Fleet was turned into smoldering hulks of twisted metal. Even before the last Japanese aircraft broke off the attack, what they had wrought was truly catastrophic. Battleships that had once projected U.S. might and prestige—the *Arizona, Pennsylvania, California, West Virginia, Maryland, Oklahoma, Nevada*—either lay on the bottom at their moorings or were too crippled to be of any immediate use.

Aerial torpedoes, armor-piercing bombs, and machine guns took a terrible toll in human life. The Navy alone lost about three times as many men—2,008—in this one attack as it had lost in the Spanish-American War and World War I combined.[1]

Yet the badly burned and wounded survivors found care and comfort. Navy medicine was already on the scene, represented by a naval hospital, a partially assembled base hospital, and the USS *Solace* (AH-5), the newest hospital ship in the fleet. Heroic round-the-clock efforts to save lives began minutes after the first Japanese bomb dropped and never waned until the last casualty had been tended to.

ABANDON SHIP

PhM2c Lee B. Soucy was a medical-laboratory technician assigned to the target ship USS *Utah* (AG-16). On Sunday morning the *Utah* lay at her moorings on Carrier Row, on the opposite side of Ford Island from Battleship Row, about three-quarters of a mile from the *Arizona*. Under the terms of the 1922 Washington Naval Treaty, the *Utah* had ceased her status as a battleship and become a mobile target vessel and later a platform for advanced antiaircraft gunnery practice.

In her role as a mobile bombing target, the *Utah*'s upper decks were lined with two layers of six-by-twelve-inch timbers intended to help absorb the impact of practice bombs dropped by both Navy and Army pilots honing their skills. "During bombing exercises, we would go below the armored deck and then they would bomb for an hour or two. Then we would come topside to get some fresh air. But during these exercises we had been bombed in the wrong place at the wrong time before," recalled Soucy. This fact only magnified the confusion once real bombs began falling at 0755 on 7 December.

---

[1]. The day was very costly for Navy medicine. Two medical officers and two dental officers lost their lives. Twenty-five corpsmen were killed in action, thirteen on the USS *Arizona* alone when a bomb hit the sick bay.

I had just had breakfast and was looking out a porthole in sick bay when someone said, "What the hell are all those planes doing up there on a Sunday?" Someone else said, "It must be those crazy Marines. They'd be the only ones out maneuvering on a Sunday." When I looked up in the sky I saw five or six planes starting their descent. Then when the first bombs dropped on the hangars at Ford Island, I thought, "Those guys are missing us by a mile."

Inasmuch as practice bombing was a daily occurrence to us, it was not too unusual for planes to drop bombs, but the time and place were quite out of line. We could not imagine bombing practice in port. It occurred to me and to most of the others that someone had really goofed this time and put live bombs on those planes by mistake.

In any event, even after I saw a huge fireball and cloud of black smoke rise from hangars on Ford Island and heard explosions, it did not occur to me that these were enemy planes. It was too incredible! Simply beyond imagination! "What a snafu," I moaned.

As I watched in amazement and disbelief, I felt the ship lurch. We didn't know it then, but we were being bombed and torpedoed by planes approaching from the port side.

The bugler and bosun's mate were on the fantail ready to raise the colors at eight o'clock. In a matter of seconds, the bugler sounded general quarters. I grabbed my first-aid bag and headed for my battle station amidship.

A number of the ship's tremors are vaguely imprinted in my mind, but I remember one jolt quite vividly. As I was running down the passageway toward my battle station, another torpedo or bomb hit and shook the ship severely. I was knocked off balance and through the log-room [navigator's office] door. I got up a little dazed and immediately darted down the ladder below the armored deck. I forgot my first-aid kit.

By then the ship was already listing. There were a few men down below who looked dumbfounded and wondered out loud, "What's going on?" I felt around my shoulder in great alarm. No first-aid kit! Being out of uniform is one thing, but being at a battle station without proper equipment is more than embarrassing.

After a minute or two below the armored deck, we heard another bugle call, then the bosun's whistle followed by the chant, "Abandon ship . . . abandon ship."

We scampered up the ladder. I raced toward the open side of the deck; an officer stood by a stack of life preservers and tossed the jackets at us as we ran by. When I reached the open deck, the ship was listing precipitously. I thought about the huge amount of ammunition we had on board and that it would surely blow up soon. I wanted to get away from the ship fast, so I discarded my life jacket. I didn't want a Mae West slowing me down.

The beach on Ford Island was rough. The day previous, I had been part of a fire-and-rescue party dispatched to fight a small fire there. The fire was out by the time we got there but I remembered distinctly the rugged beach, so I tied double knots in my shoes whereas just about everyone else kicked theirs off.

I was tensely poised for a running dive off the partially exposed hull when the ship lunged again and threw me off balance. I ended up with my bottom sliding across and down the barnacle-encrusted bottom of the ship.

When the ship had jolted, I thought we had been hit by another bomb or torpedo, but later it was determined that the mooring lines snapped, which caused the 21,000-ton ship to jerk so violently as she keeled over.[2]

Nevertheless, after I bobbed up to the surface of the water and tried to get my bearings, I spotted a motor launch with a coxswain fishing men out of the water with his boat hook. I started to swim toward the launch. After a few strokes, a hail of bullets hit the water a few feet ahead of me in line with the launch. As the strafer banked, I noted the big red insignias on the wing tips. Until then, I really had not known who had attacked us. At some point I had heard someone shout, "Where did those Germans come from?" I quickly decided that a boat full of men would be a more likely strafing target than a lone swimmer, so I changed course and hightailed it for Ford Island.

I reached the beach exhausted and as I tried to catch my breath, another pharmacist's mate, Gordon Sumner, from the *Utah,* stumbled out of the water. I was elated to see him. There is no doubt in my mind that bewilderment, if not misery, loves company. I felt guilty that I had

---

2. The *Utah*'s World War II career lasted but fifteen minutes. The old ship capsized at 0812, becoming the first U.S. ship to be lost during the attack. The rusted hull is today the site of a second Pearl Harbor memorial.

not made any effort to recover my first-aid kit. Sumner had his wrapped around his shoulders.

While we both tried to get our wind back, a jeep came speeding by and came to a screeching halt. One of the two officers in the vehicle had spotted our Red Cross brassards and hailed us aboard. They took us to a two- or three-story concrete BOQ [bachelor officer's quarters] facing Battleship Row to set up an emergency treatment station for several oil-covered casualties strewn across the floor. Most of them were from the capsized or flaming battleships. It did not take long to exhaust the supplies in Sumner's bag.

A line officer came by to inquire how we were getting along. We told him we had run out of everything and were in urgent need of bandages and some kind of solvent or alcohol to cleanse wounds. He ordered someone to strip the beds and make rolls of bandages with the sheets. Then he turned to us and said, "Alcohol? Alcohol? Will whiskey do?"

Before we could mull it over, he took off and in a few minutes he returned and plunked a case of scotch at our feet. Another person who accompanied him had an armful of bottles of a variety of liquors. I am sure denatured alcohol could not have served our purpose better for washing off the sticky oil, as well as providing some antiseptic effect for a variety of wounds and burns.

Despite the confusion, pain, and suffering, there was some gusty humor amidst the pathos and chaos. At one point an exhausted swimmer, covered with a gooey film of black oil, saw me walking around with a washcloth in one hand and a bottle of booze in the other. He hollered, "Hey Doc, could I have a shot of that medicine?" I handed him the bottle of whichever liquor I had at the time. He took a hefty swig. He had no sooner swallowed the "medicine" than he spewed it out along with black mucoidal globs of oil. He lay back a minute after he stopped vomiting, then said, "Doc, I lost that medicine. How about another dose?"

Perhaps my internal as well as external application of booze was not accepted medical practice, but it sure made me popular with the old salts. Actually, it probably was a good medical procedure if it induced vomiting. Retaining contaminated water and oil in one's stomach was not good for one's health.

Later on, a low-flying enemy pilot was strafing toward our concrete haven while I was on my knees trying to determine what to do for a prostrate casualty. Although the sailor, or Marine, was in bad shape, he raised his head feebly when he saw the plane approach and shouted, "Open the doors and let the son of a bitch in."

Events which occurred in seconds take minutes to recount. During the lull, regular medical personnel from the Ford Island Dispensary arrived with proper supplies and equipment and released Sumner and me so we could rejoin other *Utah* survivors for reassignment.

When the supplies ran out at our first-aid station, I suggested to Sumner that he volunteer to go to the Naval Dispensary for some more. When he returned, he mentioned that he'd just had a close call. A bomb had landed in the patio while he had been at the dispensary. He didn't mention any injury, so I shrugged it off. After all, under the circumstances, what was one bomb more or less.

That afternoon, while we were both walking along a lanai [screened porch] at the dispensary, he pointed to a crater in the patio. "That's where the bomb hit I told you about."

"Where were you?" I asked. He pointed to a spot not far away. I said, "Come on, if you had been that close, you'd have been killed."

To which he replied, "Oh, it didn't go off."

Sometime after dark, a squadron of scout planes from the carrier *Enterprise* (two hundred or so miles out at sea), their fuel nearly depleted, came in for a landing on Ford Island. All hell broke loose and the sky lit up with tracer bullets from numerous antiaircraft guns. As the *Enterprise* planes approached, some understandably trigger-happy gunners opened fire; then all gunners followed suit and shot down all but one of our planes. At least that's what I was told.[3]

Earlier that evening, many of the *Utah* survivors had been taken to the USS *Argonne* [AP-4], a transport. Gunners manning .50-caliber machine guns on the partially submerged USS *California* directly across from the *Argonne* hit the ship while shooting at the planes. A stray, armor-piercing bullet penetrated *Argonne*'s thin bulkhead, went through a *Utah* survivor's arm, and spent itself in another sailor's heart. He died instantly.

The name Price has been stored in my memory bank for a long time as this fatality but, at a recent reunion of *Utah* survivors, another ex-

---

3. After nightfall, as six aircraft from the carrier USS *Enterprise* that had been patrolling returned to Pearl Harbor, four were shot down by friendly fire.

shipmate, Gilbert Meyer, insisted that Price was not the one killed. I didn't argue too long because I recalled meeting two men at the Pearl Harbor Naval Hospital, several weeks after the raid, who walked around with their own obituaries in their wallets—clippings from hometown newspapers.

THE REAL THING

Nurse Ruth A. Erickson had the day off on Sunday and was having a leisurely breakfast at the Naval Hospital across from Ford Island with several of her colleagues. All of a sudden the din of aircraft engines interrupted their conversation.

Suddenly we heard planes roaring overhead and said, "The fly boys are really busy at Ford Island this morning." The island was directly across the channel from the hospital. We didn't think too much about it since the reserves were often there for weekend training.

We no sooner got those words out than we started to hear noises that were foreign to us. I leaped out of my chair and dashed to the nearest window in the corridor. Right then there was a plane flying directly over the top of our quarters, a one-story structure. The rising sun under the wing of the plane denoted the enemy. One could almost see [the pilot's] features around his goggles. He was obviously saving his ammunition for the ships. Just down the row, all the ships were sitting there—the *California,* the *Arizona,* the *Oklahoma,* and others.

My heart was racing, the telephone was ringing, the chief nurse, Gertrude Arnest, was saying, "Girls, get into your uniforms at once. This is the real thing!"

I was in my room by that time changing into uniform. It was getting dusky, almost like evening. Smoke was rising from burning ships.

I dashed across the street through a shrapnel shower, got into the lanai and just stood still for a second, as were a couple of doctors. I felt like I was frozen to the ground, but it was only a split second. I ran to the orthopedic dressing room but it was locked. A corpsman ran to the OD's [officer of the day] desk for the keys. It seemed like an eternity before he returned and the room was opened.

We drew water into every container we could find and set up the instrument boiler. Fortunately we still had electricity and water. Dr. [Comdr. Clyde W.] Brunson, the chief of medicine, was making sick call when the bombing started. When he was finished, he was to play golf . . . a thought never to be uttered again.

The first patient came into our dressing room at 8:25 A.M. with a large opening in his abdomen and bleeding profusely. They immediately started a transfusion. I can still see the tremor of Dr. Brunson's hand as he picked up the needle. Everyone was terrified. The patient died within the hour.

Then the burned patients streamed in. The USS *Nevada* had managed some steam and attempted to get out of the channel. They were unable to make it and went aground on Hospital Point right near the hospital. There was heavy oil on the water and the men dove off the ship and swam through these waters to Hospital Point, not too great a distance, but when one is burned . . . How they ever managed, I'll never know.

The tropical dress at that time was white T-shirts and shorts. The burns began where the pants ended. Bared arms and faces were plentiful.

Personnel retrieved a supply of new flit guns [insecticide sprayers] from stock. We filled these with tannic acid to spray burned bodies. Then we gave these gravely injured patients sedatives for their intense pain.

We eased orthopedic patients out of their beds with no time for linen changes, as an unending stream of burn patients continued until midafternoon. A doctor, who several days before had had renal surgery and was still convalescing, got out of his bed and began to assist the other doctors.

A Japanese plane that had been shot down crashed right next to the tennis court. It sheared off a corner of the laboratory and a number of laboratory animals—rats and guinea pigs—were destroyed.

About twelve noon the galley personnel came around with sandwiches and cold drinks; we ate on the run. About two o'clock the chief nurse was making rounds to check on all the units and arrange relief schedules. I was relieved around four P.M. and went to the nurses' quarters where everything was intact. I freshened up, had something to eat, and went back on duty at eight P.M. I was scheduled to report to a surgical unit.

By now it was dark and we worked with flashlights. The maintenance people, and anyone else who could manage a hammer and nails, were putting up black drapes or black paper to seal the crevices against any light that might stream to the outside.

About ten or eleven o'clock, there were planes overhead. I really hadn't felt frightened until this particular time. My knees were knocking together and the patients were calling, "Nurse, nurse!" The other nurse and I went to them, held their hands a few moments, and then went on to others. The noise ended very quickly and the word got around that these were our own planes.

I worked until midnight on that ward and then was directed to go down to the basement level in the main hospital building. Here the dependents—the women and children, the families of the doctors and other staff officers—were placed for the night. There were ample blankets and pillows. We lay body by body along the walls of the basement. The children were frightened and the adults tense. It was not a very restful night for anyone.

CHIEF NURSE

On Sunday morning the USS *Solace* (AH-5) lay at anchor a few hundred yards north of Battleship Row. The graceful, immaculate white hospital ship that had started her career as a passenger liner a few years earlier represented the only medical service afloat in the Pacific. The *Solace*'s skipper, executive officer, and chief of medicine had gone ashore the night before and had not yet returned. Chief nurse Grace Lally and many of her shipmates were waiting for mass to begin.

A sailor who was fishing from the ship said to me, "What is that crazy flier doing?" Then the bombs began to fall and everything went up at one time. Everywhere you looked was fire and the big ships were turning over on their sides.

Soon the casualties began coming in and it was the saddest-looking thing you ever saw. Most of the men that could get away were down to their skivvies and covered with oil.

Fearing that we would be bombed and trapped inside compartments, someone decided that all the doors should be taken off and pitched over the side. I said, "Just hold everything. We're not going to have the doors taken off." Anyway, the doors weren't removed but left open.

The whole time we were under Condition One, which was an emergency. We put life preservers on all the patients and got them ready to abandon ship, but how could you abandon ship when many of them were in body casts? But putting those life preservers on over their casts at least made them feel more secure.

After the attack, and with the changing of the tide, more bodies appeared, and they sent our boats out to get them. My nurses kept saying that I should go out to help retrieve the dead from the water. So I went out on a boat. Only one part of a body came up. It was a leg, probably from a man who had been on the *Arizona*.

And over on the beach you could see the coffins stretching all the way up. I said, "If American women could see this kind of stuff." You just couldn't imagine.

PAINTING WINDOWS

Although Lt. Cecil H. Coggins, MC, was officially health, recreation, and morale officer for the U.S. fleet in Hawaiian waters, this title was convenient cover for a physician with an uncanny knack for the intelligence business. His real job was counterespionage for the Pacific Fleet, and he reported directly to Lt. Comdr. Edwin T. Layton, fleet intelligence officer. Dr. Coggins was at home in Honolulu when the Japanese attack began.

I was up on Mikiki Roundtop in my home with my wife and two children having breakfast. We heard some planes that were trying to take the roof off our house, apparently, with landing gear. I ran out to look at them, and they were Japanese.

The children ran out to see them too, and I started for the garage, opened the garage door, and called for Dot to bring me my hat and coat. It looked like hundreds of them. They turned in unison like a big flock of seagulls and slanted downwards toward the harbor. They were carrying torpedoes under them. As I got the car out, my oldest son Pete said, "Are they are dropping torpedoes? Our planes dive lots steeper than that." This six-year-old boy said that.

I said, "You take a good, long look. You'll never see this again as long as you live. Those are Japanese planes. We are now at war."

I backed the car out of the garage and headed down the hill to the city. Through my mind ran the thought that they were not diving steeply because the water was shallow. They had to come parallel to the surface before they let their torpedoes go.

I headed down the hill, winding back and forth with one eye on the road, the other on Pearl Harbor. The din of the airplane motors and the exploding bombs seemed to be incessant. Halfway down I saw a battleship blow all to pieces. I wasn't sure that it was my old ship, the *Arizona,* but I saw a lot of white, sprinkled popcorn in the air—uniforms, people. It was a frightful thing.

I was headed for my duty station in the DIO [District Intelligence Office], which was located in the Alexander Young Hotel. I was one of the first to arrive in the office, but Captain [Irving] Mayfield was already there. He was standing, holding a can of paint and a paintbrush in his hand. As has happened since the beginning of time, when man is overwhelmed by grief and shock, his hands cling to reality by groping for some simple task to perform. We looked at each other. He was pale. He said dully, "I was getting ready to paint the windows." I could scarcely speak; my throat was full of tears, as it is now after forty-five years. He said, "There's another can of paint over there, and a brush."

So before the rest of the staff had arrived to man their posts at the telephones and other communications equipment, we were side by side painting the windowpanes a dark blue. We knew that at that moment everything that was supposed to be done was being done. We had no guns to shoot, and for a half hour there was nothing for us to do—that awful time—so we painted windows.

I said, "A lot of people are dead and a lot more are hurt pretty bad and I'm here, a surgeon. I should be in the hospital."

He said, "You know what to do. You always do your duty. Carry out your duty."

I said, "That's what I'm doing. Right now we've got nothing to do but paint these damn windows. How long have you had this paint ready for a blackout?"

He said, "We've had it here in the office for a long time now."

I said, "I read in the newspaper that there's a convention of a medical or surgical association going on now right here in Honolulu. Maybe they're beginning to bus all those doctors right now down to Pearl Harbor and they'll soon be standing in line to take care of the wounded." Just saying that made me feel better.

INTERROGATING THE FIRST JAPANESE POW

Japanese plans for destroying the fleet at Pearl Harbor included the deployment of several midget submarines. These craft, each armed with two torpedoes, were to sneak submerged into the harbor to augment the destructive power of Japanese torpedo bombers.

On the night of 6 December, five midget subs attempted to enter the channel. Two were sunk, one by the destroyer USS *Ward* (DD-139) and another by a bomb from an American plane. It is believed a third may have rolled off its mother submarine and been lost. One succeeded in entering the harbor but was later damaged by gunfire from the USS *Curtiss* (AV-4). Depth charges from the USS *Monaghan* (DD-354) finished it off. The fifth sub ran aground in the surf just off Bellows Field, and its commander was captured.

> Dr. Cecil H. Coggins, in his role as intelligence officer, interrogated the first Japanese prisoner of war, Ens. Kazuo Sakamaki.

Sakamaki seems to have been the original hard-luck kid. At the time he was launched from his piggyback position, it was discovered that his midget's only gyro compass had been out of order and [the compass] defied all efforts to fix it. Sakamaki and his engineer, Kiyoshi Inagaki, were too eager to think reasonably. They both agreed to go anyhow.

They were launched twenty-seven miles from the harbor and as long as they could see the lights from their periscope they were all right, but as they neared the entrance and the hundred square miles patrolled by destroyers, they were forced to submerge.

After an hour they raised the periscope and found they had been traveling in the wrong direction. Returning on the surface, they were sighted by the *Ward,* forced to submerge, and harassed by depth charges. Then they ran into a reef at one side of the entrance. In full reverse they managed to escape, but again ran into a reef—this time damaging their torpedoes, rendering them useless. Only by shifting the ballast did they manage to free themselves and, according to Sakamaki, they saw the burning ships, had to submerge again, and charged toward the harbor entrance, determined to "sink the *Pennsylvania.*"

As before, their compass misled them and they found themselves off Diamond Head! With their batteries failing and both suffering from nervous exhaustion, these two left-footed boys ran into their third reef of the morning, off Kaneohe, this time to stay.

They both dove off the submarine seven hundred feet from the beach. His crewman, Inagaki, apparently drowned and Sakamaki found himself lying on the sand. A soldier saw him and arrested him. He spoke poor English and was wearing nothing but a gold watch around his neck.

They brought him into the brig and called me. I took one of my nisei [acting as translator] with me and I first asked him how he felt.[4] He could scarcely answer. I asked him where his engineer was. He guessed that he had drowned. [By that time] they had given him clothing and had taken away his watch. I'd asked for it, and he saw it in my hand. I said I would come back to see him.

I went to town and had the watch cleaned and repaired. It showed that he had been number one in his naval academy class and that the gold watch had been given to him as a prize by his classmates. I came back the next day. He had put a roll of blankets in his bunk and slept under the bed, evidently figuring the Marines would reach through the bars with their bayonets and have a few stabs at him, which they might have done, too; I don't know. He expected to be killed momentarily. He was dressed, crisp and clean, and I gave him back his watch. He appeared to be grateful, and we became more friendly.

---

4. The nisei (second-generation Japanese Americans) who worked for the Office of Naval Intelligence were all hand picked by Dr. Coggins and a colleague, Bill Stephenson, and Stephenson's staff. Coggins remembered them as "the cream of the crop—good, patriotic, energetic, well-established citizens. Many were successful businessmen in Honolulu. Their ranks included doctors, lawyers, bankers, teachers, and other leaders of the community."

I started out immediately to employ a theory I had which could be called denationalization or disenfranchisement. With respect to the Japanese, I had long pointed out in my lectures that when you caught your prisoner, you ought to be able to drain any information out of him; you should have no trouble questioning him. I taught our nisei to use the prisoner's own beliefs to force him to talk freely, [beliefs such as] "I'll never be captured. If I'm ever captured I will have no family left and I will have no country left. I will be disowned by the nation and the emperor. I will be a citizen of the world, with my whole future lying in my own hands. I have been taught that if captured, I will be dishonored and must commit suicide. However, I do not wish to die and suicide is an unnatural thing. My natural instinct tells me to preserve my own life. It is not my fault that I am here." These were some of their own beliefs. The thing to do, I always thought, was to capitalize on these beliefs.

When you take a prisoner, remind him over and over of these beliefs as if they were facts. After you once make him realize that he indeed has no country, then you might begin to ask him casually, as in ordinary conversation, about his friends in his regiment, his guns, his airplanes, everything in his former country, because he would no longer feel himself obliged to keep those things a secret. His best chance in life now is to make new friends, to find a new country to belong to, and to make something worthwhile of his life.

The degree of their acceptance of their prisoner status depends entirely upon their first treatment after being captured. Remember, these people are by nature very excitable. In their homeland, they have been subjected to a rigid, tense, and fanatically religious indoctrination all their lives. Their emperor worship distorted their natural instincts to the extent that their patriotic fervor became almost pathological. A fresh-caught prisoner is often so depressed as to be completely unresponsive or so tense that, like a bomb, he needs to be carefully defused.

Sakamaki was both depressed and nervous. He not only was still alive, but he was also afraid to die. He thought his lost submarine was like a secret weapon which could be of inestimable value to America. But it was an ordinary midget submarine, seventy feet long and about forty tons, with only its underwater speed of twenty-four knots for ninety minutes distinguishing it from any other prototype. We sent it on a tour of the United States, selling war bonds.

I saw him and questioned him several times. Once he sent me a short note which was most amusing. It read, "My dear Governor General Brave, the moss killers are killing me!" He used all the honorifics that his poor English provided, but wanted to make sure that I would not be insulted by his greeting.

I rushed over to the brig to see who was killing him. I thought the Marines had given him a poke. But his tormentors turned out to be mosquitoes! I ordered a mosquito net for him to sleep under, much to the disgust of the Marine guards.

After two months Sakamaki was sent, with other prisoners, to prison camps in the United States, usually to the same relocation centers used for the internment of the West Coast Japanese.

After returning to Japan at war's end, he wrote a book about his adventures entitled *Four Years as Prisoner of War Number One*. It was a best-seller in Japan. He then went to work for the Toyota Motor Company in the personnel department and rose to a high position. It is amusing to reflect how much more successful he was in America with the midget automobile than with the midget submarine.

A BRUSH WITH THE BULL

On the eve of the great Midway battle in June 1942, commander in chief of the Pacific Fleet Adm. Chester Nimitz ordered Vice Adm. William F. Halsey to check into the Pearl Harbor Naval Hospital. Halsey, on the brink of physical exhaustion, had been tormented with such a severe skin condition that the itching prevented him from sleeping. With hives covering nearly his entire body, the admiral was in no condition to lead a fleet into battle. To replace him, Nimitz chose Rear Adm. Raymond Spruance. Heretofore known as a cruiser admiral, Spruance got the chance to prove his mettle as commander of the carrier task force that changed the course of history.

PhM2c Lee Soucy, a medical technologist recently assigned to the hospital after the loss of his ship on 7 December, tells of his encounter with "Bull."

I was ordered to go to the sick officers' quarters immediately to draw some blood from Admiral Halsey to be used for a series of tests. I knocked on the door and went in. There was a bare-chested man with just pajama bottoms on, rubbing his foot on the floor, just like a bull. The thought occurred to me, No wonder they call him Bull Halsey.

The soles of his feet were actually itching and he was covered with chalky splotches, no doubt calamine lotion. The admiral, obviously disappointed over missing the battle of Midway, looked at my tray of needles and syringes and said very gruffly, "Now what?"

I explained my mission and then asked him to sit in a chair so I could draw his blood. But he hopped on the bed and I just stood there wondering whether I should tell the old guy to move over or what. He said, "Do you want me to sit in the chair?"

I said, "Yes sir. It's not going to hurt me one way or the other but I prefer not to hurt you."

He got in the chair and never said a word. When I was finished he said, "You did that very well, son." Then he asked me how long I had been in the Navy. I replied that my enlistment was up on December 7th.

He said, "December 7th?" Then he chuckled and asked me how long I had been at the hospital.

"Ever since my ship was sunk," I replied.

"What was your ship?"

"USS *Utah*," I answered.

"*Utah!* Ah, yes. We could have used her guns."

He was right. We had the best antiaircraft guns in the world, but now they lay submerged and useless.

TWO

The Navy's War

As Pearl Harbor galvanized an unprepared nation into action, so too did Navy medicine respond to the challenge of world war. In 1941, the Navy had but eighteen continental hospitals, three overseas hospitals, two mobile hospitals, and two hospital ships in commission. Approximately 13,500 physicians, dentists, nurses, Hospital Corps officers, and corpsmen—pharmacists' mates as they were then called—manned these facilities.

By 1945 the ranks had swollen to about 169,000 personnel, a staggering growth of 1,252 percent. They were assigned to fifty-six stateside hospitals, twelve fleet hospitals, sixteen base hospitals, fourteen convalescent hospitals, fifteen hospital ships, five special augmented hospitals, and many dispensaries.

Vice Adm. Ross McIntire, surgeon general of the Navy and personal physician to Franklin Roosevelt, largely influenced this tremendous mobilization. A far abler administrator than physician, McIntire presided over the largest medical mobilization in the Navy's history. Having the ear of a president who doted on his favorite armed service certainly did not hurt the Medical Department's access to men and materiel.

With the exception of the Atlantic theater's North African, Italian, and Normandy campaigns, the story of Navy medicine in World War II is primarily the story of the Pacific war. As the Pacific theater was the Navy's war, so too was it Navy medicine's main theater of operations.

If the ferocity of the Japanese onslaught that followed Pearl Harbor left American forces reeling, isolated, and with scant hope of reinforcement, as an institution Navy medicine was equally stretched. Possessing only limited resources and with a presence only in Hawaii, the Philippines, Guam, a few small installations, and aboard the few vessels of the Asiatic Fleet, Navy medical personnel were hard pressed to treat patients as defeat became inevitable. The disease-ridden tropical environment of the Philippines only made matters worse.

THE EXPENDABLES

On 8 December 1941, World War II came to the Philippines when Japanese bombers hit Clark and Nichols Fields, destroying U.S. airpower on the ground. Two days later, high-flying bombers attacked Manila and virtually leveled the Cavite Navy Yard. Overwhelmed, U.S. Navy medical personnel and their Army compatriots ministered to the casualties as the islands prepared for a full-scale Japanese invasion.

In the weeks that followed, Americans and Filipinos fought against increasingly hopeless odds as defense lines stretched to the breaking point. Olongapo was evacuated and many of the naval personnel joined the 4th Marines at Mariveles on the Bataan Peninsula. On New Year's Day 1942, this unit left the mainland to make a last stand on Corregidor.

Days stretched into weeks, then months, as the ceaseless bombardment forced the tunnel-weary and hungry American defenders to conclude that their countrymen had abandoned them. They were expendable. By the time the siege of that tadpole-shaped island ended on 6 May 1942, Japanese might had all but extinguished American power in the Far East.

✚
BOMBS ON CAVITE

Lt. Ferdinand V. Berley had recently arrived in the Philippines, where he drew an assignment in the navy yard dispensary at Cavite. He learned that the war had started when a colleague shook him awake at 5:30 in the morning saying, "Fred, we just got word. The Japs bombed Pearl Harbor."

Berley responded with, "Good. Now we can lick the sons of bitches." And he turned over and went back to sleep.

With a Japanese attack imminent, Berley soon learned that his battle dressing station was to be the dispensary building, a wooden structure in the direct center of the yard. Realizing immediately how vulnerable the building would be to a bombing attack, he found instead an old below-ground paint locker made of concrete.

As I got down toward the paint locker, I saw a big formation of planes flying directly over Sangley Point, and the antiaircraft fire was bursting about two-thirds the way up. The planes were flying about 21,000 feet, but the antiaircraft shells were bursting about 17,000 feet or so. The next thing I knew, they were flying directly over the yard towards us in beautiful formations. And then I saw the bombs starting to fall. I ran into the paint locker and yelled, "The bombs are falling!"

Shortly thereafter we were hit, and the whole place just shook. There was a palm tree just outside that door. Later on when I came out, that palm had gone straight up in the air and back into the crater the bomb had made. It was the darndest thing I ever saw.

Then the casualties began to arrive. We did whatever we could. I remember cutting a Filipino workman's hand off because it was just barely hanging by the skin of the wrist. The whole yard was on fire and things were getting pretty rough. Trucks were arriving and picking up the wounded for transfer to Cañacao. I wound up over on the Guadalupe pier, where I found about five or six wounded. I saw a motor launch coming across and waved to the coxswain, saying I had some wounded. He yelled back that there was a boat right alongside the pier. Sure enough, looking over the side and down, I saw a launch with a Filipino coxswain just doubled up like he was hiding from everyone. I got him and we loaded the boat with the wounded and went over to the pier at Sangley Point.

I made my way to the hospital and was assigned to one of the wards where I helped triage the wounded. I administered morphine for pain, tagged them, and so on.

After a while I went up to the operating room, where they were very busy. I asked Dr. [Cmdr. Thomas] Hayes if I could assist, and he said yes. The wounded were lined up all along the stairwell, one after another.

We wore surgical gowns but never changed them. They were soaked through with blood. Those nurses were unbelievable, bringing us instruments and dressings wet even though they sterilized them as best they could. And then came the next patient. You'd amputate a leg, you'd amputate an arm. Someone would die on the table. It was just a nightmare, when I think back on it.

We operated until one or two in the morning. When we were through, my shirt and trousers were also soaked with blood. With no place to go, I just slept right under the hospital that night.

TUNNEL RATS

Just days later, Dr. Berley and his comrades evacuated Cavite, and, when Gen. Douglas MacArthur declared Manila an open city, the Americans began a harrowing retreat down the Bataan Peninsula toward the port of Mariveles. On the night of 29 December, Berley and his 4th Marines sailed the short distance across Manila Bay by barge.

We went to Middleside Barracks, where we stowed our gear. They told us the barracks were bombproof. The next day we could see all the Army personnel with their starched khakis, ties, and everything. It just didn't look like a war was taking place on Corregidor. A buddy and I went to the officers' club and had lunch. On the way down, we saw what looked like the kind of field gun you'd see from World War I. A couple of Army personnel were working on it. We said to them, "We understand you have some 5-inch antiaircraft guns here on the Rock."

They said, "We don't have any 5-inch antiaircraft guns. They're 3-inch antiaircraft guns."

When he told me how many batteries he had, I thought, Oh boy. We're going to have a repeat of what I saw at Sangley Point. Shortly afterward, the air-raid alarm went off. In case of a bombing attack we were to go down to the first deck and stay in the building. I did just that, winding up in a room with Colonel [Don] Curtis. I was right in front of a door lying flat on the floor with my tin helmet.

When the first string of bombs came across, the third one hit the barracks about a hundred feet to my left. It went through the roof, through all three decks, and landed in the dining room, blowing the walls apart in the room I was in. Bombproof! You talk about being shell-shocked! I was shell-shocked. I could hear these bombs coming down and every one sounded like it was aimed for the back of my neck. At the end of that raid, we all knew that Middleside Barracks was anything but bombproof.

Afterward we were told to move down to James Ravine, a kind of a little hollow area with a concrete tunnel dug in the side. This was the most terrible thing I ever went through. I've never been more scared in my life. Following that experience in Middleside, if you heard anything at all that sounded like bombs, you ran for that darned tunnel.

After about a week, the Marines were dispersed around the island for beach defense. My old company, F, needed a doctor so I went to Wheeler Point on the end of Corregidor that faced Batangas. And that's the best thing that ever happened to me because had I stayed at James Ravine, I think I would have gone nuts.

Getting out in the open away from that tunnel made all the difference in the world. If a bombing attack occurred, you could jump into a foxhole. To become a tunnel rat was the worst thing that could happen to anyone. You would develop a psychological aspect of fear you just couldn't get rid of. I think that's what happened to a lot of those people who holed up in Malinta Tunnel. There was a Filipino scout battery stationed just about 150 feet from us. They had a 155-mm battery facing Bataan and had built a tunnel which they used as their plotting room. It went straight on in from the road. The tunnel then took a right turn and was extended maybe 50 feet or so to run parallel to the road that came to Wheeler Point. That's where I had my battle dressing station and sick bay.

We were on rations of two meals a day and they got skimpier and skimpier all the time. We got a stew of some sort and a type of porridge for breakfast and for supper. I know we ate up all the horses and mules. And we ate some sort of cereal in the morning for breakfast and maybe some toast. We were hungry all the time. I got to know some of the Filipino scouts. They took some sort of weed and when they threw it out in the ocean it stunned the fish. Then they collected the fish and had themselves a fish fry.

The scouts also found wild camotes, a type of sweet potato. I asked how to find them and then walked around my sector looking, but was never successful. I probably wouldn't have recognized a camote if I saw it at that time.

One morning we were surprised at breakfast. The Japs opened up with artillery from Batangas. If that barrage had been a hundred yards short, it would have cleaned us out. But it went right over our heads. They had been aiming at the guns above us. From then on, we never had any warning at all. It was really scary. With the bombing you could at least see the planes. But with artillery, there was no warning at all. If all of a sudden you heard the shells whizzing by, at least you were safe. If you didn't hear them and they landed, that was it!

We also saw some Jap planes get shot down. We had the same fuse problem we had at Sangley Point. But eventually the submarines brought us some fuses that enabled the shells to reach up to their altitude. As a matter of fact, we got two planes one day. We later heard a couple of big-shot generals were aboard inspecting the Rock. I saw the shells burst right beneath the planes and they went down over Bataan. We just stood on our heads and cheered. It was terrific!

We also learned about the bombing of Tokyo on April 18th by Doolittle, which also was a real morale booster, and we got our first news of what had happened at Pearl Harbor. One of the submarines brought some pictures from *Life* magazine showing what had happened there. When we saw those pictures, we knew then the war was not going to end in six months.

Of course, we could hear the guns on Bataan creeping closer and closer toward us. Eventually we heard that Bataan had fallen. Whoever could escape came over to the Rock as best they could. We incorporated them into our beach defenses about a week or ten days before the fall.

As far as casualties were concerned, we had a few shrapnel wounds, mainly from the shelling. We treated them and then brought them in by truck to Malinta Tunnel hospital. I used to make a run to the hospital about once a week or once every ten days to replenish my supplies and report to Hayes.

We knew the fall was imminent. About a night or two before the main landing, the Japanese had a dress rehearsal and it was unbelievable! The sky was lit up half the night—shells from all over the place rained down in a constant bombardment till well after midnight. My commander made me turn in my sidearm and my rifle. He said, "You can't have that. Put your Red Cross brassard on."

I argued with him. "Look, at least I can defend myself a little bit." We knew that if they landed where we were, there was no place to go. We just had a narrow road next to the water and then a drop down through some woods about twenty-five feet to the shoreline below. If they landed there, we knew that was it. But he was adamant. I took my two guns and put them behind a wall in this tunnel. I was hoping one day to get them back.

The morning of the landings we got word to take our stations. I went to my battle dressing station. Nothing was happening around us but we heard a lot of firing going on—machine guns, rifle fire, and so on. Finally we were ordered to destroy all our equipment and report back to Wheeler Point. That was the closest I ever came to crying. Hiking all the way back to Wheeler Point you could hear small-arms fire, especially on top above us.

When we got back, everyone congregated there. We didn't know what to do. Communications were cut off. We stayed for a day or so and saw the Japs up above raising their guns and yelling "Banzai!" But we were pretty secure because we were right below the sheer wall that went on up to the top.

After a day of this and no food, we finally talked the major into marching on in to Malinta. He wasn't in any hurry to do it, saying, "Let them come and find us," but he finally gave in. We got a sheet to use as a white flag and then marched all the way back to Bottomside.

Just before we got there, we met our first Japs. They were looking for rings, watches, anything they could take from us. I hid my watch and ring in my shoes. When we got to Malinta Tunnel, I still had my Red

Cross brassard on. They pointed for me to go to the tunnel and I told them I didn't want to go. I wanted to stay with my group. When one of them shoved a bayonet right at my stomach, I changed my mind.

Everything was just a chaotic mess. There was no order of any kind whatsoever. I went into the tunnel and reported to Hayes.

✛

A CORPSMAN'S STORY

PhM2c Ernest J. Irvin was attached to C Battery, a U.S. Marine antiaircraft outfit that manned four 3-inch guns.[1] The battery had set up in a turnip patch on the edge of the little village of Binakayan. "We were so far off the beaten path even the Navy couldn't keep track of us," recalls Irvin.

On December 10th the Japs bombed Cavite. We counted eighty bombers go right over us. We couldn't reach them but we kept them from getting down too low. They said we got two of them.

On the 22d [of December], our battery abandoned our position and a destroyer took us from Sangley Point to Mariveles. It was one of the old four-stackers, the USS *Pillsbury* [DD-227]. It went on to Indochina and then was sunk off Java with all hands lost, including the division doctor. We headed for the hills north of Mariveles and joined up with the 4th Marines, who had been dumped in Olongapo after arriving from Shanghai in October or November '41.

They moved the 4th Marines to a bivouac area in the hills above Mariveles and they went over to Corregidor right after Christmas. I guess it was the 28th or so when our guns went through Manila by truck. We went by ship to Bataan. They found this flat place between the Navy section base and the little village of Mariveles and we set up our guns up

---

1. C Battery, of which Irwin was a member, was initially deployed across Bacoor Bay a mile south of the navy yard. The Battery was manned by two officers and seventy-seven enlisted men. It was armed with four 3-inch 50-caliber dual-purpose guns (surface or air) of World War I vintage. They had been salvaged from the scrap heap at the navy yard and mounted on makeshift metal bases. The fire-control system consisted of an altimeter of that same vintage. The battery also had five .50-caliber, water-cooled machine guns. C Battery attracted very few visitors or guests.

there. They were naval guns. They had strips of steel with the barrels sitting on top. Normally these strips were welded to the deck of the ship. Imagine them sitting in a rice paddy that had the consistency of jello. When the guns fired they would sink right in and the ground all around shook.

We were also supposed to defend a position in the hills near Longoskawayan Point against Japanese landing parties. Our boys on Corregidor began shelling the point with their 12-inch mortars to discourage the Japs. They'd drop one in the water, and the next one, and about the third would knock trees down not far away from us. You would hear what sounded like a freight train coming in. Whenever we heard the noise we said, "Tojo, count your men, we're going to take a few."

We thought for sure they would get us. The five or six of us pressed into service to hold the line on the ridge had decided that if we heard another shot from Corregidor, we'd haul ass out of there. On the night of 25 January 1942, we felt sure one would land and explode in our midst!

But we stayed there until the bitter end on Bataan. Before we were through, C Battery was credited with nineteen enemy aircraft. Some of those we hit we saw trailing smoke. They bombed us like crazy once they finally figured out where we were. They bombed the Navy section base a few times and the Dewey dry dock in Mariveles. They hit the *Canopus* a few times.[2]

The night Bataan fell, the Filipino army boys went by single file, kicking up dust as they staggered along. They were all dejected and beat up without their guns. They looked like hobos—a little stick and a kerchief with all their belongings. I would ask them, "Where ya going, Joe?" We called them Joe and they called us Joe.

All any of them would say was, "I'm going to the probince [*sic*] to see my companion." Every one of them had the same answer. They formed in a flat area our P-40s had used as a landing strip. By then we had no

---

2. After the bombing of the Cavite Navy Yard on 10 December 1941, the yard ceased to be operational. The few Navy ships that were in Manila Bay escaped to regroup in French Indochina and Australia. On 29 December 1941 and 1 January 1942, the old submarine tender USS *Canopus* (AS-9) received direct bomb hits. One, an armor-piercing bomb, penetrated all the way through to the sick bay, rendering the ship unable to withstand heavy seas. It was then beached and moored in a cove at the Navy section base at Mariveles, and it continued to provide meager repairs and support to submarines that came into Manila Bay under cover of darkness. The vessel also provided its crewmen as fighters in the improvised naval battalion that fought the Japanese invaders. The *Canopus* was scuttled following the surrender of Bataan.

P-40s left. They just congregated there and flopped down waiting for something. Then the Jap fighter planes came in and began strafing. It was like shooting fish in a barrel.

About two weeks before Bataan fell, we were assigned to the 60th Coast Artillery, which was an Army outfit. That's what saved us from making the Death March. When Bataan fell, our lieutenant, a guy named [Willard B.] Holdredge, called the Marines over on Corregidor and asked if we could join them. They said sure, but they had no way of getting us over there. "You're on your own." He then called the Navy but with no luck. He then got a bright idea and called the colonel in the 60th Coast Artillery, who said "Get your men down to the quarantine station in Mariveles at eleven tonight. I've got a tug. You can join my men and we'll get over there." So we did.

We destroyed what we could of our guns. They loaded about seventy of us in this tiny little room in the tug's hold, where I could scarcely breathe. Right about then someone asked if there was a doctor aboard and I responded. There was a Filipino who was very badly hurt. Just before we boarded the tug, our boys were blowing up everything they could on Bataan. A rock had actually torn his arm off and he was going to die. I applied a tourniquet and stayed with him all night long up topside, where it was cool. We didn't leave until seven the next morning, when Jap planes began strafing the huge huddle of Filipino soldiers on the airstrip.

When we got over to Corregidor, I was assigned to beach defense in Government Ravine, at a lower level near the water's edge. At Bataan I learned that when enemy planes came over I could spot them and decide whether they could drop their eggs on us. If they were headed right over us I knew that if they opened their bomb bays at the right time, they would get us. Only then would I take cover. Otherwise, they wouldn't bother me. When I got to Corregidor they'd sound the siren when the planes took off from Nichols field or from Clark, twenty miles or so away. And then all these people would head for a hole. You would go nuts with that kind of crap.

One time as I was sitting on a rock during a raid, a truck came whizzing by. A chief, Jack Kirbow, was riding on top. He yelled, "[Jeremiah] Crews wants to see you in the tunnel!" So after the raid I bummed a ride over to Malinta. That happened six days before Corregidor fell.

I had been pulled off beach defense in Government Ravine to work in the Malinta Tunnel hospital. When I got to the tunnel, Crews said he was bringing me in for a rest. I said, "Hey, I'm not tired. I'm ready to fight." In Government Ravine there was an Army captain, a mean, wild SOB with long hair and covered with oil. He swam from Bataan to Corregidor clutching his .45-caliber pistol in his mouth. He and I planned to repel the entire Jap army when they decided to land. I certainly didn't want to be a tunnel rat.

I saw [nurse] Ann Bernatitus the night before she left. She wanted me to write a letter to my mother and she'd mail it for me. I said no. It might give her false hope. I really didn't think the Japs would let us live. I'd seen what they'd done in China. Hell, they chopped off more heads than you could shake a stick at. I figured they would just wipe us out and go fight somewhere else. We all knew it was a matter of time. We thought the Japs would either gas us in the tunnel or march us out and shoot us.

PIGBOAT DOC

On the eve of war in the Pacific, PhM1c Wheeler Lipes was stationed at the Cañacao Naval Hospital but found the routine less than exciting. Although not considered a glamorous assignment, service aboard a submarine seemed just the ticket. Since physicians were not assigned to submarines, such duty enabled an ambitious young corpsman to make his mark.

The duty at the hospital was excellent and it counted as sea duty, but I wanted to go into submarines and had talked to the personnel officer. He thought I was insane for wanting to give up the good life to go to pigboats.

The squadron medical officer I spoke to out on the *Canopus* [AS-9] told me there were just no submarines out there for me. I said, "If I find one, may I have it?"

He told me I could but said again that nothing was vacant. A second-class, Lester, and I went out to a bunch of moored submarines and went aboard the USS *Shark* [SS-174]. We went down the hatch, through the boat, and out the other end. There was a fellow aboard who was ready to be transferred. When we came out the after engine-room hatch and up onto the deck, he said, "Do you want this one?"

I said, "I don't want any part of this Shark." The ship was dirty. I'm impressed with things that are neat, sharp, and clean. I just didn't feel comfortable.[3]

I continued out over the subs that were tied up till I came to the very last one. It was the USS *Sealion* [SS-195]. I went down the hatch and back in the after battery area. The *Sealion* was sparkling, it was clean, it was new, built in '39. It just had a good feeling about it. I said to the pharmacist's mate, a guy named Richter, "Do you like this ship? Do you like submarines?"

He said, "I hate submarines, I hate anybody in submarines, and I hate anybody that knows anybody in submarines."

"Do you want to get off this thing?" I asked him.

He said, "That's my greatest wish, but . . ."

I said, "I'll take it."

So we went to see the squadron medical officer, and that's how I got assigned to the *Sealion*. It was a good move.

Then the bombing took place [10 December 1941]. In fact, I had been at the dispensary [at the Cavite Navy Yard] when the bombers came. You could hear them roaring, and the sirens were going off. I ran several blocks to get back to the ship and had to cross a barge that our torpedoes were on.

I went down the after torpedo room hatch and started through. When I got to the engine room, there was a guy sitting up there in the hatch watching the bombers. I climbed up the ladder and said, "Let me take a look."

He put his foot against me and said, "No, this is my seat."

So I went on forward, stepped into the control-room area, and turned left into the radio shack. Just as I stepped in—Blammo!—a bomb came down the after engine-room hatch where that guy was watching those bombers.

The next bomb hit our conning tower and its nose came through into the radio shack. It was the shrapnel from that explosion that got

---

3. The *Shark* was lost at sea in early 1942.

the conning tower of the *Seadragon* [SS-194] and killed the engineering officer, just chopped his head off, and wounded several people.[4]

After the bombing, I tried to get out of the ship but found I was trapped. As I exited the steel hatch from the forward torpedo room, I found the wooden hatch in the teak deck just above jammed from one of the bombs that had hit us. I began yelling, "Get me out of here!"

It happens that the skipper of the submarine, a guy named [Lt. Comdr.] Richard Voge, was up on deck. He used something to pull that hatch loose, then took me by the hand and pulled me out of there. By this time the *Sealion* was settling, and it was every man for himself. Everybody was doing what they could to salvage the submarine but there was nothing anyone could do.

I was exhausted but I did what I could to render aid. There were wounded men all over the place. I saw one of my friends who usually wore a big, wide four-inch belt. He was blown in half right at the belt line. And there was a lot of confusion. Everybody was trying to report to Manila or get back to the submarine tender. I was still taking care of the wounded.

Sometime about eleven that night I was on the far perimeter of the base, away from the submarines, when I heard a motor launch idling along. I yelled at the guy aboard. He happened to be a coxswain who had been on the *Sealion* with me. He had been in the water and found the launch adrift, and now was going around picking up survivors or anyone he could. He pulled up close to the pier and I jumped down into the launch. After we picked up six or eight other people, we took off across Manila Bay to where the *Canopus* was moored.

They had towed the *Seadragon* over there from her slip and tied it up to the stern of the *Canopus*. All the *Seadragon*'s main engines were down. In fact, the only engine still functioning was a small auxiliary, just a donkey engine. Since it had been in overhaul, everything was a mess—parts were out, and there were holes in the pressure hull and some in the conning tower.

I went aboard the *Canopus* about midnight and ate the best meal I ever ate. It had been a long time since I had eaten. They gave me hotdogs and sauerkraut. They also gave me a cot and a towel, and I took a bath and stretched out. Just as I sat on that cot, they paged over the loudspeaker for me to report to the sick bay.

---

4. The *Sealion* and *Seadragon* were sister submarines and at the time of the Japanese attack were tied up side by side at a Cavite Navy Yard pier for overhaul.

The pharmacist's mate on the *Seadragon* was injured and was transferred off the submarine to the hospital, leaving no pharmacist's mate, no Medical Department representative aboard that ship.

When I arrived in the sick bay, there were three or four first classes around trying to convince the senior medical officer to let one of them be assigned to the *Seadragon,* which was now without a corpsman. He then said to me, "How would you feel about another submarine?"

I said, "I'm ready now, sir." And that's how I got on the *Seadragon.*

The next morning after I went aboard, they took the *Seadragon* out in the bay, rolled it over on one side, took a wooden box, and made a cofferdam. Then they took little pieces of steel and welded them in place over the holes. We always had a conversation during depth-charge attacks concerning those patches; we had the utmost confidence in them. We thought they were better than the original hull.

There was no adjustment period. The crew welcomed me as a part of the team. All of us had whatever our jobs were, and we did them, and you did them with one another, because you couldn't do anything in that ship without the other guy being a part of it. When you were out on long patrols in those days, torpedomen stayed in their compartments for long periods of time and never came out. The guys in the middle section of the ship, in the control room, in the after batteries, or forward batteries didn't go into the torpedo rooms. I took that trip of maybe 150 feet and saw people I hadn't seen for two or three weeks.

I guess one of the first bits of indoctrination for me was a guy who got his finger caught in the combing when somebody slammed the hatch, and it popped off part of the thumb tissue. I managed to put that back, and his thumb worked fine.

Submarines were not built for fleet work that would last over long periods of time. They were not intended for thirty-day and forty-five-day patrols. So the only storage you had for food was to put all the canned foods on the deck. You could tell when it was time to go home because you could see the deck. And if you still had torpedoes and no food, you still had to stay on station. That was the way it was.

They would bring aboard corrugated cardboard cartons filled with cans of food, and they all had labels on them. After a short incubation period, the ship would be filled with cockroaches. They came aboard in the interstitial sections of the corrugation and they ate the glue on the cans. Eventually it got around to the point where the cans didn't have labels. Sometimes I awoke with my legs black with roaches.

The air-conditioning system didn't work after the first week. It was just standard because Freon leaked out. They had installed a copper tank and hooked it up to the drain lines. When they operated the system, the condensate collected and ran back into this five- or six-foot copper tank, and that's what we used to brush our teeth. It was just perspiration that had been condensed.

We never had enough bunks. Everybody had to have a turnover of the bunks on watch. The mattresses were soaked with perspiration and they were mildewed. I guess they hadn't accounted for this because the air-conditioning was supposed to take care of much of that. Eventually we got permission to discard the mattresses. Everybody was willing to help get them out of there. Afterward we slept on open springs. You spread your shirt out over the springs as if you were in the finest hotel in the world and got in the bunk.

Once the war began, we were part of the submarine force feeding Bataan, or attempting to. We'd go into Cebu, leave our torpedoes, take on food, and run it to Corregidor for use at Bataan. They had to get it over to Bataan on lighters [shallow-draft barges used to transport cargoes short distances]. After a while the situation had deteriorated to such a point on Bataan that they were firing on Corregidor and Corregidor was firing on Bataan. We had started to unload, and they decided we just couldn't do it. There was no way we could get that food off, and we had many tons of food. So we had to negotiate the minefield and get out of there. On the way out we picked up people who were to be evacuated.

On one of the trips out of Corregidor, the minesweeper *Pigeon* [AM-47] came alongside, and I remember the guy who was on it—his name was [Richard L.] Bolster.[5] Bolster was a hospital corpsman. He also was a diver and a wrestler—a big, big guy. He leaned over the rail and yelled, "Have you got any morphine or anything for pain?"

I had two tubes of eighth grain or quarter grain, and I gave him a little tiny tube, half of what we had. You could see that we were losing the battle and there was no resupply. I think it hit me dramatically that here

---

5. See Bolster's excerpt—"Rice Is Life"—in chapter 3.

we couldn't get a tube of morphine for pain. All we had were twenty little tablets in those little tubes. And it was a drop in the bucket for what he would need. But corpsmen were determined to do whatever they could to ease pain and suffering, and they did a great job.

YANGTZE PATROLLER

Lt. Alfred L. Smith joined the Navy in 1938 and received his orientation in military medicine at the Naval Medical School in 1939. He then became a Yangtze Patroller, stationed aboard the USS *Luzon* (PG-47), one of many shallow-draft river craft that patrolled the Yellow and Yangtze Rivers defending Uncle Sam's interests in China.

As the Japanese menace grew and the Yangtze Patrol was disbanded along with its parent command, the Asiatic Fleet, the Americans withdrew to the Philippines. Smith arrived in Manila shortly before Pearl Harbor and, like many of his comrades, was trapped by the outbreak of war.

My first assignment after reporting to the Asiatic Squadron in 1939 was the Cavite Navy Yard dispensary in the Philippines. I was there about six months before being assigned to the U.S. naval hospital at Cañacao near Manila and then the 4th Marines in Shanghai. Then I was transferred to Camp Holcomb in North China. In August of 1940 we evacuated to Shanghai, where I went on river-patrol duty aboard the USS *Luzon*.

To be truthful, there often wasn't much to keep us occupied. I was on a ship with a hundred sailors, all rough and ready and well tattooed. I would hold sick call and find that nobody was sick. My workday began at 8:00 and was over by 8:05.

We patrolled up and down the river until I knew the Yangtze better than the back of my hand. I saw things I had never seen before. One time I went ashore, not far from where the *Panay* was sunk.[6] There was

---

6. On 12 December 1937, Japanese aircraft attacked the USS *Panay* (PR-5) as she cruised the Yangtze. Three men were killed and forty-three sailors and five civilian passengers wounded. After the United States lodged a formal protest, Tokyo accepted responsibility and paid indemnities.

a little Chinese hospital that had a ward filled with about thirty people. It seemed very strange that no one was sitting up or showing any signs of life. "What's wrong with them?" I asked.

They all had leishmaniasis. I had never seen a single case in my life and suddenly there was a whole ward full.

The Japanese were very much in evidence. When we patrolled the river we went through territory they controlled. And it was the same when we played golf. To get to the golf course we had to stop at a Japanese checkpoint. When they saw the American flag and stars on the bumper, they usually waved us through.

In November of 1941 a telegram came ordering the 4th Marines and river gunboats to proceed to Manila. By then, the *Luzon*'s sides had been raised and reinforced with planks. When we passed Formosa, we could see Japanese ships waiting. They signaled for us to stop and head back to China. But Rear Admiral [William A. Glassford, Jr.] Glassford replied that he was proceeding south. One of the cruisers aimed its guns but didn't fire. I didn't know it at the time but one of our submarines was accompanying us. I never saw it until we approached Luzon and it surfaced nearby. Later I learned that had the cruiser opened fire it would have been torpedoed.

It took us through the worst weather I'd ever seen. The *Luzon* had never been in the ocean before and even though we had boarded her up, she took water and rolled like crazy. Once she tipped forty-five degrees one way and forty-six degrees the other. Dishes on shelves with a side rail came over the rail and smashed all over the deck. When we got to Manila someone pointed out that the sides of the boat had bent between each rib.

I had been out in the Far East two and a half years and should have been back in the States. Transportation was sitting right there in Manila Harbor. I think Admiral [Thomas C.] Hart [commander in chief, U.S. Asiatic Fleet] knew what was up. I think he knew the war was coming. My orders and many others' were on his desk waiting to be signed. On Sunday, the day before Pearl Harbor, a Commander Harris and some other officer went out to the golf course. After the eighteenth hole everyone came into the clubhouse for a drink. Harris sat down nearby Admiral Hart and asked him about the orders. Hart said, "Your orders are on my desk with a stack that high. If everything is all right tomorrow at ten o'clock, come by and I'll have them signed."

The next morning at 4:10 the pharmacist's mate came down, tapped on my door, and said, "Doctor, don't turn on the light and don't light a cigarette. We're at war with Japan." Needless to say, no one went to the admiral's office to pick up any orders. Then the American President Lines ship with my stateroom shoved off and went back to the States. And there I was.

About twenty-four hours later, things began getting rough. We saw them bomb Nichols and Clark Fields. Two days later, bombers flattened the Cavite Navy Yard in less than an hour. I was sitting on the *Luzon* about two hundred yards offshore. We were a small target and obviously not worth hitting.

Around Christmas I recall the skipper standing on the bridge with a pair of binoculars. He saw two bombers coming toward us and shouted, "Full steam ahead, right hard rudder." The ship took a nosedive forward and the bombs dropped where we had been.

Not long after that, we were ordered to sail to Bataan and patrol the coast at night. The Japs would wait until dark and land behind our lines on barges. In a few weeks we ran out of fuel oil for the gunboat. With what was left we sailed out into Manila Bay and moored just off Fort Hughes to help with beach defense. Hughes was on one of the small islands.

Once the Japanese took Bataan, they set up their artillery on the beach and began hitting Fort Hughes. We hid in the bushes, in foxholes, or wherever we could find cover. The range was about four miles and they could hit wherever they wanted. Their aim was very accurate. They could easily see where the shells landed from a spotter balloon. By then we had only one P-40 left. It was pretty beaten up and wired together so it could just barely fly.

About that time we were told a submarine was leaving Corregidor, and we were all expected to write a letter home. It didn't matter who you wrote to just as long as there was mail for that sub to take. One old sailor protested, saying he had no one to write to. They said, "You'd better find someone because the captain is not gonna like this."

So he sat down and wrote: "Dear Mr. President, Please send us another P-40. The one we've got is all worn out." And I understand that Roosevelt got it.

A NURSE'S STORY

On the eve of Pearl Harbor, twelve Navy nurses were serving in the Philippines at the Cañacao Naval Hospital.[7] When the Japanese first bombed the airfields around Manila and afterward destroyed the Cavite Navy Yard on 10 December 1941, these women not only had ringside seats but got a firsthand taste of the horrors of modern war as well. Suddenly they were forced to deal with hundreds of casualties. Nurse Dorothy Still tells how it was.

In 1939 I received orders to the Cañacao Naval Hospital in the Philippines. I traveled across the Pacific on the *Henderson* [AP-1]. It was a festive trip. We first stopped at Honolulu; I can still see the people on the dock there with their lais, and the hula dancers. Then we spent two or three days going around the islands.

Although the Philippines was not quite as spectacular as Hawaii, I became very fond of the base there anyway. The navy yard was just across Manila Bay, about a half mile away. It was a very active social life. There were always parties and, of course, the nurses got involved along with everybody else.

Our social concerns were put on the back burner when the dependents were sent home around the first of 1941. While we heard about the Rape of Nanking, nobody thought the Japs would be silly enough to try and do anything to Uncle Sam.

Pearl Harbor shocked me as it did everyone else. I and the other nurses were awakened in the middle of the night and told that Pearl Harbor had been hit. We were ordered to go to the hospital as soon as we got dressed. Since the hospital was right in the target zone, we sent all the ambulatory patients back to duty and the rest to Manila. Arrangements were made to admit the patients to what had been a dependents' ward at the Sternberg Army Hospital.

---

7. Chief nurse Laura Cobb, Bertha Evans, Helen Gorzelanski, Susie Pitcher, Eldene Paige, Edwina Todd, Goldia O'Haver, Mary Rose Harrington, Margaret Nash, Mary Chapman, Dorothy Still, and Ann Bernatitus.

On Wednesday the 10th, the [Cavite] navy yard was bombed. We could hear the planes roaring overhead. When they had finished wiping out the navy yard, they came around and hit one of the radio towers and down it came, crash bang. The raid lasted about an hour; then all of a sudden it was quiet. The quiet after so much noise was a shock in itself. It was a loud quiet.

We came out from under the building where we had taken shelter and there was the navy yard all flattened, and black smoke coming up everywhere.

We rushed to the hospital, and patients were all over the place. There were Filipino women, children, and men, and our own people from the navy yard. It was really a shocking scene.

The power to the hospital was knocked out. It was a pretty hectic afternoon. Triage was impossible; you just tried to find out which were the worst ones to go to surgery, and so on.

One patient called me over and said, "Nurse, I'm dying." I thought he was talking through his hat. I said to him, "Oh you're going to be fine."

And he responded, "Oh no, I know I'm dying." He told me that when he was in surgery, he'd heard the doctor tell the corpsmen and nurses that there was no use in trying to operate because his entire stomach and intestines were exposed. So they just put a hot blanket over his abdomen, covered him up, and sent him back to the ward.

I told him they must have been talking about somebody else. He said, "Oh no. They were talking about me." I told him I didn't think that was true and I would check to clear up the confusion. When I pulled back the covers there was a horrible odor. And there wasn't enough skin to connect. I was just sick. I asked him if he was comfortable and was there anything he needed. Would he like a sip of water? I told him I would be right back. You couldn't tell a patient he was dying; that just wasn't done.

I went back to making my rounds but it kept bothering me. I just felt so guilty about not being able to do something for the guy. Finally I got the courage to go back and ask him if there was anything else I could do for him. His bed was empty. He was dead. I went out and had myself a good cry.

We weren't the only ones overrun with patients. Sternberg Hospital too was quickly swamped. The only place available was Estado Mayor, an old Army base. We used the barracks as a temporary hospital. In the meantime they decided to set up joint surgical teams [with Army and Navy Medical Corps] throughout the city.

I was with the group assigned to the Jai Alai Club. Our purpose was to care for anyone that was hit, civilian or military, that would come into these emergency centers. We set up a little receiving station near the front of the building, but didn't get any patients. After spending a few weeks there, we were told to move to the Santa Scholastica school, also in Manila. The Army had already converted it into a hospital. Actually, we had more hospital personnel than patients. On 31 December the Army evacuated all the Army patients on a hospital ship and took them to Australia.

Meanwhile, the Army was retreating toward Bataan to make a stand there. The military declared Manila an open city and retreated, but the medical personnel remained.

THE ONE THAT GOT AWAY

As the Japanese onslaught continued unabated and American and Filipino resistance ended, eleven of the nurses became prisoners of war. One escaped. Assigned to an Army unit that fought a losing battle against the Japanese invaders on Bataan, Ann Bernatitus ended up on Corregidor and was the only Navy nurse evacuated by submarine just a day before the island bastion surrendered.

Ann A. Bernatitus joined the Navy in 1936 when that service had only 325 nurses. Following her second assignment at the naval hospital in Annapolis, she received orders to the Cañacao Naval Hospital. She arrived there in July 1940. "All I can remember about Manila is the smell of copra, which seemed to be everywhere," she said. "The nipa huts, the kids running around naked. The houses on stilts, the carabao. But life was very good out there too. We went to work at eight o'clock. You went to lunch and then didn't have to go back on duty. We had the afternoons off."

The exotic surroundings and tropical duty, with its houseboys, shopping, golf, and endless receptions, would soon become a cherished memory. A few days following the outbreak of war in the Pacific, Bernatitus and her nurse colleagues were divided into teams and assigned to remote locations in Manila, where it was thought their services would be needed. When Gen. Douglas MacArthur declared Manila an open city, Bernatitus, attached to a Navy surgical team, joined an Army convoy heading to Bataan.

There were twenty-four Army nurses, twenty-five Filipino nurses, and me, the one Navy nurse. As we passed through the villages, the natives came out and cheered us, giving us the V for victory sign. Many times during the trip the bus would have to stop and we would dive into gutters along the roadside, because the Japanese planes were overhead.

When we arrived at Camp Limay, Hospital Number 1, we found twenty-five wooden, one-story buildings, fifteen of them wards. A water pipe outside each ward provided water. The utility room for the bedpans was the back porch. The buildings were in a rectangle, with the operating-room building at the upper end with a generator and water towers alongside. At the farther end was the building housing the nurses' quarters and the officers' mess hall. The remaining buildings were along each side. Behind the buildings on the left side of the beach was a warehouse in which were stored the equipment and supplies for the hospital. In the center of this area were grass and trees, and foxholes dug everywhere. We were assigned two to a room.

Everyone was involved in setting up the hospital. All the supplies and equipment were crated and stored in the warehouse on the beach. The crates were neither marked nor stored as units, so the Navy crates had to be opened before you found the items for your particular unit. In one of them, there were surgical gowns wrapped in newspapers dated 1917.

The operating room was a long narrow building with approximately seven or eight tables set up in the center. Along the window openings were the cabinets with supplies. There were shutters with a stick to keep them open. I'm a bit vague on how we sterilized the gauze and linen, but it seems to me it was done in pressure cookers operated by kerosene. The instruments were sterilized by placing them in a foot tub filled with Lysol, then rinsing in alcohol. The period of sterilization depended on how fast they were needed. As the patients were brought in they were assigned to a table by Dr. Weinstein of the Army Medical Corps. The team assigned to that table took care of the patient regardless of what type of surgery was indicated. Casualties were heavy and the operating room was an extremely busy place.

We got there on December 24th. On January 23d 1942, Camp Limay moved to Little Baguio, farther down the peninsula. We had two meals a day—9:00 A.M. and 4:00 P.M. The wards were just concrete slabs with corrugated roofs. They were open on the sides. The operating room was on a little knoll.

On March 30th the hospital was bombed, even though the warehouse on the beach had a big red cross. There was a bench outside the operating room; I almost killed myself trying to get under that bench. When the alarm sounded you could hear the bombs coming down—a whistling sound.

On April 7th, the following week, they bombed us again and hit one of the wards. It was terrible. That hospital was right next door to the ammunition dump. There were patients who were tied in traction. The nurses had to cut the ropes so they could fall to the deck. There were many killed and wounded and pajamas in the treetops.

Every operating table was filled. The casualties would come in from the field all dirty. We did what we could. There were lice; I kept my hair covered all the time. We did many leg amputations because we had a lot of gas gangrene out there. We were washing the dirty dressings that they used during an operation. We washed them out, refolded, sterilized, and used them again.

On the 8th, when the front lines collapsed, we were transferred to Corregidor. It was after supper. We ate at four o'clock. About eight o'clock they told us to take what we had—and we didn't have much—and put us on buses. I left Dr. Smith and Dr. [Claud] Fraleigh there. Later on Dr. Smith showed up on Corregidor; Dr. Fraleigh didn't.

I think I had all I owned in a pillowcase. To get to Mariveles, we had to take a road they called the Zig Zag Trail, with a drop-off on both sides. We met the fellows coming up, going to the front lines.

We got down to the dock at Mariveles and had to stay there for a while waiting for a boat. Finally it arrived; it must have been a ferry. I sat in the passageway on a wicker chair, carrying my camera; I never gave that up and brought it home with me. They were shooting back and forth over us.

When we got to Corregidor I don't think the people there knew we were coming, because that night we had to sleep two in a bunk. The following morning, the Army chief nurse came to me. She took me out to what we called the hospital exit to show me what Bataan looked like with the ammunition dumps going up. You wouldn't believe the fireworks.

But I'd been less scared on Bataan than I was on Corregidor. When the Japanese bombed, the whole place just shook. We were in the hospital tunnel. The Malinta Tunnel ran straight through and the laterals branched off of it. The main tunnel was where MacArthur and [Gen. Jonathan] Wainwright had their headquarters. The hospital was in one of the laterals. Off the hospital lateral were other laterals. One was the nurse's quarters; another was the mess hall. Another was the operating room. It was not a clean tunnel; it was just rock.

I didn't do much work when I got to Corregidor because I had dysentery. Of course the Army was in charge, so Dr. Smith wasn't working either. I remember only doing one amputation with him.

I got to Corregidor April 8th and left on May 3d. I don't know how I was selected to be evacuated from Corregidor. The planes came in first to evacuate people. Two Navy PBYs took several Army nurses and fifteen other passengers on April 29th. How they picked them, I don't know.

Then on May 3d, they called us to the mess hall and told us we were going to be leaving that night. They stressed that weight didn't matter as much as size. All I had was a duffel bag. I'd always said that I didn't want to go out of there on an airplane; I would rather go by submarine. We hoped that would happen. They told us we would meet after dark in front of Wainwright's headquarters, but then the Japanese started shelling us so they canceled.

Then they told us to meet two or three hours later. Your name was called and you stepped out of the crowd, because everybody was gathered around to see this. Wainwright shook your hand and wished you Godspeed and he said, "Tell them how it is out here."

And then I got in a car and they took us out of the tunnel down to the dock. Everything was pitch-black, just some trees standing with no leaves, no nothing, everything charred. When we got down there we boarded a boat that was even smaller than the one that took us to Corregidor. Then we shoved off. We had to go through our own minefields to get to the submarine. We learned later that it was taking us so long to get out there that the submarine wasn't sure Corregidor hadn't already fallen.

Finally we saw a dark shape and came alongside of it. You could hear the slapping of the water between the two objects. Someone said, "Get your foot over the rail." And then someone pulled me. The first thing I knew I was going down the hatch. I got down there awfully fast. I had landed in the control room. Everything was lighted up and there were all these valves.

Besides me there were six Army officers, six Navy officers, and eleven Army nurses. There was also one civilian woman, and two stowaways—a Navy electrician's mate and a man who'd been with the Army transport.

When we were safely aboard the *Spearfish* [SS-190], they told us the voyage would last seventeen days; I thought I couldn't make it. First they took us into the officers' mess. That's where we sat, and they gave us tea and chocolate cake. We hadn't seen chocolate cake and tea in a long time.

The chiefs gave up their quarters for us. It was just a cabin with a sink in it. And our luggage came in there with us. We had to sleep in shifts—hot-bunking. I was one of the four picked to go to bed right away. The next morning when my eight hours were up, four others went to sleep.

You just had to kill time any way you could. The only thing we heard down in that submarine was the sound of the screws turning. We spent most of our time in the crew's mess. Someone had a Victrola that was playing all the time, and the crew came with magazines they had stashed away someplace. We sat and talked. And of course, the boys loved it.

The crew ate first. Anything they served was wonderful for us. We hadn't seen food like that. You know, after a while the gals were cooking for the boys.

For bathing and washing, each of us got one bucket of water when we went to bed. And each nurse got a bucket of water to go into the john and take a shower. If you don't think that was a treat. It was wonderful.

While we were on that submarine we remained submerged during the day, and at dusk we would surface to charge our batteries. When we came up, we came up at an angle. And then someone opened a hatch and we felt this gush of nice fresh air come through. We had hardly done this when *whish,* down we went again. Well, that was an experience.

Once they thought they sighted something. They turned everything off and everybody was sitting around doing nothing. We watched the men. Those who had shirts on dripped with perspiration. You could just see those shirts gradually turning from tan to brown with it. We must have been submerged for several hours, just barely crawling. But everything turned out okay.

When we got in to Fremantle [Australia], everybody from the admiral on down was there. The Navy had a hotel where people stayed, and that's where they put us up, a Navy wife and I. And the Army just took their nurses. I saw some of them when we were going home.

One day I realized that I had just had it. I wanted to go home. And nobody objected. Arrangements were made for me to fly to Melbourne to get the *West Point* [AP-23] troopship back. The Navy really took good care of me. When we got on that ship, they gave me just about the best stateroom in the house.

Ann Bernatitus returned to the United States and received the Legion of Merit for her heroic service at Bataan. She also traveled extensively, speaking about her experiences and promoting the sale of war bonds. After several shore assignments, she returned to the Pacific in 1944 as chief nurse aboard the hospital ship USS *Relief* (AH-1).

THREE

Guests of the Emperor

For most veterans who served in World War II, homecoming was a joyous occasion. They jumped back into the mainstream and picked up life where they had left it. For those who had been liberated from prisoner-of-war camps in the Pacific, though, the homecoming and recovery were long and difficult. The disease, torture, and deprivation they had suffered had robbed most of their health, and their lives would never quite return to normal.

A half century later, survivors of the Bataan death march, Corregidor, Camp O'Donnell, Cabanatuan, Davao, Tarlac, Bilibid, Woosung, Bicycle Camp, Changi, the Siam-Burma railroad, Umeda, Zentsuji, Fukuoka, Shinagawa, Tsumori, Omori, Ichioka, Kobe, Manchuria, and the infamous Japanese hell ships remember vividly the early days of 1942, when a seemingly invincible Japanese war machine quickly extinguished U.S. power in the Pacific. With the attack on the Philippines, they were among the first Americans to fight against hopeless odds until forced to give up, abandoned by a nation whose priority was liberating Europe from the Nazis.

For some, the days, weeks, and months of brutal captivity, forced labor, starvation, and boredom became a distant blur as time tended to sift out the worst of the horror. Others would never forget their days as prisoners of war. The sinister brutality inflicted upon these unfortunate men by their captors is almost beyond comprehension. Torture, sadism, beheadings, death ships, and starvation were routine.

In his book *Prisoners of the Japanese: POWs of World War II in the Pacific,* Gavan Daws vividly describes atrocities unparalleled in their singularity: "POWs, civilian internees, and Asian natives starved, beaten, tortured, shot, beheaded. The water cure. Electric shock. Vivisection. Cannibalism. Men strung up over open flames or coiled in barbed wire and rolled along the ground . . ."[1]

At very least, nearly all POWs experienced starvation. Many others witnessed barbarity inflicted by an enemy whose culture dictated that a soldier should die for one's emperor. The soldier who surrendered was beneath contempt. American POWs suffered accordingly.

When Guam and Wake fell in December 1941, the Japanese conquerors shipped the Marine, Navy, and civilian defenders of Guam to prison camps in Japan.[2] The Wake survivors went first to Shanghai and then Woosung. For the approximately 17,000 Americans and 12,000 Filipino scouts who surrendered in the Philippines, the real ordeal had barely begun. Although the Corregidor defenders had been spared the infamous Bataan death march, they still faced a grim future. It is estimated that 30 percent of the American captives and 80 percent of the Filipinos died during the first year.[3] Some were held in such notorious hellholes as Cabanatuan and Camp O'Donnell. The "lucky" ones ended up at Bilibid.

Built by the Spanish in 1865 as their main prison, Bilibid for the Japanese served as a central receiving station from which they transferred American prisoners to and from forced-labor camps throughout the Philippines. Later in the war it became a way station for prisoners on their way to Japan. When POWs became too weak from starvation and disease to work in the labor camps, their Japanese guards brought

1. Daws, *Prisoners of the Japanese,* 363.
2. Five navy nurses were stationed at the naval hospital in Guam when the war broke out; Virginia Fogarty, Marian Olds, Lorraine Christiansen, Doris Yetter, and Leona Jackson. Interned in Japan until the summer of 1942, they were exchanged for Japanese diplomats and nationals held in the United States.
3. Bird, *American POWs of World War II,* 141.

them to the hospital at Bilibid for treatment. Often they were already in such poor condition that the end could be measured in hours.

Bilibid had massive twenty-foot-high walls covering a city block in downtown Manila. A tall guard tower rose from the prison yard, and cement cell blocks radiated outward like spokes of a giant wheel. The cell blocks resembled cages in a row for housing large zoo animals, each cell holding about fifteen men, and each block having six such cells on a side.

When the newest prisoners arrived from the recently conquered Corregidor in late May 1942, they found a primary hospital already functioning, staffed by the medical personnel from Cañacao. But overall, Bilibid was a jarring sight filled with a filthy mess of humanity. Even at the outset, disease and malnutrition were widespread.

BILIBID POW

When the island bastion of Corregidor fell in May 1942, Lt. Alfred Smith, MC, became a prisoner of war. For nearly thirty-four months he languished in Bilibid. When MacArthur's troops rescued him in February 1945, he was ill, malnourished, and nearly blind. Yet, he pointed out, it may have been his poor condition that kept him off the death ships. In fact, he was the only officer from the *Luzon*'s crew to come home.

For the rest of his life, Smith asked the question repeated by others who somehow survived the camps, "Why am I here and not my buddies?"

The day we surrendered I was determined to get back to the States. That was not the attitude of everyone there. Many of them had already given up hope. I figured that someday the Yanks and tanks would be back and when they came I'd still be around.

The Japanese brought us to what was called the 92d Garage Area. It was a mass of humanity with scarcely any room to lie down. During the day, we'd bake in the sun with no shelter. There was no sanitation. We'd have a line waiting for water two or three hundred long, just to get a canteen of water. You got a mess kit full of rice with flies so thick on it you would take a spoon of it and before you would get it to your mouth you'd blow the flies off and eat the stuff. You had no choice; there wasn't anything else. We were there over a week before they took us by ship to Manila and from there to Bilibid. From that day on I never got outside that prison.

Bilibid was pretty bad. The only good thing I could say about that place is that we had running water. And rice was not the main course but the only course. We were fed moldy, musty rice that had been swept up from the floors of warehouses. The Japanese boiled it and it had a very sour taste. You could smell it a mile away. They put it in buckets set on rollers. Those who wouldn't eat it are still out there.

Sometimes we got camote tops. The camote is the Filipino equivalent of a sweet potato. The tops were boiled in rock salt. That was the extent of our greens. On rare occasions we had fish. The Japs didn't clean them, just fried them whole. At first we would pick out the bones, but after a while we ate them from end to end like a cookie.

Some of the prisoners had Filipino contacts on the outside and got us mongo beans. Mongo beans look like peas, no bigger than birdshot, but are rich in protein. One time a dog got caught in the wire surrounding the camp. We skinned it and boiled it in rock salt. Dogs are not bad eating. Another time the Japanese brought ducks into the prison to eat the garbage we threw out but they got beriberi and starved to death.

Every day was pretty much the same. Between work details, we played chess and cards. We bought a deck from another prisoner for fifty dollars. U.S. currency wasn't worth anything anyway. Fifty bucks for a deck of cards was a real bargain.

Before I got sick, I saw patients in the hospital we set up. We had practically nothing to run it with—no medicine and few instruments. We did have a makeshift operating room, but sterile facilities didn't exist. Heck, we had every disease you could think of in there—malaria, pellagra, dengue, beriberi, xerophthalmia, yaws, scurvy, elephantiasis, tuberculosis, and general malnutrition.

I was sick in bed most of the time with swollen ankles, painful feet, nausea, vomiting, diarrhea. It was at that point that many people said, "Oh hell, I'm not gonna eat that moldy stuff anymore." And they didn't, and went right downhill and died. We buried a lot of men behind that prison.

I had been having some trouble with the sun. My eyes seemed more sensitive than usual. But the blindness came suddenly. I think it was in September of 1942. I was reading a book about the presidents, the life of Andrew Jackson. I was on page forty-two and put it aside for the night. The next day I couldn't even find the page number, let alone the page. We had an ophthalmologist there at the time. He took one look at my eyes and said I probably had optic neuritis but now showed signs of optic atrophy. The nerve endings had almost completely disintegrated.

It was caused by vitamin B deficiency—thiamine hydrochloride. Lack of vitamin A causes xerophthalmia, ulcers on the corneas. We had plenty of those cases. When I got back to the States they poured vitamins into me every which way but it didn't do much good.

Even though we were isolated in that prison, we knew how the war was going. Down at the other end of the hall were four warrant officers. One of them appeared to be a little on the stupid side. He had built himself a stool to sit on. Underneath was a compartment with a radio he had assembled from scavenged parts. The Japanese appointed these warrant officers to take a head count every day. Often the counts took place after dark and so the Japanese had to furnish flashlights. Needless to say, the batteries didn't last very long in those flashlights.

Anyway, they would get news on the radio. They knew the Americans had landed in Bougainville and the southern islands but they didn't tell us. They would wait until the Japanese sent out a working party or there would be a transfer of men. About four hours after the newcomers arrived, the "stupid" one would say, "I heard a good rumor. Americans have landed in Leyte." Never would you get the news right away, only after some group was sent out on a detail to clean up a street or something and they'd come back. Nobody knew where the rumor came from.

After the Americans came, the warrant officer set his stool out on the ground and opened up the top and there was the radio. That was the best-kept secret in the camp and the stupid routine was one of the best acts I've ever seen.[4]

---

4. The radioman was Lt. Homer T. Hutchinson, a former mining engineer.

DOWN WITH THE STARS AND STRIPES

At Bilibid, work details often interrupted the monotony of a POW's daily existence. A truck required unloading, a road crew needed additional men, a Japanese officer decided his quarters had to be spruced up. In most cases a prisoner could dread the consequences of laboring all day in the broiling heat of a Philippine summer without adequate food or water. But there were some who welcomed any opportunity to leave the loathsome surroundings of Bilibid, if only for a day.

In November 1943 the Japanese ordered Comdr. Thomas Hayes, commanding officer of the Bilibid Prison hospital, to provide a draft of men for several days. Actors and extras were needed for a film depicting the Japanese victory in the Philippines. The script was simple. For the camera, Japanese soldiers and Americans playing themselves were to reenact Gen. Jonathan Wainwright's surrender of Corregidor. Scenes shot there would be spliced to others filmed at Bataan in what would become *Down With the Stars and Stripes,* a propaganda motion picture to be shown to Japanese audiences.

> PhM2c Chester K. Fast had his acting debut in the film, playing the roles of a soldier guarding one of the tunnels, General Wainwright's chauffeur, and his military aide.

I think they sent about a hundred of us to the Rock for the movie detail. Although there were other prisoners, Commander Hayes made the choice of what corpsmen would go. There was a bunch of us. Hayes wrote something about the fact that we were forced to do this.[5]

We all went over on a boat. Prior to leaving, a couple of prisoners not assigned to be in the movie brought maps and diagrams to show some of us where they thought money and jewels were buried. Some of us had

---

5. Robert Kentner's journal for 12 November 1943 notes: "The 37 corpsmen were commended at Senior Medical Officer's Mast for the splendid manner in which they conducted themselves during this trying and undesirable duty."

ideas of a treasure hunt, but to no avail since the guards would not let anyone wander away from the group.

There were about eight guards for each group. When we arrived at Corregidor and got off, we went up on the roof of one of the tunnels. I knew nothing about Corregidor because I had never been there before. We were standing there when a Japanese officer came up to us and in perfect English said, "Hi guys, how you doing?" He explained that he had been to school somewhere in the Los Angeles area and had gone back to Japan to visit his grandparents when the war started. He told us the only way he could stay out of the fighting was to join a troupe to entertain the soldiers, the equivalent of our USO. He was the star of the film. The director was also trained and had worked in Hollywood. That's all we knew about him.

As for uniforms, they gave us khakis to put on. I don't know how they kept track of everybody because there were very few guards; it was very loose. There were no threats or anything like that.

They had a script. In one scene, they had a bunch of us running out of one of the caves. I was standing in the cave with a rifle. They lined us up in one of the tunnels and then had a group come out. Jim [PhM2c James F.] Bray played the part of "Skinny" Wainwright. I was his aide and a major. The big scene was Jim and I walking out of the tunnel waving a white flag. Then they filmed a scene where we all marched up with the American flag and met the Japanese officers. Of course, we had to speak English. Whatever they said was in their language. In another scene I was driving the big limousine. Showing the same face playing different roles didn't seem to make any difference to them.

There were also some action scenes. There was one where the main Japanese actor and whoever was following him were coming across some water. It was actually a little creek. At the right time, all kinds of little bombs, or whatever they used for effects, exploded as they came across. You could see the water spray.

They had some level of expertise as far as knowing how to put a film together. The actor was good. And the director apparently knew what he was doing. It wasn't a slipshod job by any means. They had the dynamite set to explode at the proper time.

We were over on Corregidor about three days and then returned to Bilibid. And then ten of us went down to the studio in Manila a few times. I played a major holding a staff meeting. They brought in special food for us and we were treated all right. And we got to watch what was going on. Of course, my attitude was, anytime I could get out of camp and go on a working party, I'd go. It was my recreation.

None of us ever saw the movie, but our Bilibid guards did and teased me about it. One recognized me and said, "Ah, cinema, cinema." It was very amateurish, but an interesting adventure.

OHASHI

After his capture at Corregidor, Dr. Ferdinand V. Berley had a variety of prison experiences. His odyssey took him first to Bilibid, then to the farm camp of Cabanatuan, and finally to Japan itself, where he worked in the prison hospital at Tsumori Camp in Osaka, caring for American and Dutch POWs. Shortly thereafter, the Japanese sent him to Ichioka, a nearby hovel masquerading as a hospital. While there he established a relationship with the Japanese hospital commander, a man named Ohashi, who had been a prominent surgeon in civilian life.

Ohashi's sense of fairness and compassion contrasted sharply with what the prisoners had become accustomed to. It was then that Berley decided to learn Japanese. "Prior to that I thought anyone who learned how to speak Japanese was a traitor and I wouldn't do it," he said. "But now the idea seemed to be a good one."

I shouldn't even call Ichioka a hospital. It was underneath the stands on one side of an athletic stadium. A long passageway divided the place in two and was about six feet wide, and on either side were wooden platforms about one and a half feet high. These were divided by partitions which formed bays, about twelve feet square. The patients lay on their straw mattresses in these bays with their feet toward the center. The ceiling slanted down so that on the right side you couldn't stand up. There was no ventilation, no windows.

Another doctor had been sent to Ichioka besides myself, an Australian named Ackroyd. He had been at Zentsugi, a camp on the Inland Sea, where they had sent all the officers. He arrived at Ichioka about three or four days before I did. Many of the sick in this camp were British. Just a few of our men were there.

Ackroyd and I settled down and got acquainted. Our office was a small room at the back end left side. He and I slept up forward on the right side, where you couldn't stand. Everyone had two grayish-brown Japanese-issue woolen blankets you formed into a sleeping bag that you could crawl into on top of a straw mattress. There was a washroom and toilet at the back end, but most of the sick were too weak to bathe and some were covered with lice. There was nothing there but a bunch of scarecrows—horribly diseased, sick men.

The new doctor, Ohashi, sent for Ackroyd and then for me. Evidently he could understand me better than Ackroyd. I had trouble understanding him myself. Ohashi wanted me to come every afternoon for an hour and teach him English, which I did. I became his tutor.

We had plenty of cigarettes and Ackroyd smoked and coughed constantly. And he never turned his head or put his hand in front of his face. We slept next to one another and he coughed all night. Later on he was diagnosed with TB. There was TB all through the place. With Ackroyd coughing in my face all the time, it was a miracle I didn't get a severe case as well.

The food was pretty terrible. Once a month we were supposed to get a ration of fish. I remember seeing fish come in one day, and when we got our meal that night I didn't see any fish, so I asked the cook where the fish was. He told me the Japs had taken it. He said that was one of the things they did. I went to Ackroyd and said, "Look, you are senior to me. They stole our ration of fish. What are you going to do about it?" He replied that there wasn't much to do about it. I told him if he was unwilling to go see Ohashi, I would. I shamed him into going.

Every night the Japs came in to hold tenko [roll call]. Ackroyd stood at attention; I stood at attention next to him. That night there were three of them. One was named Kato. He had his hands behind his back. And there were two other guards behind him on either side. They too had their hands behind their backs. Ackroyd spouted off the tenko, which told the Japanese how many patients were there and so on. And right after that they started on us. They had long leather belts and they beat the daylights out of all of us. They even went to where the sick guys were lying on their straw mats and, yelling and screaming, they beat them. Then they warned me, "Don't you say anything to Ohashi." It was the fish protest that caused all this. I learned a lesson the hard way.

My tutoring of Ohashi progressed to the point where he was getting pretty good and we could understand one another pretty well. I asked myself how I could possibly get him to go back where the sickest patients were and see what we had. He had no idea about all those horrible, stinking bodies with lice, TB, and whatnot, emaciated men just like the pictures you see from Buchenwald and places like that.

Finally we got talking about medicine, and I said to him, "We have several cases back there and we just don't know what to do with them. They're quite complicated and beyond our scope. I was wondering if you might take the time to come back with us and examine some of them." And he agreed.

We had those who could walk come back in that little office, one after another. He sat on a stool and all he said was "Sah, sah." He couldn't believe what he was seeing. A few days later, we had the biggest damn feast you've ever seen. It was unbelievable!

BOMBS ON KOBE

Shortly thereafter Berley was moved yet again, to what the Japanese euphemistically called the Kobe International Prisoner of War Hospital. There he was to be the senior medical officer in charge. The new hospital, staffed by Australian, British, Dutch, and American personnel, was the Japanese response to international outrage over their treatment of POWs. It occupied a former American school in the hills above Kobe. "It was a beautiful location. We had a nice clean air and a wonderful view of part of the harbor," said Berley.

From their vantage point, he and his comrades watched the war come home to Japan. Hope that freedom was not far off was tempered by fear that American bombs might end their suffering first.

In February 1945 we experienced our first air raid. They hit the shipyard plant right below us. These bombers came in and what a sight that was! We saw one fighter going up to hit a B-29 from behind and as he was climbing above it from behind, all of a sudden he just flipped and spiraled on down into the sea. I saw two planes shot down that day by B-29s. We also saw one bomber hit and drift smoking out to sea.

The bombing raids became more frequent and, to help build our morale, we organized a pool as to when the next one would take place. Everybody got into this thing. You put in a yen or whatever you wanted and picked the time of the next raid.

One day I saw the Japanese tow an aircraft-carrier hull they had been working on into the harbor. Evidently they had launched it from one of the shipyards. Just about the 17th of March, around St. Patrick's Day, planes suddenly appeared out of nowhere. The Japs had an elaborate system of air-raid warnings. They rang bells when planes were first spotted, and you would hear the bells getting closer and closer. These planes came in so fast there was no time to ring bells, and the bombs were falling when the bells finally sounded. They were Navy dive-bombers. That was a sight to see! They were just like a bunch of bees buzzing all over trying to find targets. I saw them level off and make several direct hits on that aircraft carrier. I waited all day for that darned thing to sink but it never did. We knew then that things were getting mighty close.

During that time, we saw some interesting cases at the hospital. We had several patients brought in from the work camp below—the stevedores. One was a young army boy born and raised in the Philippines who had never received any tetanus antitoxin. He had injured his toe and had a very bad infection. We tried to get the guards to allow him to stay in the hospital, but they wouldn't and carried him back. Two days later they brought him back. To make a long story short, he came down with tetanus. John Bookman treated him. Ohashi was able to get some tetanus serum from another hospital. John gave large doses of the serum and heavy doses of sedatives to deal with his tremendous seizures; his back would get almost like an arch. The only way to combat them was with the sedatives; we had plenty of those. And the man survived!

We also had an Australian major brought in from Zentsuji, the officers' camp on an island in the Inland Sea. He had a tumor on his cheek that had invaded the bone. A British doctor named Page was the surgeon, and I assisted. John Bookman gave the anesthesia, a mixture of chloroform. It was just a miraculous thing John did. We were able to operate on him for five or six hours and the surgery came out fine. We ran into some pretty tough bleeding at times but were able to stop that. Working right underneath the brain, we removed the tumor and half his maxilla, and then closed a flap over it. A lot of personnel and even some patients donated part of their powdered-milk ration we had gotten from

Red Cross supplies so that we could nourish him through a nasogastric tube. We sent him back to his camp, where he recovered. I think he actually made it back to Australia.

On the morning of 5 June, about 5:30 or so in the morning, the alarms went off. We didn't see anything imminent at the time, so we went ahead and had our breakfast at 7:30. About fifteen or twenty minutes later, the attack on Kobe began. We moved all patients downstairs to the main floor and most of them into a ward. We also took whatever stores we had—about ten bags of grain, soy butter, medicine—from the storehouse and put it in a shelter we had dug in front of this ward for safekeeping. We also had pulled some first-aid kits together, with bandages, morphine, stethoscopes, and things like that.

I went running around through the halls yelling, "This is it. This is the big one!" We looked up into the sky, but by that time you couldn't even see the sun, which was pretty well blotted out by the smoke from below. By then the planes were flying directly over us. The first wave came in below and then the next wave followed. Then the next would move over. They were pattern-bombing. Pieces of tin, bullets, and wreckage were floating down and hitting the compound.

Fortunately we moved over in front of I Building, and all hell broke loose. Later I counted about ten large oil bombs that hit our compound. When they hit, they exploded with a great big *whoosh* and a tremendous flame. One hit right in the room where we had taken one of our patients, a man named Hammelgard. I was about fifteen feet away. There was a tremendous explosion of just fire, nothing like a bomb blast. Later on we figured that five of them hit the buildings. Fortunately, none struck the ward where we had taken most of the patients.

Before the attack we'd put many of the patients in another shelter we had dug, and had also taken as many blankets as we could and thrown them in the little pond. I remember running back and forth bringing patients out. Nearby, flames were erupting out of a hole in the ground where a bomb hit a storage shelter we had dug for our grain. It was on fire. I was just lucky I didn't fall into that thing.

The fires had become so intense it was unbearable to stay in the compound. I was one of the last to leave. As I went out, patients, staff, and many Japanese civilians were lined up along the road. Some were lying there, some were sitting. Some were moaning and crying. With our emergency kits we administered aid to them too. Although we didn't have much to treat them with, we had plenty of morphine, which we administered for pain. By then it was almost completely dark from the smoke; the sun was invisible.

After everything subsided, we moved back into the compound to assess the damage. Hammelgard and two TB patients had been killed, and there were about seventeen patients burned and about three others with severe injuries. About twenty others had been slightly injured by falling timbers.

So there we were with everything in ashes, to the cement foundations. Later we found Hammelgard's torso; the rest of his body was completely burned. We also found just a few bones from the other two victims. They had been completely incinerated.

Because of the destruction, the wind had kicked up and was just blowing like all get out. Ohashi's room in his building was still standing, and he turned it over to us. We then tried to build a temporary shelter near the morgue, but could only put about five or six of the badly burned in there. All patients that could walk and staff were lined up and ordered to leave. I was left with about thirty-five of the severe cases, including seventeen badly burned. I chose John Bookman and four corpsmen to stay with me. So we were left there by ourselves.

We worked till about midnight with what few medical supplies we were able to salvage from the burned-out storage we had built. Practically all the grain and other food had burned. I think we had seventy sulfanilamide pills and some bandages, but not very many, certainly not enough to take care of the injured, but we did the best we could.

✚

RICE IS LIFE

PhM1c Richard L. Bolster was on duty aboard the minesweeper USS *Pigeon* (AM-47) when the Japanese invaded the Philippines. On the afternoon of 4 May 1942, ordnance from a Japanese dive-bomber hit the *Pigeon*'s starboard quarter and the old ship sank in eight minutes. Bolster escaped but was captured two days later, when Corregidor fell.

He spent the next thirteen months in Manila's Bilibid prison. The Japanese eventually transferred him and a draft of prisoners to another POW camp in the countryside—Cabanatuan—and then to Japan. There he and his comrades became slave laborers, chipping sand from castings in the foundry of Osaka's Mitsubishi shipyard.

Following his liberation in September 1945, Pharmacist's Mate Bolster was commissioned a Lt. (jg) in the Hospital Corps. He later wrote a moving account about an incident that occurred near the end of the war.

In the Orient everything is subordinate to rice. Rice is life! After thirty months of duty in Asiatic waters before the war, I knew this. After forty months of imprisonment by the Japanese, I understood this. There is a difference between knowing and understanding.

In the first year of imprisonment in the Philippines, 50 percent of the deaths could be traced to "I just can't eat dry rice." Even our captors used to say, "Ah—(with a hiss through their teeth) but the Americans don't eat enough rice."

The Japanese were right, for once—our doubting resulted from our proof (on paper) that the human body could not be sustained on rice alone. That was in 1942. In 1947, those of us who have returned are living evidence that rice is life. In the long months in prison camps, there was not enough rice for those of us who had learned to *like* rice.

Many of us were selected from the prison camps in the Philippines for the "Japanese Far Eastern Excursion"—destination Japan. Most of us thought our traveling to be of the one-way variety. And for the many who died en route and those who survived the trip only to die in the Japanese homeland, it was a one-way journey.

Japan, early in 1945, was in its death throes. At Kobe, on the south end of Honshu Island, the Japanese had collected large numbers of Allied war prisoners. We had been selected to help staff the Kobe International Prisoner of War Hospital. Comprised of medical department personnel, both officer and enlisted, from among the British, Australians, Dutch, and Americans, the hospital was operated as commensurately as possible in accordance with rank and rating.

The United States Navy was represented on the staff of the hospital by three medical officers, one dental officer, and six pharmacists' mates.

The Kobe prison was a Japanese enterprise of propaganda—an institution designed to please the expected victorious Allied troops. Considering the state of poverty and rationing in Japan at the time, the Japanese were as lavish in equipping the hospital as their means and supplies would permit.

The building had formerly been a missionary [Presbyterian boys'] school. While not large, it was capable of housing more than a hundred patients. It included a small operating room, a dental unit, a portable X-ray unit, a laboratory, and three wards.

A pharmacy, adequate in size and surprisingly well stocked, completed the facilities available. The pharmacy's stock was surprising because it is difficult to picture, with words, the extreme shortage of all materials in Japan during the last days of the war.

While the hospital was totally incapable of providing for all the sick in the prison camps in the area, much good was accomplished from the time of the commissioning in the spring of 1944 until it was destroyed by Allied bombing on the morning of 5 June 1945.

The wooden buildings were a pile of smoking ashes in a little more than thirty minutes after being struck by incendiary bombs at about 9:30 A.M. Three patients died during the raid, and a half dozen more who suffered third-degree burns died as a result. We were able to salvage some supplies and equipment, but the Japanese guard prevented us from entering the burning building for more than a pitifully short supply.

On the evening of the day following our loss of the hospital, we were ordered to move. The new camp location was about eight miles away. We salvaged nails and improvised litters from boards removed from the high fence that had encircled the hospital area. The litters were for the sicker patients. Others we carried piggyback part of the way.

At about 10:00 P.M., a light rain which had been making movement unpleasant turned to a raging downpour with heavy gales of wind, adding to our misery and discomfort. There we were, leaving the outskirts of Kobe, half-starved specters of men, some walking, some carried, some half-carried; the smoldering ruins of the hospital, reagitated into flames by the wind; pieces of roof suspended at odd angles across telegraph wires; stark outlines of building left partially standing; homeless people seeking shelter in abandoned streetcars; a fantastic, overwhelming sense of ruin and helplessness on all sides. I thought at the time that this was, in truth, the valley of the shadow of death. It appears even more so in recollection.

By morning we had arrived in our new camp (new to us), in the Maryama district of Kobe. The camp was vermin-infested, and the Japanese cut our ration to two meals a day, less than an estimated eight hundred calories. This was when rice was really life. It was measured to the last gram. It was doled out the first time around with a bowl and a paddle, then with a spoon, then practically by the grain.

If one man had a noticeable bit more in his bowl than another it meant a quarrel. The man who doled out the rice was a public figure indeed. He was generally selected by his fellow prisoners as a person of forthright honesty coupled with an uncanny sense of equality in his ability to standardize and equalize all rice rations. He gambled his reputation with each meal on the possible slip of a spoon or too much pressure on one man's bowl with the paddle and not enough on another's. All these were resultant circumstances because there was not enough rice, and we *understood* that rice was life.

Our new camp location was on a high elevation where, even in July, the nights were cold. One day the Japanese quartermaster took five of the enlisted staff, procured a hand-drawn cart, and informed them that they would go to the site of the former hospital to see what could be salvaged. As one of the five, I was very happy to make the eight-mile trek, because it meant a change of environment, if only for a day; also, the quartermaster had promised us a noon meal somewhere along the way.

Of the group, two were American, two were British, and one was Australian. There was little talking among us; we grated somewhat on each other's personalities. This is always the way when men are hungry. Furthermore, we knew each other too well. Each knew instinctively what another would say concerning almost anything.

We stopped once to smoke some of our precious tobacco. Tobacco was the second most vital item after rice. Much as we irritated each other, we always shared our tobacco, because there was no telling who might have tobacco when you had none. It was a sort of investment in the future. We rested, smoked, then went on again, dragging the heavy cart in turn, silently relieving one another in relay. At two o'clock we arrived at the old site. Hopefully and hesitatingly we questioned the quartermaster regarding the promised meal.

Maybe because it was a lovely summer day, maybe because he knew things we didn't, I'm not sure. I prefer to believe the former, and I still believe I'm right. In any event, he bared his teeth in a jagged grin. "*Ima* (eat now) messy-messy," he said.

We asked the logical next question: "How much?"

Then he uttered the word that threw us into ecstasy. "*Toxon,*" he said. *Toxon* means plenty, or all you want, or a great deal, or whatever one prefers to call it.

Though the once-beautiful Kobe was a rubble, the day was more lovely already. Evergreens on the slopes were sharp in panoramic relief against a soft afternoon sky. The harbor glistened in the distance. A beautiful rosebush clung bravely to a trellis, both adjacent to a tree that had been scorched. I thought then how inseparable are life and death, but it was still a rosebush and still alive and therefore still beautiful.

The quartermaster showed us where to get a cauldron and sack of rice. The cauldron was rusty and the rice full of gravel and sand. What did we care how much gravel was in the rice? It could be washed. I found myself looking at the Australian and he at me. Then we found ourselves laughing. Then we noticed the other three laughing in unison, and there we stood, laughing like little children, laughing because there was no other way to express ourselves, maybe laughing partly at our ludicrousness. I don't think I quite know yet. Then it came upon us simultaneously, as thoughts do when men know one another too well— we didn't hate each other anymore. The long-pent-up emotions of laughter and love had been freed by one sack of gravelly rice. We were closer to each other then than we had been in long, long months.

We turned to, built a fire, cleaned the rice, scoured the cauldron, drew some water, put the rice in the cauldron, measured the water in proportion to the rice, then poured it into the cauldron, and the cooking commenced. We shared our tobacco around. It was all too wonderful. We watched the water start to boil in the bottom of the cauldron. We watched the grains of rice swell. The first small bubbles turned into larger ones as the water came to a full boil. When the rice had absorbed the excess of water and the surface grains had steamed to dry, flaky kernels, we knew that the rice was done. We would have our stomachs full—truly full for the first time since last December, and this was July. We had tobacco for two more rounds yet. We would have enough rice to take some back with us, the quartermaster being willing. Oh, life was good that day; and even now when I think about it and write about it, I still feel a remnant of the ecstatic twinge that I felt so keenly then.

We stood over the cauldron and heaped up the bowls that the quartermaster had borrowed for us. We didn't have to measure it, all we had to do was heap it up, just heap it up, and then start on another bowl full. We didn't talk until the first bowl was gone. Seldom did prisoners talk while eating. It proved a distraction from the pleasure of eating. On the second bowl, the talk started. Our talk didn't bore us; not today. The Australian was witty. The Britishers were not dull either; not anymore. Rice was life and we had *toxon*.

We had rice left over. We found a wooden bucket and put the rice in it. We hoped that we might take it back to camp. We set it at one side so it wouldn't be conspicuous. We didn't want to make the quartermaster angry by having him think that we were wasteful with the rice when he had truly been generous. We loaded the cart with salvaged, half-burned blankets. At 5:00 P.M. we were ready for the long haul back to camp. Our stomachs were still full. We laughed and swapped stories. The sun was still high in the west. The green mass of pines on the slope had known peace and seemed quietly waiting for its return, appeared to know—yes, it even appeared to know that we, all five of us—had had enough rice.

We started back to camp. The road was rough and hilly. The blankets were an awkward, cumbersome load, making the cart difficult to pull. The wheels grated for lack of oil. Three pulled and two pushed from behind. Still, it was all right; we worked willingly. Our bodies and minds were agile and alert. Our clothes stuck to our bodies and we were dirty, but all this was secondary because for once we were not hungry. Life was good again.

At dusk we stopped at the halfway mark to rest. We brought out the bucket of rice. The quartermaster told us that we must not eat when a Japanese civilian passed, because it might cause talk. He informed us that such an enormous amount of rice among five men would cause trouble in a small suburb where rations were short. He stated that he himself might have to answer for it. Two civilians passed in the deep dusk. We hid the bucket and ceased mastication, our mouths still full, until the quartermaster said that we might eat again.

It was fully dark and the moon was high when we topped the last hill before entering the camp. A dog bayed somewhere, and night birds were audible in the pines. It was as beautiful a night as the afternoon had been; not a night for a prison camp. I remember musing that somewhere, people walked arm in arm and found love and beauty in each other, things that we had all but forgotten. The camp seemed right for us. It was a dim dream that we had ever been free men. It was an even stranger fantasy that we would ever be free again, though we sensed that enough, as the time was drawing close.

Right then we had had enough and still had enough rice. That was the important thing.

A DOCTOR'S STORY

Just hours after the first Japanese troops arrived in Manila, the conquerors showed up at the nearby Cañacao Naval Hospital. Navy physician Capt. Lea Sartin later recalled that "a detachment of guards under the command of a petty officer set up a guard post at the front gate. A machine gun was set up at the gate, surrounded by a barricade of sandbags and aimed at the front door of the hospital."[6] After physically abusing staff and patients and looting the hospital's precious supply of medicines, the Japanese took the Americans to Bilibid prison. Thus began a nightmare for Sartin that would last three years.

Because he was the senior officer present, the Japanese designated him commanding officer of the hospital that the Americans were allowed to set up within Bilibid's forbidding walls.

Conditions in Bilibid were as extremely bad from every standpoint as can be imagined. This notorious prison had been abandoned a few years previously, because it was no longer considered a suitable place to imprison criminals. And in the intervening time the buildings had deteriorated from neglect and decay. Some of them had been used as storehouses and work offices of some of the Philippine departments. Most of the plumbing fixtures and electric light wires and connections had been removed. The roofs of all the buildings leaked during rainy weather. Equipment for cooking was primitive in the extreme.

There was a kitchen under a shed and a mess hall that would possibly accommodate forty to fifty persons at a sitting. The only cooking

---

6. Sartin, "Report of Activities of the United States Naval Hospital in the Philippines," 47.

utensils were twelve or fifteen fifty-gallon *callas* [cauldrons], in which rice could be steamed or the watery soup boiled. The unscreened kitchen was infested with clouds of flies. The long open latrine, emptying into an open cesspool, which was literally teeming with myriads of maggots, was not more than fifty feet away. The mess hall was partially screened, but its capacity was so small that it had no value to us as a place to eat.

Many critically ill patients were found in Bilibid. One Army captain, suffering from the clinical signs and symptoms of cerebral malaria, dysentery and pneumonia, died during the first night. Eight other patients were found in a small chapel building, where they were lying on Army stretchers fouled with dysenteric feces and covered with swarms of flies. Three of these men were suffering from pneumonia and five from dysentery.

Into this filthy and degrading hellhole, American prisoners of war were herded and housed with no semblance of regard for the rules and regulations of the Geneva Convention or the International Rules of Warfare.[7] Officers and men were herded together and no attention or recognition was given to our chain of command. These were the conditions the officers and men of the U.S. Naval Hospital Unit confronted when they entered Bilibid.

On 1 October 1943 the Japanese transferred Sartin and a draft of men to Cabanatuan, a notorious series of camps about ninety miles north of Manila. By the end of the war, Cabanatuan was said to be the largest American POW camp in Asia. Because it was in a low rice-growing region, monsoon rains often turned the ground into a fetid swamp, which bred swarms of malarial mosquitoes and flies. Crudely built, overflowing, and overused latrines added to the general misery and death toll from dysentery. Hundreds of sick, emaciated men died here each day.

Nevertheless, by the fall of 1943 the Japanese allowed the prisoners to augment their almost-nonexistent rations by growing vegetables. Sartin and his men also had the prospect of seeing old friends and comrades.

---

7. Although the Japanese had signed the Geneva Red Cross Convention, Tokyo was not a signatory to the convention relating to the treatment of prisoners of war. Nevertheless, in early 1942 Japanese officials assured Swiss diplomats that Japan would make every effort to adhere to the latter convention. This was an empty promise.

There were about 3,500 Americans at Cabanatuan. The camp, under the leadership of Lt. Col. Curtis T. Beecher, USMC, was well organized. The food served there at that time, while poor and insufficient in quantity, was much better than it had ever been in Bilibid. The quantity and quality of the food issued continued at this level until about December 1943, when the American Red Cross boxes arrived. Each man received as his portion four and half Red Cross boxes, which was a Godsend.

However, coincident with the receipt of this food, there was a sharp decrease in the food issued by the Japanese. The food issued by them was slowly and relentlessly decreased, until the personnel of the camp were on rations which were far below the maintenance level in calories, protein, fats, and vitamins for the last five or six months.

The hospital buildings at Cabanatuan were not as good as those at Bilibid, and the sanitary arrangements were very crude. However, the doctors and corpsmen made up for the deficiencies of the buildings by careful and painstaking attention to the details of their work. It must be said that excellent medical care was given to the sick, even in such poverty and squalor of housing and hospital equipment.

A typical day began with reveille shortly before dawn, followed by bango or tenko. All persons had to assemble in groups and count off. Working parties assembled about 0730 to 0800. Each group was assigned to do a particular kind of work that day, some to work on the farm, some to go out in the woods to cut firewood for the kitchens, others to do construction work and the work of sanitation around the compound. After the groups were formed they were marched to the gate, where they were met by Japanese guards with rifles and fixed bayonets. These guards accompanied the working parties everywhere they went. Some of them were good-natured and apparently human, but many of them were vicious, cruel, sadistic individuals and scarcely a day passed but some American was viciously beaten for a trifling or fancied infraction of Japanese rules.

Sometime about July or August 1944, during the noon hour, we heard the crack of a rifle. A few moments later another shot was fired. We all ran from our barracks to see what was happening, but were ordered to get back in by some of the senior American line officers who'd seen what had happened.

Lieutenant Hufcutt, USA, was working in his little private garden, located inside the inner fence of the compound. A Japanese sentry, stationed in one of the towers outside the compound, began to scream in Japanese. This was a common occurrence, and as Lieutenant Hufcutt was working with his back to the enemy, he never knew that the sentry was screaming at him. The sentry rested his rifle on a railing of the tower, took deliberate aim, and fired. Lieutenant Hufcutt fell to the ground, struggling. When the Japanese sentry saw that he was still alive he took deliberate aim and fired again.

A few moments later, Lieutenant Colonel Deeter, the medical officer in charge of the dispensary of that area, took a stretcher and, accompanied by a Japanese interpreter who had been summoned, went to the aid of Lieutenant Hufcutt, but I think he was dead before they got to him, the second shot having ended his life almost instantly. It is doubtful if he ever knew what happened to him.

FOUR

Island Warfare

In light of the Pacific theater of operations, Navy medicine had to reinvent itself. Necessity and adaptability were the watchwords. The nature of island-hopping through a far-flung and often tropical environment required a new medical strategy. Navy medicine had to overcome both the environment and the Japanese.

Medical personnel encountered exotic diseases they had never seen before. For example, in the early campaign to subdue the Solomon Islands, malaria caused more casualties than did enemy bullets. Two months after the initial landings on Guadalcanal, the number of patients hospitalized with malaria exceeded all other diseases, and some units even suffered 100 percent casualty rate. Throughout the war, that dreaded disease accounted for 113,256 cases and 90 deaths among naval personnel.[1]

Navy medicine moved quickly to reduce malaria's impact. Medical personnel trained in preventive medicine spread oil on malaria-breeding

---

1. Christine Beadle and Stephen L. Hoffman. "History of Malaria in the United States Naval Forces at War," 320–29.

areas, physicians and corpsmen began dispensing Atabrine as a malaria suppressant, and the Navy's research effort increased manyfold.[2]

But Navy medicine faced its greatest challenge in dealing with the aftermath of intense, bloody warfare fought in remote Pacific islands, far from fixed hospitals. This put enormous pressure on medical personnel closest to the front and forced new approaches to primary care and evacuation.

Those corpsmen serving with the Marines participated in all stages of their medical care, from preventive and emergency battlefield aid to definitive medical treatment at rear-area base hospitals. The most dramatic and demanding duty a corpsman could have was with Marine units in the field. Because the Marine Corps has always relied upon the Navy for medical support, corpsmen accompanied the leathernecks and suffered the brunt of combat themselves. Many of them went unarmed, reserving their carrying strength for plasma and medical supplies. The corpsmen's devotion to duty translated into their being the most highly decorated rate in the Navy. During the Iwo Jima and Okinawa campaigns alone, corpsmen earned seven Medals of Honor.

Besides providing daily care, they were the first critical link in the evacuation chain. From the time a Marine suffered a wound in a Guadalcanal jungle or on an Iwo Jima beach, his company corpsman braved Japanese fire to render aid. He applied a battle dressing, administered morphine and perhaps plasma or serum albumin, and tagged the casualty.

In a briefing to his corpsmen before the landings on Iwo Jima, a young medical officer reminded them of the dos and don'ts.

> If the wounded Marine is in pain, give him morphine. But don't give morphine in case of head injuries. Sprinkle sulfanilamide crystals on head wounds and get the men to the ship as quickly as possible.
>
> It is possible you may find a tracheotomy necessary at some time. If no other instruments are at hand, use your pocketknife and make the opening into the trachea, so as to permit air to enter the windpipe.
>
> Don't expose yourself to rush to the aid of a wounded man if it means you are going into the direct line of fire from the same rifle that brought him down. This would only make two of you to take care of, instead of one.[3]

---

2. Spreading oil on stagnant pools where mosquitoes breed prevents the larvae from getting oxygen; the larvae then suffocate.
3. Levin, "Briefing for Iwo Beach," 35–36.

If he was lucky, the corpsman commandeered a litter team to move the casualty out of harm's way and on to a battalion aid station, or collecting and clearing company, for further treatment by both physicians and corpsmen.

This care would mean stabilizing the patient with plasma, serum albumin, and, later in the war, whole blood. In some cases the wounded Marine was then taken to the beach for evacuation. In others, the casualty was taken to a divisional hospital, where doctors and corpsmen performed further stabilization, including major surgery if needed.

Meanwhile, LCVPs (landing craft, vehicles and personnel), LSTs (landing ships, tank), or LVTs (landing vehicles, tracked) carried the injured from the beach to a waiting hospital ship, troop transport, or a troop transport with hospital facilities (APH). During the 1942–43 Guadalcanal campaign, specially equipped C-47s enabled the first air evacuation of casualties to rear-area hospitals, and by early 1945 the first class of specially trained flight nurses was ready to help care for the first American POWs recently liberated in the Philippines. In March, these skilled women began accompanying C-47s on their evacuation flights from bloody Iwo Jima.

Once a wounded patient was safely aboard an evacuation vessel, physicians could provide more definitive care, which might include surgery. If at this stage the patient's wounds were less serious, he might be returned to duty. Otherwise he would be sent on to a base or mobile hospital (later called fleet hospital) some distance away. The Navy deployed base and fleet hospitals throughout the Pacific to solve the problem of providing definitive care for Navy and Marine Corps personnel close to the battle areas.

Base hospitals were non-mobile facilities usually set up in preexisting buildings. Mobile or fleet hospitals were supposed to be mobile. They consisted of tent shelters, Quonset huts, wooden frame structures, or a combination thereof. They were assembled, packed, supplied, and staffed in the United States and then shipped to the Pacific. Once in theater, physicians, corpsmen, dentists, and, nurses, who arrived later, provided the primary care. Corpsmen operated X-ray units, served as preventive-medicine and lab technicians, dental assistants, and, early in the war, even performed duties usually reserved for nurses. Working hours were long, and there were few liberties and even fewer places for personnel to spend them.

The following accounts tell the story of the island campaign through the eyes of a flight surgeon who witnessed the jungle hell of Guadalcanal; three corpsmen on the front lines at Peleliu, Iwo Jima, and Okinawa; and two flight nurses who witnessed combat close up.

BLACK TUESDAY AT GUADALCANAL

If the long road back in the Pacific war began with the victory at Midway in June 1942, the first offensive of that war began with the battle for Guadalcanal.

The first Allied thrust into the Solomons, code-named Watchtower, called for the seizure of the tiny island of Tulagi, adjacent to Guadalcanal. However, a Japanese airfield on the latter made Guadalcanal a much more important objective. Still armed with bolt-action Springfields and conveyed from troop transports by outmoded and rampless Higgins boats, Marines of the 1st Marine Division waded ashore on both islands on 7 and 8 August 1942. Facing minimal Japanese resistance, the Marines had no clue that within days the "cake walk" would become one of the longest, costliest, and most bitterly fought campaigns of World War II.

American fighting men had never encountered a place like Guadalcanal. The stinking, wet, equatorial jungle, often drenched by torrential rains, was lousy with crocodiles, snakes, lizards, tree leeches, rats, land crabs, and a menagerie of insects identifiable only, perhaps, to an entomologist.

The odor of rotting coconuts soon mingled with the stench of rotting bodies. And in a climate where dysentery, jungle rot, dengue, and malaria created more casualties than hostile fire, the outcome of the campaign was never a foregone conclusion.

Dr. Victor S. Falk joined the Navy in January 1941. After practicing medicine in a Marine artillery battalion in San Diego for a few months, he found the work neither exciting nor medically challenging and took the first opportunity to apply for flight surgeon training at Pensacola, Florida.

Following his graduation from the School of Aviation Medicine, he returned to San Diego, where he was assigned to the 1st Marine Air Headquarters at North Island. Shortly thereafter he received orders to a Marine dive-bomber squadron headed for the Pacific theater.

We went out on the luxury liner *Lurline* and stopped in Samoa. There were eight or nine of us and we were a bit crowded in a cabin designed for two people in peacetime. But the sad part was that after about six weeks, only two out of that group were still alive.

When we got to Samoa we transferred to the *Matsonia,* the *Lurline*'s sister ship, and from there we sailed to New Caledonia, where we boarded a Navy transport and sat in the harbor for a few days.

Then we set up a camp outside of Nouméa, New Caledonia. The understanding was that the pilots I was with, who had very little experience with dive-bombers, were going to have a period of training at Nouméa. But they never got it and we ended up going to Guadalcanal just a few days later on the USS *Zeilin* (APA-3).

These pilots never got their share of training before they were thrown into the thick of the fight. And they were not well integrated. They did not go up to Guadalcanal as a squadron. They went a few at a time as transportation became available. It was probably over a period of a month before they all got there. I arrived at Guadalcanal on October 13th. I no sooner got ashore when my commanding officer told me that we could fly out of there in any direction and find Japanese ships.

It was about noon when the Japanese bombers came over with a fighter escort. About an hour or two later there was another strike, which hit the airfield and gasoline dump. Shortly thereafter, sporadic artillery fire came from the hills beyond Henderson Field. It was that night when all hell broke loose, and this became the worst day they would ever have. We always referred to that event as Black Tuesday. My recollections of that night are quite vivid.

As soon as it got dark, I turned in with the senior members of my squadron, in our bivouac area between Henderson Field and the beach. I no sooner got settled when someone came to tell me it was my turn to leave at dawn with a load of casualties from Henderson Field. I had no choice but to go—back to where I had just come from. Anyway, I left and got about halfway there.

The artillery fire continued and then suddenly a Japanese plane dropped some brilliant green flares. All hell suddenly broke loose. As we learned later, the battleships *Haruna* and *Kongo* began shelling Henderson Field, but a lot of the shells fell short, and these 14-inch shells burst in the coconut trees right in our bivouac area. I heard later that those ships fired nine hundred 14-inch shells at Henderson Field. Three senior officers in the squadron were killed and another was mortally wounded.

There was no protection whatsoever but for a foxhole in the ground. I was not in the bivouac when the shelling started, but closer to Henderson Field. I could hear the shells coming in, and they made an awful racket whistling overhead. And at the same time planes were dropping bombs, and artillery shells were coming in from the other direction. Most of our planes were hit, our aviation gasoline went up, and ammunition dumps exploded like huge fireworks. I took cover in a foxhole while the ground shook from the bombardment like a continuous earthquake.

The shelling lasted maybe two hours. And then someone came and said they needed help back in the bivouac area I had just left. I commandeered an ambulance and went back to pick up the casualties so I could take them to the 1st Marine Division hospital at Henderson Field.

I found them on the ground or in a foxhole. One of them was a medical officer, Dr. [Lt. Henry R.] Ringness. He was paralyzed from the waist down but was still lucid enough to tell me exactly what had happened to him. He described a spinal-cord injury at such-and-such level. He was very clinical about it. But he was unaware that a shell fragment had sheared off one of his buttocks. Before I arrived, he had been able to drag himself around and help some of the injured.

I got him on a stretcher and took him to the so-called hospital at Henderson Field. There were only two or three survivors. One, our intelligence officer, had been a World War I aviator named Capt. Basil McDuffie. He had been on Guadalcanal less than twenty-four hours. He broke his leg scrambling for a foxhole. The rest were all dead, beyond help. There was still aerial bombing and artillery shelling, but I can't recall if the naval bombardment was still going on.

The 1st Marine Division hospital was a very crude wooden structure built by the Japanese. Adjacent to the hospital was an underground shelter where we took the casualties, because the shelling was still going on. Even fifty years later, I still have vivid recollections of how dank that place was.

I recall another incident that night I will never forget. Our squadron adjutant, who had been very badly wounded, was brought in and I was attempting to start plasma on him. Someone came up behind me and demanded to know what I was doing and who I was. I identified myself and told him what I was doing. He said he was commander so-and-so and ordered me to stop treating the man. I couldn't believe it. Anyway, the adjutant died.

We left at dawn with a full load of casualties, but Dr. Ringness was not among them. He was not in good-enough shape to be evacuated. The patients were loaded in litters about three or four deep. I recall there were about thirty of them, plus several war correspondents who wanted to get out of Guadalcanal. And the field was pretty badly cratered by shells. There were only one or two planes that were flyable at that point. Even our plane had a few holes in it.

We stopped at Efate in the New Hebrides, where there was a base hospital. After we unloaded the casualties, we went down to Nouméa, spent a night there, and then started back to Henderson Field again via Espíritu Santo. We had quite a lot of cargo on that return trip—ten fifty-five-gallon drums of aviation gasoline, oxygen tanks, bombs, and two tanks of gasoline that had been installed as auxiliary fuel for over-water flights. I sat wedged between these two tanks. As we got ready to depart for Guadalcanal, they told us communications were out there, and we would find out who controlled Henderson Field when we attempted to land.

From then on there was plenty of action at Henderson Field. It was pretty constant but there was no naval shelling for another month—until November—and when it came, it was not as bad as what we had experienced on Black Tuesday.

But we did have "Washing Machine Charlie," a lone Japanese bomber who appeared nightly and disrupted everyone's sleep. He was just a nuisance. He would drop a bomb periodically but was overhead most of the night. And we were sitting in a hole in the ground being nibbled on by mosquitoes.

Malaria was a big problem. About 75 percent of my squadron had it. I treated it with quinine. Atabrine came along later on. If the patients were really bad we would evacuate them.

But being a flight surgeon, my main concern was my aviators. The squadron never really functioned as a unit, particularly with the number of commanding officers we had. I think I had eight of them in a couple of months. The pilots who were left were not in very good shape, between diarrhea, lack of sleep, and very little food. The morale wasn't very good either, because every day we'd lose another two pilots. We got down to less than 50 percent, and the survivors were not very eager. I talked to our air-group commander, a lieutenant colonel, about it. He said he could not ground the men but if I felt it medically necessary, I could do so. I finally grounded the whole squadron and it never flew again at Guadalcanal.

THE CORAL OF PELELIU

To many historians, Peleliu represents a bloody distraction—the unnecessary battle of the Pacific war. They argue that the tiny island in the Palau chain had little or no strategic importance either in retaking the Philippines or island-hopping to Tokyo. Peleliu, they point out, should have been left to wither on the vine.

Peleliu also symbolizes one of the most serious miscalculations of World War II. The campaign that was supposed to take but four days began with the first landings on 15 September 1944 and ended seventy-three days later, when Army troops overcame the last Japanese resistance. As naval historian Samuel Eliot Morison noted, "There was nothing wrong in American planning for Peleliu except something exceedingly wrong—a woefully inadequate knowledge of the terrain."[4]

Prior to the landings, aerial reconnaissance had failed to detect coral ridges honeycombed with caves and tunnels and buttressed by concrete casemates and pillboxes, features that provided the Japanese defenders with an immense advantage. For the invaders, on the other hand, Peleliu was flamethrower country.

What every survivor remembers about Peleliu was the heat, the humidity, and the thirst. But above all, they remember the coral—the porous and jagged remains of long-dead sea animals that made the island what it was.

---

4. Morison, *History of United States Naval Operations in World War II*, vol. 12: 36.

PhM3c Beryl A. Bonacker patched up his share of shrapnel and gunshot wounds, while the malevolent coral sliced through shoes, ripped clothes to shreds, and lacerated the flesh.

We were the eleventh wave to hit Orange Beach, the beach right opposite the airstrip. But we didn't make it clear in. Our boat got hung up on some coral which prevented us from beaching. So we went over the side or out the front gate into about three feet of water churned up by the boat's engine. I'm glad it wasn't any deeper, because there were pieces of coral sticking up out of the water. And since the water was all roiled up, you didn't know what you were stepping in or on. Fellows were falling and tripping.

The beach was comparatively narrow and just ahead was a rise of about four feet. If you raised your head, you looked right down a runway. We lay crouched for what seemed like hours. Then we finally got word to move out. One by one we got to our feet and moved forward. Someone or something had stopped the shelling and we moved up on the airstrip and began running.

I don't remember any casualties from hostile fire going across to the airfield, but we did have an awful lot of casualties caused by coral. Guys were falling and scraping themselves on it. I remember wrapping a lot of arms, legs, fingers, and knees. I still have scars on my right arm from coral; I'll always have them.

There was no protection running over open ground across the airstrip. We could see buildings at the far end but they still seemed a long way off yet. When we got to the cement buildings, there was a feeling of protection. The Navy had shelled these structures the day before. They were still standing but were pocked with holes and gave off a sulphur smell.

We really thought we'd gone far enough for one day, but the higher-ups thought otherwise. After a short rest and readjustment of gear on our backs and hips, we started inland.

Our canteens were getting lighter, which meant we were getting low on water. And the temperature was running around a hundred degrees with the humidity in the nineties. As it turned out, we didn't see the water truck until the next afternoon.

For food we had K-rations, which included a little chocolate bar; it was horrible. There was also powdered milk. When you added water it was lukewarm. Then there were eggs in a can, meat in a can, and Sterno to heat it. But in combat we weren't usually hungry. When you finally settled down and were safe where you were, then you got hungry. Otherwise, your stomach was secondary. You were thinking about staying alive.

But you can't go without food very long and fight at the same time. One of the biggest problems we had was trying to get men to eat who wouldn't. I don't remember what our exact words were. I think I said, "We're not going to get anything better, fellas, so you might as well eat what you've got." There were always rumors that more K-rations and C-rations were going to be brought in or something better was coming up to us. I think these rumors did more damage than anything. Something better didn't come along and we had to eat what we had.

By now we had extra water brought to us in five-gallon cans. We filled our canteens with water we took out of a small tank mounted on a two-wheel trailer and pulled by a jeep. These water tanks had been loaded aboard the troop transports before leaving Pavuvu, possibly a week or two prior to the Peleliu campaign. The tanks hadn't been cleaned properly and so we drank rusty water with an oil taste. It was also lukewarm and, as I recall, we took an Atabrine with the water.

It was the beginning of the third day before I first saw death, a Japanese soldier who had probably been killed either by a grenade or fragments from the previous shelling. His body had many wounds and was partially hidden by dirt and coral.

Of course, I treated my share of wounded. One Marine had been shot through the flesh of his right shoulder and didn't even know he had been hit. He was on my left when the bullet hit him. If it had been a little more to the right, my left shoulder would have been hit. I applied sulfa and bandaged him. One of our corpsmen got hit in the stomach. His name was Kenneth L. Blewitt, from Oklahoma. He came overseas with me in the 40th Replacement Battalion. There wasn't a thing we could do for him. He was a smoker and wanted a cigarette. We gave him one, put him on a litter, and took him to an ambulance about a block away from the aid tent. He was gone before we loaded him aboard.

Yet what stands out in my mind is the coral damage. It was just tremendous! It might sound silly but I took care of more coral wounds than anything else. With all the climbing up and down, abrasions and cuts were inevitable. In most cases a simple scratch wouldn't show up until days later and then it would be infected no matter how minor it was.

Often mortars and shells would send coral fragments flying in all directions at a zillion miles an hour, causing jagged, horrible wounds. And then the men got coral poisoning, ran a temperature, and their wounds would fester very badly. We had to clean those wounds every day. We gave them a medication but I don't recall what it was.

At night, there were no trees to speak of or chunks of coral large enough where we could take shelter. You usually slept in a shellhole. We occasionally got rain, mostly at night. You covered yourself with your poncho and tried to get as comfortable as possible. You laid your head on your pack but couldn't take your helmet off. They wouldn't let us. And you wanted to take it off, because it was so hot under that helmet. A bullet could penetrate the helmet from quite a distance, but it did protect the head from coral.

And, of course, there were no clothes to change into. We had to wear what we had. We all wore those clothes for thirty-one days. The only baths we got were out of a helmet, and that was to wash your hands and sometimes just your face. We were so filthy, I can remember rolling up my sleeves and there was so much dirt and crud on my arms that when I ran my fingernails up my arm, I made furrows. Of course nobody shaved. Some guys perspired more than others, so we stunk to high heaven. It was downright miserable.

CLEAN SHEETS AND THREE SQUARES

If one had to choose a single image from World War II depicting valor and the triumph of the American fighting man, Joe Rosenthal's immortal photograph of the flag-raising on Iwo Jima would be that picture.

In February 1945, the strategic bombing campaign against Japanese cities was in full swing. To get there and back, B-29s based in the Marianas faced an almost-3,000-mile round trip. For a bomber with battle damage or mechanical trouble, the odds of making it all the way back were not good. Iwo Jima, approximately halfway between Guam and Japan, would provide the "superforts" a much-needed base and improve the odds considerably. The island had to be taken.

Planners anticipated a three-day operation to capture the tiny eight-square-mile island. They were wrong. Instead, it took nearly a month of some of the bloodiest and most vicious fighting the Marines had ever experienced. And when they were through, the American flag atop Mount Suribachi would become the enduring symbol of the U.S. Marine Corps.

PhM2c Stanley E. Dabrowski accompanied the Marines ashore and stayed with them until the end. From New Britain, Connecticut, Stanley Dabrowski was seventeen years old and just out of high school in 1943. Like other young draftable men, he decided the infantry was not for him. With an interest in medicine, he decided the Hospital Corps was a good choice.

After an eight-week course at the naval hospital at Portsmouth, Virginia, he reported for duty at the U.S. Naval Hospital in Charleston, South Carolina, where he was assigned to the contagious ward. Finding the work routine and unchallenging, he requested a transfer. Soon his name was on the list for the Fleet Marine Force and he was to report to Camp Lejeune, North Carolina, for Field Medical Service School. "Fleet Marine? This must be sea duty," he thought—but it would not be the kind he expected.

We got off the bus at Camp Lejeune and I looked around and said, "Gee, there's no Navy here. It's all Marine Corps green. Everything is USMC." Standing there on the asphalt was a Marine corporal with a Smokey the Bear hat and his duty belt, starched shirt with the creases right down here, very neat.

"All right you guys, fall in." He impressed me tremendously and was our DI [drill instructor] throughout our training. We were no longer in the Navy. Everything from then on was Marine Corps, including the dress green uniforms. The insignia was khaki. We didn't even have white underwear; everything was green.

Our training included all the things that one has to know about field medicine, but more important than that it was just like going through Marine boot camp—close order drill, infiltration courses with live machine-gun fire, crawling under barbed wire, hand-to-hand combat. We spent two weeks on the rifle range—M1 Garand, M1 carbine, .45, machine gun, hand grenades, even a bayonet course, would you believe.

They had to prepare us for what we were going to face, but nobody ever told us what combat was going to be like.

After about ten weeks of training at Camp Lejeune, we were assigned to the new 5th Marine Division being formed at Camp Pendleton, California. So after we graduated from Field Medical Service School, we went aboard a Pullman train for a seven-day trip to the West Coast. This was quite an adventure. It was my first time away from home. We would leave the train once a day for calisthenics, naturally. Other than that you either sat there and read, napped, or there would be card games, a little bit of crap shooting, or what have you. It was a long troop train. They weren't just transferring medical personnel, but Marines also. Before we got to the great divide in Colorado, they hitched another steam engine onto the huge beast of a steam engine that was already pulling us. And then they hitched another one behind to push the train over the divide. The whole thing seemed to be going just by inches and you could hear the chug of those engines straining. Once we got over the divide, we traveled through the deserts of Utah and Nevada. I saw my first coyote out there.

We stopped at a place in California called Needles, in the Death Valley area. Those trains were not air-conditioned in those days. When we got outside the train the temperature was 115 degrees, like a blast of fire in your face. But typical of the Marine Corps, we got off the train and did calisthenics. They gave us time to wash up. There was a big tank to fill the boiler on the engine. That's what we got to shower under. The water was cold and very pleasing.

Every time we stopped, there was a truckload of sandwiches. They fed us on the train but it was never as you see in the movies, with tablecloths and stewards asking you what you wanted. They threw a sandwich and an apple and something we called bug juice at us. Breakfast was a stand-up type of situation. If you sat down to eat your powdered eggs and toast, or SOS, it was too much like luxury.

But we survived and got into Camp Pendleton. I remember coming out of that desert part of California, over a mountain, and seeing the lush greenery which was southern California. This seemed like it was going to be great duty.

I was assigned to Company C of the 5th Medical Battalion of the 5th Marine Division. And as a medical company in a medical battalion, C Company was assigned to an infantry regiment, the 28th Marines. A medical company consisted of about ninety-eight corpsmen, three surgeons, two internists, a dentist, and an administrative warrant officer. I was part of a pool of corpsmen that would staff the battalion aid stations or regimental aid stations. Parts of the company would also staff division or regimental hospitals.

I was assigned to a thirteen-man medical collecting team. Our job was selecting casualties that needed attention first. We were to transfer them to better facilities as soon as possible, [and] we had four stretcher teams assigned to us. The corpsmen were to do the histories and tagging and to administer first aid. The training was fantastic, and everyone knew exactly how we were going to do all these things. We did it repeatedly until we could do it in our sleep.

After six months of intensive training at Camp Pendleton, including amphibious assaults on nearby beaches, we went overseas on 19 September 1944. Our first stop was Hilo, on the big island of Hawaii, and then on to Camp Tarawa, [which] the Marines put together after they came back from the Battle of Tarawa.

Then we got into intensive training. And we trained and trained—amphibious exercises along the beaches and infantry assaults. Our job was to set up the aid stations, apply battle dressings, administer medications properly, tag and evacuate the wounded, the whole bit. One thing always stood out in our minds. Every time we went on these so-called field problems—the Army called them maneuvers—there was always a hill involved. One battalion would turn to the right, another battalion would go straight across, and another battalion would assault the hill. It wasn't until we saw the first picture of Iwo Jima that it dawned on us why. That hill was Mount Suribachi! And the 28th Marines would be the conquerors of Mount Suribachi.

We left Honolulu in January of '45 to go to Eniwetok, in the Marshalls, for a few days of rest and relaxation and refueling. I was assigned to LST-758, which was Coast Guard–manned. We had our final dress rehearsal off Saipan and Tinian on February 12th; we then started steaming toward our destination.

It wasn't until we were out to sea, when nobody could get off, that we were told officially that our objective was Iwo Jima. That was on February 13th. They broke out maps and models of the island made of rubber or clay. It showed us our assault beaches where we would land, the airfields, the mountain, the whole bit. They also told us that D-day was February 19th, less than a week away; H-hour was 0900.

We were off Iwo Jima on the eve of the 19th, but everything was black. We didn't see the island. Reveille was about 3:00 A.M. We had the typical breakfast of steak and eggs, but not many people ate an awful lot because your heart was up in your throat. We had no idea what to expect. When we had been briefed on the operation, they'd told us it would be a three-day operation. Well, that didn't seem so bad.

I carried a carbine and a .45. Unlike the Army in Europe, the medical people were armed. At Guadalcanal, corpsmen still wore Red Cross brassards on their arms and a red cross on their helmets. They were the first ones to be knocked off by snipers. In the Marine Corps, nobody wore any kind of insignia on their helmets or clothes. Even in subsequent campaigns, corpsmen would be singled out simply because they looked different from others because of the equipment they carried. We carried kits which I didn't like at all because they marked us as corpsmen. It was like a lieutenant or a captain carrying a map case, as opposed to an infantryman, who had only had a rifle and a canteen on his belt. We were told to carry sidearms not as offensive weapons, but for self-protection.

I had a medical kit on each shoulder. In the left pouch we carried all our battle dressings, sulfa powder, burn dressings. In the right pouch were morphine Syrettes, tags, iodine pencils, ammonia inhalants, hemostats and scalpels, and other assorted equipment.

We got down to the tank deck and got aboard our vehicles, the LVTs [landing vehicle tracked]. Their engines were already running and in spite of huge fans, there were an awful lot of fumes. The engines ran on an aviation grade of gasoline. People started getting sick. When they realized what was happening, they shut down some of the engines.

There were fourteen men plus equipment in my LVT. We were taking medical equipment—stretchers, and so on. We got off at 0800, just drove off the ramp into the sea. We were about a mile off the beach bobbing along with many other ships, mostly LSTs, APAs [attack transports] right behind us, small LCIs [landing craft, infantry], small gunboats with rockets. Someone quipped, "What a beautiful day to die." You could see the smoke and the fire, and with the fantastic amount of noise, you wondered how anything could survive something like that.

We bobbed around while they formed the assault waves. This was very important. You had to get in line. On paper it was a beautiful thing and if you had been up in the air it must have been a thrilling sight. But as soon as we got on that beach, everything fell apart. It was just mass confusion and units got scattered. The thing I noticed immediately was the tremendous amount of noise, concussion, small-arms fire, explosions of artillery and mortar shells.

As we were coming into the beach, we were under a rolling barrage of the 16-inch guns of the battleships. You could just feel those shells going over your head. My unit, part of the 28th Marines, landed in the third assault wave at 0907 on Green Beach, right under Suribachi. When we landed the only thing we heard was the incoming, the stuff we were throwing at them. The beaches were relatively quiet but for heavy small-arms fire. Occasionally a mortar or artillery shell would land, but it seemed as though the Navy had done a good job of knocking out their big guns.

But then, about an hour or hour and a half later, we started getting hammered with the most intense fire, to most everybody's surprise. We just couldn't believe the kind of fire that began coming down on us—mortars, artillery, rockets, the whole bit. It was so intense and the carnage and the wreckage on the beach was so fantastic, that subsequent waves could not get ashore that afternoon.

The beach was very narrow because the winds and the waves had terraced the volcanic ash. There were two or three terraces. Just trying to crawl up this thing was like trying to crawl through buckwheat in a bin. Iwo Jima was a volcanic island and the beaches were not sand but ash, very soft. We stepped off and were in up to our ankles.

I lost a very dear friend right there on the beach, Stan Sanders. He was sewed through by machine-gun bullets. It was the most shocking thing you could experience. Here you were talking to the man just a few minutes ago. I ran to him and his eyes were glazed over and he was dead. It was devastating.

Everyone was yelling, "Move, move, move." And then from everywhere were these pleas, "Corpsman, corpsman!" Once we began to take heavy fire, casualties mounted tremendously. My first was a sergeant with a sucking chest wound. He had taken a machine-gun bullet right through the lungs.

One of the paramount things we had trained for were sucking chest wounds. You had to do something immediately or else the man would drown in his own blood. You had to close off the wound so he would not get air through it. You had to ram this big battle dressing into it and compress it as much as possible and tie it off. Give him a shot of morphine, write out a tag, and mark him; this was another thing that was very important. You had to put a big M on his forehead to indicate that he had already been given morphine. And then someone would have to drag him off the beach. I could not do this. I had to advance with my unit.

As it was, we had to catch up with our units. The Marines were trained to move—to push to reach an objective. They just went and we had to go along with them. My battalion was assaulting across the narrow neck of the island and we were catching all our fire from Suribachi. The people who were entrenched up there could see all over the island. The 28th Regiment was supposed to cut Suribachi off from the rest of the island. By the end of the first day, the Marines had gotten across to the other side of the island, cutting it in two.

The first night and second day on Iwo were nightmares. Not only were we under constant heavy fire, but it started to rain and was cold, so we were all really miserable. However, things slowed down because we had ceased advancing and were in defensive positions.

By this time there was some semblance of order. We didn't have an official aid station as such. We chose the deepest shell hole we could find and started taking care of the severely wounded. At the beginning, the battalion aid stations were never very far away from the beach. As we moved inland, they remained close to the front line. So evacuating casualties was a short trip. But when we started experiencing heavy casualties, it was almost impossible to comprehend.

The first thing you had to do was assess the casualty. Almost certainly they had immediately gone into shock. Combatting shock and hemorrhage were the first priorities. We used tourniquets and hemostats. There were so many cases where there were traumatic amputations—no arm, or both legs. And then there were abdominal injuries—torn-out intestinal tracts. Often I was beside myself trying to decide what to do with these people. And surprisingly, sometimes these young men—of course we were all young—would be covered by a poncho and lying on a stretcher. And I'd say, "Hey Mack, how are you doing?"

"Pretty good, Doc."

"What's the problem?"

"Oh, my left arm got it." So you'd lift the poncho and you'd see a stump. My God, you'd think, He's still lucid and he still can talk.

First I had to tourniquet it, give him morphine. We had these huge battle dressings about the size of an 8½-by-11 page of paper with ties on them. You would sprinkle sulfa powder on the stump, and almost immediately it would be washed out by the oozing blood. But you did it nevertheless. And then you'd put the dressing on as tightly as possible. These men, the resolve they had . . . You'd tag them, get their name and number off their dog tags. You'd put the man's unit down if you could find out what it was, because they always took statistics down at the end of the day as to killed and wounded and what units they were from.

Our fight was preserving life. You did all this automatically. It was just so natural to do these things even though you were never, never, never primed for the things you saw. The injuries to these men were traumatic; so were the experiences.

Nevertheless, we did what we had to do and then we got the stretcher teams to get them down to the beach as soon as possible. At that time the regimental aid station was not set up to take care of them. Things were too fluid. The beach was the best place to send them so they could be evacuated offshore.

As you know, Iwo Jima was not a three-day affair. I don't think we were at the middle of the second airfield by the third day. The 1st Battalion of the 28th Marines was by this time put into reserve and the 2d Battalion began assaulting Mt. Suribachi.

You know the world-renowned photo Joe Rosenthal made of the flag-raising. There were two flag-raisings on Iwo Jima. The first patrol that went up had a small flag brought ashore by the battalion adjutant. I recall very well because we were at the bottom of the mountain at the aid station and I saw that team going up. They met resistance but made it to the summit and put up the flag. Of course everyone cheered, because this was the most important piece of real estate they could take. Once they'd deprived the Japanese of that observation post, things down below got a little cooler.

After the 23d, the battalion had a few days' rest. We got a little reprieve to resupply, collect the wounded, and get some food. Then we started again toward the north part of the island. We were right beneath Suribachi. We had bisected the island, and the 4th Division was already pushing north from their sector. By this time two regiments of the 3d Division had been brought in due to the tremendous number of casualties both the 4th and 5th Divisions had suffered. They ran into some very fierce opposition, and it got to a point where it was inch by inch, foot by foot, rather than yards at a time.

The terrain above the airfields was pocked with caves, pillboxes, labyrinths of tunnels, and such a crossfire that it was a murderous situation. You can read this in the historic accounts of the battle—Turkey Knob, the Meat Grinder, and Hill 362, the one that will stand out in my mind forever. This is where our regiment was pinned down by murderous fire. The most terrifying and devastating aspect of combat were the mortar barrages. They came straight down on you due to their trajectory, and when they registered, you were in for a terrible beating.

Of course, as corpsmen, we advanced with our troops. On the 3d of March I was administering a unit of serum albumin to a very severely wounded Marine in a shellhole, where we had some semblance of safety. I was about six inches above ground with my hand holding the serum albumin bottle, a bottle a bit smaller than a Coke can. I caught a piece of hot shrapnel which shattered the bottle and almost took the tip of my finger off. The shock of being hit flipped me over and I lost my helmet, and another chunk of shrapnel grazed my scalp. Neither wound was severe enough to take me out of commission, but I did have a helluva headache and one big bandage on my finger. And I just continued my duties. Later on I was showered with the blast from a phosphorus round and was hit in the left knee. Again I was lucky enough not to have gotten a wound that put me out of commission. However, I did have the latter wound attended to by a surgeon back on the beach.

In another instance, I had a wounded man not fifty feet away. Some of the Marines told me he had been there for about a half hour. "Hey Doc, go out there and bring him back in." He wasn't moaning, but you could see movement. So I figured I would go out and take a look at him. I started across this area and right behind me someone said, "Hey Doc, where the hell do you think you're going?"

I said, "I've got a man out there I have to bring in."

He said, "The hell you are. You're in the middle of a minefield. Freeze." Talk about traumatic experiences.

Usually the engineers would indicate an access path with tape or white streamers. They would probe for the mines with a bayonet and clear the area. Apparently this hadn't been done yet and I hadn't realized it. I was halfway through, so I continued and got my man.

My most traumatic experience on Iwo Jima occurred in the Hill 362 sector. I was about to get out of a shellhole when I was knocked back down by a mortar round that hit my shoulder pack but did not detonate! It was a dud. It was agonizing terror to try to get out of that hole. To this day I shudder when I think of it.

We made trips almost constantly, evacuating the wounded. By the time we had advanced farther, the battalion aid station was in full operation. Understand that it was always mobile. As the troops moved up, we had to follow, otherwise there would be too big a gap between the line companies and medical help. We evacuated the wounded with the LVTs. You couldn't use trucks; there were no roads. The LVTs could go anywhere, just like a tank. And we used another little vehicle we called the Weasel, a small tracked vehicle about the size of a jeep. You could do anything with this little thing. We could get two severe casualties on a Weasel.

When we had to do it by hand, our stretcher teams were under constant fire. And the stretcher teams were always singled out by the snipers. Frequently you would hear these things, *pft, pft*. It didn't register until after a while that you were being shot at.

The first LST to land on Iwo Jima I think did so on the 21st. The only way we could get the wounded off the beach initially was with the alligators—the LVTs. On that first day there was no way Higgins boats could get ashore, because of the tremendous amount of wreckage.

Most of the evacuation was done by hospital ship. The *Solace* [AH-5], the *Bountiful* [AH-9], and the *Samaritan* [AH-10] were at Iwo Jima. Once they were loaded, they would steam back to the Marianas. At night they were fifteen to twenty miles offshore, fully illuminated.

I also saw the first hospital plane come in from Guam or Saipan on the 3d or 4th of March. It had a big red cross on it. We delivered a group of severely wounded to the airfield for air evacuation. The first Navy nurse came on this plane [Ens. Jane Kendeigh].

Was Iwo worth the kind of casualties we suffered? Was it all necessary? Well, yes. Taking Iwo Jima was a brutal necessity. I remember the first B-29 that landed on Iwo Jima. We were up around Hill 362, which wasn't too far away from Motoyama airfield. It was on March 4th or 5th, or thereabouts. It was the first time I saw a B-29. It was fantastically large. It came around circling and you could tell he was in trouble. Apparently he got the okay to land, but the back end of the field was still under Japanese fire. He came down in a hell of a cloud of dust because the field wasn't finished; the Seabees were still working on it. He went as far as he had to, but as he taxied the Japs bracketed him with mortar fire. However, he was able to get to safety at the Suribachi end of the runway.

I understand when the guys came tumbling out of that plane they kissed the ground and some of the Marines said, "My God, what's the matter with those guys, kissing this hellhole. I want to get on that ship to get the hell out of here with them." I heard later that they asked this crew if they wanted to spend the night and they said no thanks. Was Iwo worthwhile? Understand that if the island hadn't been there for these people, probably more than 25,000 airmen would have died.

My unit left Iwo on March 26th. What was left of our division went back to Camp Tarawa to regroup mentally and physically. And we were getting our replacements of raw, young people. Mind you, we were old salts as eighteen- and nineteen-year-old combat veterans. The replacements looked at us with great awe. After all, we had been on Iwo Jima.

Many of those who had been hospitalized came back to duty. I remember running into the first casualty that I took care of on Iwo. One day we were sitting around when I heard a voice say, "I'm looking for Doc Dabrowski. Dabrowski, where are you?" I recognized him immediately. He gave me this big bear hug and said, "Doc, I just wanted to thank you for saving my life."

Now that one thing was worth Iwo Jima to me. It just does something to you. One of the things you constantly had on your mind when you were up to your elbows in grime, dirt, and blood. You were constantly asking yourself, Am I doing the right thing? Am I doing enough for them?

How many I saved I don't know. I don't know to this day. But that's what we were trained for and that's what we did. When I look back on it, as gruesome as it was, I have a lot of satisfaction knowing that I was part of something that was meaningful. The 5th Marine Division is no more than a memory, but it is a memory I will carry all my life.

Following the Iwo Jima campaign, Doc Dabrowski's Marine division was assigned to Operation Olympic, the planned invasion of Japan. Even though the Japanese surrender made that last campaign unnecessary, Dabrowski went to Japan in September 1945 as part of the occupation force. He was discharged in December 1945.

FIRST FLIGHT NURSE
ON A PACIFIC BATTLEFIELD

Proud of the sacrifice and heroism of sons and daughters who were fighting in the Pacific, Americans were always thirsty for news from the front. And the Navy, always eager to oblige, provided copy and images whenever possible. As one of the most vicious battles in the history of the Marine Corps was running its course in late February and early March 1945 at Iwo Jima, a very newsworthy event took place there. On D-day plus 12 the first C-47 transport equipped for air evacuation landed on a newly secured airfield. Aboard the plane was photogenic Navy flight nurse Ens. Jane Kendeigh.

Fortuitously, Lt. Gill DeWitt, one of Edward Steichen's skilled photographers, was also there.[5] Not long afterward, the Naval Air Transport Service public-relations office made available to the press quality photographs of that mission. In later years DeWitt affixed some of those images into a personal scrapbook enhanced by the following commentary.

It was several days after D-day on fiery, little Iwo Jima. Probably the bloodiest battlefield in all history was this small volcanic island of only eight square miles.

My superior officer at the time, Capt. Edward Steichen, USNR, had assigned me to photograph the first Navy flight nurse in action. Several days elapsed after the assignment before news was received on Guam that the first airfield had been "secured" and was reasonably safe for operation. Late one afternoon I was notified to leave from Agaña Airfield Guam at 2:00 A.M. the following morning with the chief flight nurse, Lt. (jg) Ann Purvis.

---

5. The famed photographer had joined the Navy at age sixty-three to document the war on film and had assembled some of the most gifted photographers of the time. "Photograph everything that happens. Concentrate on the men," was Steichen's dictum.

At ten minutes to 2:00 in the morning I reported to the field only to learn that the first plane had departed five minutes previously and the second plane was about to leave.

My disappointment was keen for I felt the news value of the story would be lost by being with the second such plane to arrive, but I climbed aboard the C-47 transport plane to find the chief pharmacist's mate and pretty little Jane Kendeigh awaiting the takeoff. All of us wore the required "Mae Wests" in case we might be forced down in the 700 miles of sea that lay ahead. The plane was loaded with cots, blankets and medical supplies, and very soon after takeoff Jane piled the blankets high and tried to rest. There was a grueling fifteen hours ahead and it wouldn't be pleasant.

A few hours later she awoke to find hot coffee and sandwiches ready. It was still dark and she took a lesson in celestial navigation from the plane's navigator. Afterward she returned and began to acquaint herself with the boxes of medical supplies, Syrettes, bandages, and items she might need with the load of casualties we were to bring back.

At the break of dawn she was called forward by the pilot, Lieutenant Burns, who showed her our present position and pointed out the few Jap-infested islands we passed along the way.

Shortly afterward the radioman came back and said, "There's Iwo!" and then he told us that an offshore bombardment was in progress and we had been ordered to circle the field for ninety minutes until it was over. It was a thrilling sight to watch some thousand ships shelling the half island still doggedly held by the Japs.

We circled and circled the small island and watched the bursting shells beneath us like firecrackers on a Fourth of July. The front line was so easily distinguished by the trail of smoke and dust across the north end of the island.

When the bombardment was completed we received landing instructions and as Mount Suribachi swished past us we settled to a perfect three-point landing and taxied up to the casualty tent and climbed out for a long-deserved stretch as the pounding of the nearby guns and mortars made conversation impracticable. We quickly walked to the nearby evacuation tent as litter bearers began to bring us our load of casualties.

Once in the tent we asked about the "first" plane carrying Lieutenant (jg) Purvis, and learned they had become lost and were due in very soon. Strangely enough, ours *was* the first plane, and Jane Kendeigh the first nurse to land on Iwo Jima.

Jane comforted those she could. Her presence and soft voice on this faraway battlefield did wonders to the morale of these broken men. Every man received her individual attention and cheering words of encouragement. She carefully checked each patient as they were lifted or climbed aboard the plane that would take them away from this hell on earth.

Aboard again—and after a precarious downwind take-off to prevent crossing the Jap line at low altitude, Jane and the corpsman began studying case histories, giving injections, making each patient a bit more comfortable. The most serious cases received the most attention and records were scrupulously kept to aid the waiting doctors at the fleet naval hospitals on Guam.

Back on Guam, Jane [checked] her broken cargo off the plane to the attending flight surgeon. Anxiously, she [watched] each patient removed from the plane to the waiting ambulances.

Everyone was dead tired. It had been a long and exciting fifteen hours and now a good bath and a night's sleep were uppermost in our minds. Thirty-six hours later Jane would leave again for Iwo, and soon all of this would become routine.

Ensign Kendeigh would also be the first Navy flight nurse to land at Okinawa.

A FLIGHT NURSE AT IWO

Kathryn Van Wagner was twenty-three when she joined the Navy in 1944. Her last civilian job had been as an assistant supervisor of a suite of operating rooms at the Jersey City Medical Center. At the time, local factories had already switched from manufacturing civilian goods to aircraft parts and other war materiel, and industrial accidents were common. As a result, the young nurse got quite a bit of experience helping to treat serious trauma. That education would put her in good stead when she confronted battlefield injuries for the first time.

Ensign Van Wagner was stationed at the Naval Air Station, Norfolk, Virginia, when she volunteered to become a member of the first class of twelve flight nurses about to undergo training at Alameda, California. "I don't think they knew what to train us for, because they didn't know what we were getting into," she recalls.

Van Wagner and fellow graduates of this first class would be the first women to evacuate wounded by air from an active battlefield in the Pacific.

In order to qualify for flight nurse, I had to swim the length of a swimming pool in green coveralls and boots, which I managed to do, and then get out of the pool on a free-swinging rope ladder. However, I had twelve years of acrobatics and ballet and toe-dancing lessons, so I was very muscular. Otherwise, I would not have been able to do it. It was quite a feat.

We used the Link Trainer [aircraft cockpit simulator]. We learned about artificial horizon, direction, altitude. We were also instructed how to utilize the four Mark VII life rafts which were on each plane, and reminded of the dangers of positive air pressure on chest wounds which have negative air pressure. They taught us basic first aid—perhaps a little more than basic. I knew a lot of it already because of my operating-room experience. But at that time, nurses didn't do what they do today. Nurses really were very low on the totem pole in the medical hierarchy, and they were trying to bring us up a rank by giving us certain information we might need in pressure dressings and that sort of thing.

I don't remember much of the other training until we were assigned to Guam. We were outfitted in flight nurse's uniforms—green elastique, lightweight pants, gray cotton dresses and pants. Elastique was a type of material that fit beautifully. It was a heavy wool that was able to stretch. It had a diagonal zipper going from upper right to lower left. We had gray cotton uniforms issued as well as flight boots, and flight jackets with our names and wings on them. These jackets looked like elephant skin. It was a very heavy, crinkly leather. This was the gear we were sent with.

The twelve of us really felt very special and were treated very special. I must say that in my entire Navy career I was always afforded respect. There was no wink with a salute, which a young woman in a Navy uniform might have expected.

We flew to Honolulu, then to Johnston Island, to Kwajalein Island, and then landed at Guam. When we got there they were not prepared for us at all. They quickly set up a tent, brought in some cots, and barbed wire. Our compound was enclosed in rows and rows of barbed wire at Agaña air base, which was close to the cliffs and not far from the B-29 landing strip. In order for a nurse to leave the compound you had to be accompanied by two men, both wearing sidearms.

My flights to Iwo Jima were on the 8th, 12th, 16th, and 18th of March 1945. We flew in what the Navy designated an R-4D. It was a C-47. The C-47s had huge auxiliary gas tanks in them. They were as large as four water heaters and took up an enormous space in the cabin. These two tanks were right behind the pilot's cockpit and then began the area where we had our patients. There was just a corpsman along with me on these flights. His name was Emerson Brown and he was a very big man. He and I worked exceptionally well together.

I had never heard of Iwo Jima. We knew we were going to an island where an airstrip had just been established that would support the weight of an R-4D. Perhaps they said Iwo Jima, but at that time my geography wasn't good enough to know where that was.

That very first flight was unreal. As we approached the island I stood behind the pilot, looked down and saw a destroyer blown up. We could see munitions from our ships on one side of the island going over to the other side of the island. It was like an umbrella. And there was enemy fire going out and hitting the ships—the destroyers and the LSTs. I just couldn't believe I was seeing what I was actually seeing.

I was never afraid. At twenty-three one doesn't think of one's mortality. Nothing could happen to me or anyone I knew.

Anyway, we came in under that barrage and landed on the beach. The fighting was going on very close to the plane. On one of my missions when I was standing next to the plane, a Marine handed me a trench mortar and said, "Do you want to shoot the Japanese?"

And I said, "Sure." So I just dropped the mortar round in the slot and it shot right over a hill.

The medics brought the wounded men to the beach and put them in a tent. I was given some kind of rundown on the types of wounds the men had. Everything was done very quickly; they wanted to get us out of there very fast. So I really didn't know exactly what I had. We walked down these rows of men. Someone said, "These twenty-four will be on your plane." The auxiliary tanks took up the space of at least eight or more litters, so we could only carry twenty-four patients in litters.

We had on board a huge wooden box with whole blood and medications, mostly sulfa drugs. Although penicillin was in existence at that time, I only knew it at St. Albans [Naval Hospital] where it was given by injection every three hours in doses of about 50,000 units per cc [cubic centimeter]. Now it's given in the millions. But all we had was just the sulfa drugs in powder form.

As soon as we took off, the corpsman and I made very quick rounds to see what we had. The patients had the original bandages that the medics had applied where the men were injured. That's the condition we received them in when they got to the beach.

When I got them they were not stabilized. Some of them had injuries only twenty minutes old. The corpsmen were bringing them in in droves. There were some doctors there who took a quick look to decide whether the injured were going on this flight or the next one. And those men were dirty. Iwo Jima was all black sand and dust. When the propellers kicked it all up, the wounded were bandaged with that dust in their dressings. I knew I would have these men from six to eight hours. When I got them I attempted to clean out the wounds and sprinkle them with sulfa powder and re-bandage them.

As I took off each of the bandages, I realized I had more than I could handle. For many of the men, there was little I could do except to sprinkle sulfa powder into the wounds and re-bandage them. I would put pressure dressings on if necessary. I remember making Montgomery straps. A Montgomery strap is a wide piece of adhesive tape folded over on itself. You would poke three holes in it and you could make a kind of corset with a set of these. In the holes you poked the bandage to make a string to tie it tight to use for an abdominal wound, for example. They made dressing changes more efficient and quicker.

I also splinted and gave morphine with Syrettes. A Syrette looks like a tiny tube of ophthalmic ointment. Each one carried a quarter or a half grain of morphine, and each had its own needle. I carried a handful of them in my pocket. You injected and then squeezed out the contents. If I wanted to give less than the quarter grain, I had to guess.

Guam was our home base. Between flights we worked in tents at the base hospital there, on many of the same men we had evacuated. This was before they got the Quonset huts up.

On all the flights the space between the litters was very narrow, so the men couldn't lift their heads to look at their feet. If I were doing a dressing on a foot, they would say, "How does it look, Lieutenant?" If I was looking at a complete traumatic amputation I would say, "Well, it's pretty badly messed up, but fortunately they have inducted the best doctors that we have and they're all in Guam waiting for you." And then I'd go on to the next man.

It happened several times that I was absolutely shocked when I took the dressings off and realized what I was looking at. When these men asked me about their condition, I became an actress no matter what they asked me. I would look and then say, "Well, it's a mess but it can be fixed," knowing full well that nothing could be done. My knowledge of anatomy and physiology was very good and my operating-room experience allowed me to picture what was going to happen when these men got there.

I remember one patient who had dived into a foxhole. He broke his jaw and clavicle, and ended up with his rear end up. His buttocks were peppered with shrapnel. I couldn't lie him on his stomach. I couldn't lie him on his back or his side. I couldn't make him comfortable. For his fractured clavicle, which was an open fracture with bone protruding from the skin, I rolled up a jacket, put it in his armpit, and hyperextended his arm so that the broken bone would go back under the skin. Then I bandaged the wound and applied a sling with an elastic bandage to keep the arm in that position.

On one flight I encountered phosphorus wounds for the first time. I had never heard anything in my training about phosphorus until I got a man who had tracks all over him that kept spreading. From high-school chemistry I remembered that phosphorus burns only in the presence of air. And I wondered how the hell I was going to stop this. So I smeared all those phosphorus burns with Vaseline. That was one of my dilemmas. I had never encountered phosphorus burns before. But I guess I did the right thing.

On one of the Iwo Jima trips a Marine major came to me and said, "We have four Japanese Imperial Marine prisoners. I'm sending them back on your flight."

The plane was already loaded. I went back to the major and said, "What does that mean?"

He said I would have to have two guards for each prisoner. These Imperial Marines were six feet tall. They were the tallest Japanese I had ever seen. It meant that I would have to bump twelve patients who were already strapped into their litters and ready to go. I said, "Major, I can't do it. Can't the prisoners go on the next plane?"

He said, "I've ordered you to take these men now."

My reply was, "You go aboard and pick the twelve men that will have to be bumped."

He then said, "Go ahead and go."

On those six- to eight-hour flights we had canned turkey, C-rations, K-rations, canned butter, canned peanut butter, and fresh bread that was baked at Guam. I fed them from the cans or gave them sliced-turkey sandwiches. We also had a lot of juices in huge GI cans.

As for the whole blood, it was in a box lined with what looked like fiberglass for insulation. I had qualms about using it. The men had dog tags which indicated blood type, but there was no designation whether it was positive or negative. I only remember giving three units of blood because the two patients to whom I gave the blood were hemorrhaging badly and it appeared they wouldn't make it, and they didn't. I had my heart in my mouth.

Those two patients and a third Marine were the only ones I lost in my few trips, and [the deaths] resulted from a single event. While we were on the ground loading patients, a Zero came over. I heard a terrible noise and chatter. I was away from the tent at the time and out of the plane, possibly on a hill not far from where we had landed. The plane strafed the tent holding the patients we were about to evacuate. A bullet also pierced our wing tank, which did not explode because it was full and there were no fumes to ignite. It's fortunate it wasn't a tracer round.

We were detained there for many hours until that hole could be repaired. I stayed on the plane with the men during that time, never thinking that another Zero could come by and strafe the plane, and none ever did.

They loaded all the patients on the plane right after the attack, so when I had to evaluate them on the plane, three were in very bad shape. They had been wounded again as they lay in the tent. They were put on the plane during the confusion which followed the strafing of the tent. Triage had been practiced until this incident.

One was an abdominal evisceration. Another had a severe head injury. Part of the man's skull was gone and his brain was exposed. The third had a sucking chest wound. I turned that man over and could see the exit wound. He was bleeding profusely. I knew his pleural cavity was filling with blood so I turned him on the side that was bleeding in an effort to keep the lung that wasn't affected, possibly aerating. These were real quick decisions. I had covered both the entrance and exit wounds with just adhesive tape in a futile attempt to stop the loss of pleural air.

On the way back to Guam, the pilot came back and said that because of very strong head winds we would have to jettison something. I told him that the only thing I had to dump was the very heavy medicine cabinet with the whole blood in it. So we just pushed it out of the plane. He then said that wouldn't be enough and we would have to land in Saipan. He asked me if there was anything else that we could get rid of and I told him I had three deceased Marines, but I didn't want to push them out. I jettisoned most of the large cans of fruit juice.

On the way to Saipan I never covered their faces. When I made rounds and checked each of the Marines and sailors, I stopped at their litters and spoke to them even though I knew that they were dead, because I didn't want the others to know that anyone had been lost.

The morale of the men getting on the plane was sky high. They were in what I would call psychological shock and didn't complain about their wounds. They were just glad to get the hell out of that place.

When we landed in Saipan, the corpsman and I offloaded the three [dead] men. The pilot had radioed ahead for an ambulance from the base hospital, but it hadn't arrived yet. So we put them under the shade of the wing and I stood there with the corpsman thinking that I wasn't finished. I had to do something. I asked him to bring me a glass of grapefruit juice. He went in the plane and poured a cup of juice. I had him take off his hat; I wasn't wearing one. Then I sprinkled the juice on them and said "In the name of the Father, the Son, and the Holy Ghost," and baptized all three. Even though I wasn't particularly religious, it was something I had to do.

When the ambulance came and we got back on the plane I had to become an actress and probably deserved an Oscar. The morale of the men leaving Iwo Jima was very high, as I said, and they had been joking back and forth. But when I got back on the plane at Saipan, there was dead silence. And I said, "Okay guys, next stop is Guam." They didn't answer me. It seems the middle row of patients could see what I had done through the portholes and they told everyone else.

Then one of them called me over and said he wanted to tell me something. When I leaned over to listen he put his arms around me and gave me a kiss on my cheek. And then, one by one, each grasped my hand or pulled me to him. It was the most emotional thing I have ever experienced.

I have to say that on all the flights I felt so close to each of the patients. It wasn't a bonding; it wasn't love. It was a combination of apprehension for their disabilities, the fact that I was the professional responsible, and that they depended on me at a very critical time in their lives. They must have felt it too, because as they deplaned almost every one gave me a kiss or a hug. Each one was very special to me.

One of them gave me a green bag and said, "I want you to have this."

I said, "No, I don't need anything." But he insisted. I opened the bag and there were gold teeth and bloody, dried-up Japanese ears inside. These were his souvenirs of Iwo Jima. I said they looked very interesting but I couldn't imagine using them and insisted that he keep his souvenirs. Those trophies were all he had to give me.

MEDAL OF HONOR

As the Pacific war reached its climax in April 1945, Okinawa, the last battle of World War II, became the dress rehearsal for the invasion of Japan. Defending the sixty-mile-long island was a refinement of strategy the Japanese had used at Peleliu and Iwo Jima, the so-called defense in depth. Not having the means to defend Okinawa in its entirety, Lt. Gen. Mitsuru Ushijima chose to make his stand in the south.

The plan was to grant the invaders the beach, then lure them inland. Force their soldiers to confront defenses of concrete and steel with interlocking fire zones. Compel them to worm their way into networks of subterranean ant farms packed with fanatical men willing to sell their lives dearly.

If the landing on 1 April 1945 and the days immediately following seemed a breeze, American forces would soon bog down as they approached Ushijima's main defenses in the south, named the Shuri Line for the nearby thirteenth-century castle. There the topography gave the defender every advantage while presenting the attacker with steep escarpments, deep ravines, rolling hills, limestone ridges and caves, and even fortified tombs of the native Okinawans.

As the rains began to fall and the offensive stalled in a sea of mud, the battle began to mimic the nightmare stalemate of World War I trench warfare. Despite air attack, naval gunfire from battleships and cruisers, and large-caliber howitzers, it would take the resolute soldier armed with Browning automatic rifle (BAR), Garand, carbine, and grenade to flush the Japanese from their fortified holes.

Although HA1c [hospital apprentice first class] Robert E. Bush was a newcomer to combat, the eighteen-year-old corpsman had encountered death soon after coming ashore on 1 April. While attending one of the few fatalities that first day, he had found himself literally looking down the barrel of a Japanese rifle. "He was so close, I could tell the caliber," he said, adding that he probably was spared only because his comrades had held their fire a few moments earlier as a woman emerged from a nearby cave to recover a wounded Japanese.

About a month later as his unit engaged the Japanese, Bush again was called upon to tend a fallen Marine. The events that followed earned him the Congressional Medal of Honor.

On the morning of 2 May we were assigned the task of securing a relatively low hill which connected in some manner to the China Sea. I'd be surprised if it was fifty feet high. I was in our command post. The company commander was in a rather heated discussion with our platoon sergeant, who was suggesting that we get a battleship to hit that hill a few times before we went up. He pointed out that it might be heavily defended.

Despite the sergeant's concern, the platoon leader decided to take a squad to look at the hill. My opinion, as humble as it was sitting in the command post that morning, was that this was not a good decision.

As soon as they got to the base of the hill, the Japanese emerged from the ground and all hell broke loose. Many of our guys were killed and wounded, including the lieutenant, who took cover in a shellhole.

In those days, if someone was wounded in front of the lines, as a corpsman you had some important things to consider. If you exposed yourself and they nailed you, the rest of the Marines lost their corpsman.

So they were not too happy to send you out, any more than we were too happy to go out.

But that decision lay with the corpsman, not with the platoon sergeant. I looked where the lieutenant was and said, "Okay, I'll go out there. Give me a guy in front of me and another behind me. We'll bust ass across the field to get to him and I'll see what I can do."

So that's what we did. As we crossed the rice paddy, which was about a hundred yards wide, the Japanese started in on us from the top of the hill. They killed both men who were protecting me, but I was unhurt. I got to the lieutenant and jumped into the hole with him. It looked like his left shoulder had been hit with a mortar shell, and there was a lot of blood.

I immediately noticed that his eyes were dilating, and I knew I was losing him. I put a battle dressing on his shoulder, opened a can of albumin, and put the needle in his vein. I will never forget what he said to me. "There ain't no Nips here, Doc."

"Jim, they're all over the place!" I replied. "Just be quiet. They'll hear us. I'll get you out of here." It was customary to call our lieutenants by their first names. This way if the enemy heard us, they wouldn't recognize them as officers. He kept jabbering and I knew he was out of it. After a few moments, I finally shut him up.

In the meantime, I looked on that ridge and was scared to death. I grabbed his carbine and dropped the clip into my left hand. I pushed down on the [follower] to see how many rounds he had left. It was tight so I knew he hadn't fired a single round. I jammed it back in, took the safety off, and set the carbine down beside him. As I again reviewed the hill, suddenly a head popped up. I could see a star on his helmet.

I was still holding onto the albumin can. Behind us were our two squads watching all this. They had a light machine gun set up but didn't dare fire, probably for fear of hitting us.

Suddenly I felt a tug on the can. I let go of it and up jumped the lieutenant out of the hole and across the rice paddy back toward our lines, dragging the can behind him. The albumin must have given him a high and he was gone. When he took off, the top of that hill just opened up. I didn't bother looking back at the lieutenant because I had immediately written him off.

I grabbed the carbine and, with the help of God, was able to see the Japanese sticking their heads up. As scared as I was, I knew I had to fight or die. There were no other alternatives. Every time a head came up, I'd drop the carbine just below the protective berm on the hill and send one round out, always considering how much ammo I had left. I figured such an insubstantial berm wasn't going to stop a bullet at that close range. There were fifteen rounds in the clip and I had two extras strapped to the stock. That gave me forty-five rounds. I'd send out just one or two at a time, and when a head wouldn't come back up I knew I was hitting them. I could see the whole thing in that little round peep sight.

I kept that up for awhile; I don't know how long, probably two or three minutes. I hadn't kept track of the number of shots I had fired so I put a fresh clip in when I had an opportunity. Now I had fifteen rounds again.

Right about that time, the hand grenades started coming in. They knew where I was. As the first one hit I threw my arm up over my face, but my right eye was already gone. The only thing that saved my life was my .45 in the shoulder holster. That's what stopped most of the fragments. I got some in my heart, which are still there, and many, many fragments around my left shoulder.

There was also a hell of a big hole under my left arm into my lungs. When I tried to breathe, air was leaking in down there. I knew this was a serious wound. I put a compress over it and then tried to lower my left arm, but something in my shoulder was sadly disconnected up there. I could move my elbow and left hand and was still able to use my weapons.

But I was really in trouble. This all happened so quickly that these are the only things I remember. Other grenades started coming in; one hit my butt and another my belly, but these didn't cause serious damage. However, I knew I had to get out of there.

There weren't too many options. I didn't dare follow the lieutenant's example and go out in the field. I couldn't go straight up the hill because it was just too steep, especially in my condition. So I grabbed the carbine and headed off to the left of the hill, which wasn't so steep. I found I could ascend the hill from that direction.

I fired the carbine until it was empty, then emptied my .45 and threw it away. That pistol was my pride and joy. When I carried it I thought I was John Dillinger. I then picked up an M1 laying near a dead Marine and kept going.

It seemed curious the Japanese didn't see me. They were looking straight ahead down toward the hole where I had been and never did come down from the hill. They were tunneled under the ground. Picture a hole in the ground about so many feet deep and then lateral holes about three or four feet from the surface. They were in these lateral holes. They had allowed our Marines on the scouting mission to go on by and then came out of the hole and opened fire.

The next break I had—and I had quite a few breaks on this thing—was when I went around the hill. Things were really fuzzy because one eye was gone and the other was a little blurry too. The Japanese just didn't know where I was and so they had quit shooting and were throwing grenades down at an empty hole. When I got to the top of the hill, I wondered why they weren't sitting there with guns pointed at me.

I learned why thirty years later. Four Marines from the original patrol had jumped into the hole with the enemy and drawn their attention. They had been there the whole time. My sniping had also diverted the attention of the Japanese. Finally the Marines jumped out of the hole and down a steep part of the hill to get away. One was killed in the fall. And that explains why they were looking for the Marines and not for me.

When I got around the hill and to the top, their backs were to me, four of them lined up like dominoes in a row. They didn't have a chance in hell. I had the element of surprise and I needed all the advantage I could. Just holding that rifle in my condition was a real effort. I walked along the ridge and winged every Japanese I saw.

Suddenly I didn't see another soul. I was the only one standing on the skyline of that hill. And so I left, going right down that hill, and kept right on going back the way I came.

I carried the M1 all the way to our lines, where I ran into a guy named Cass, one of our Marines. There was a wall that looked as though it was used to house pigs. It was about three feet high and in no way could I get over it. I said, "Cass, give me a hand here." And he helped me over that thing.

Then Fred Hollier grabbed my left arm and took me back. The next thing I remember was a corpsman patching me up.

On July 26th, 1945, I was discharged at Oak Knoll Naval Hospital. They pinned a little "Ruptured Duck" [eagle pin given to all honorably discharged veterans] on my lapel, gave me a few bucks, and I was on my way home.

Some time later I was back in high school and living with my mother. One day just as I was leaving the house, the phone rang. It was James

Forrestal, secretary of the Navy. He told me I had been selected to receive the Medal of Honor from President [Harry S.] Truman the following Wednesday. I told him it was hard for me to believe. I had done nothing more than I had done the whole time I was over there. The only thing different this time was that I'd had a weapon.

My mother said, "Why don't you get married and take your wife? You're going to get married anyway." I said, "Okay," and my honeymoon was that train trip to Washington.

When my wife and I got to Washington, we met President Truman. Fourteen people were being decorated at the same time, people like Pappy Boyington, Louis Wilson, and a lot of famous men who had done a lot of things during the early part of the war. After Truman announced that he had raised everyone's rank one notch by executive order, he said to me, "You'll now be a third-class pharmacist's mate."

"No, I'm out of the service," I replied. I had been recommended for pharmacist's mate third class but was discharged before the paperwork had come through. Therefore I was still a hospital apprentice first class.

"Well," he said, "you don't get anything then." That was just like Harry Truman, a great sense of humor.

I don't think I was a hero by any stretch of the imagination. I was out there doing what I was paid to do and trying to protect a man's life. And I did it with some very fortunate breaks, good training, and help from God.

Robert Bush eventually cofounded a lumber company in his native Washington state and also served as the company's pilot for twenty-five years. How did he get a pilot's license with but one eye? "Will Rogers's pilot, Wiley Post, was a one-eyed pilot. I figured if he could do it, I could do it. Anyway, I never told anybody I had one eye and nobody ever asked me." Bush has since served as president of the Congressional Medal of Honor Society.

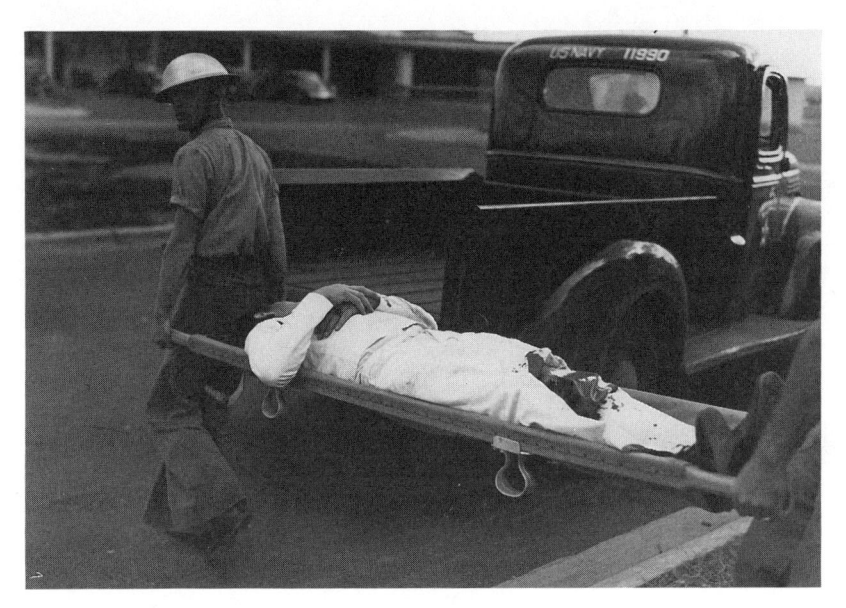

Pacific theater, act one. Even as the bombs fall on Pearl Harbor, a wounded sailor is carried to safety.

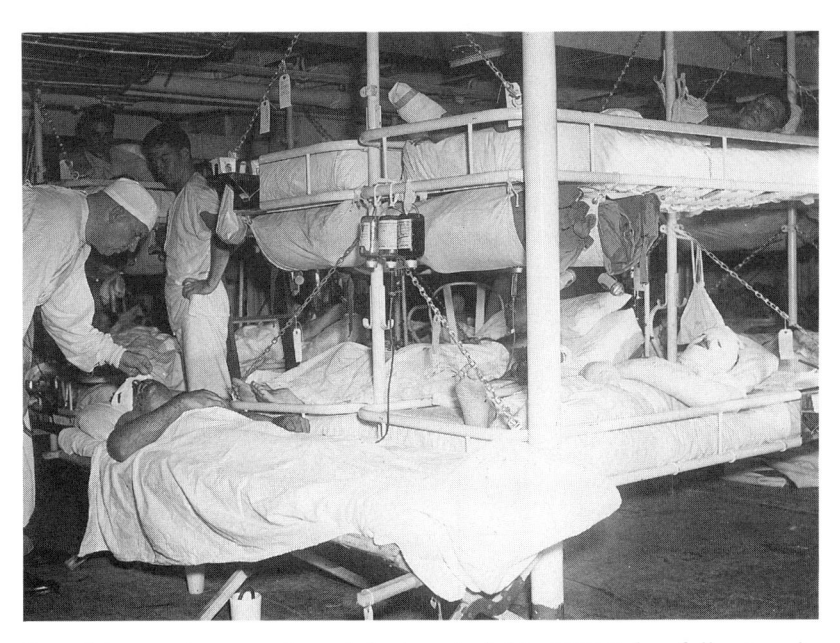

Casualties receive care aboard the hospital ship USS *Solace* following the Pearl Harbor attack. Men with flash burn, shrapnel, and concussion injuries inundated the *Solace*'s wards, the naval hospital at Pearl Harbor, and nearly all military and civilian medical facilities in the Honolulu area.

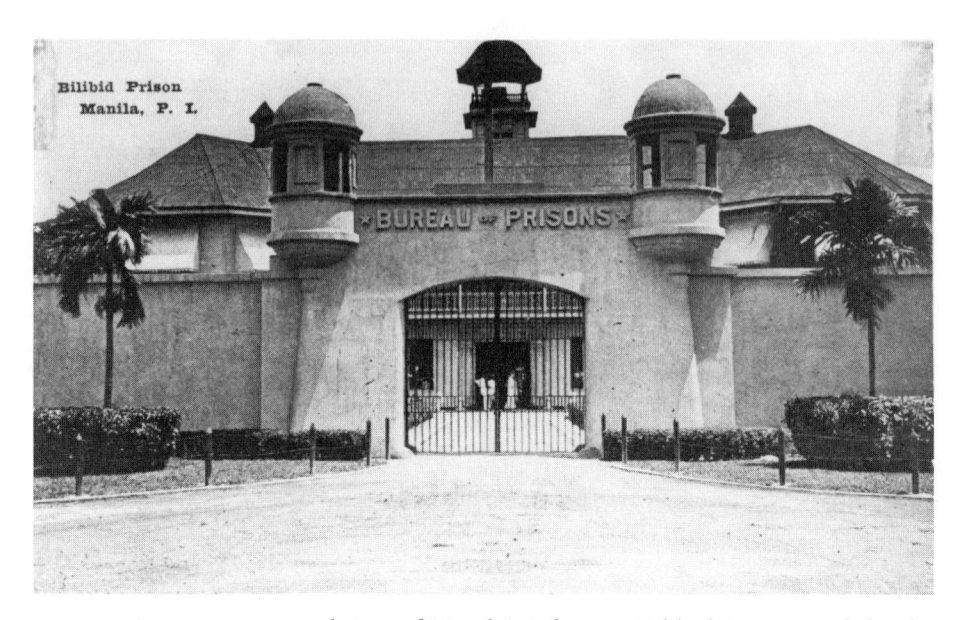

A prewar postcard view of Manila's infamous Bilibid Prison. Built by the Spanish in 1865, Bilibid had become the main criminal prison in the Philippines by the eve of war. Even though it had recently been condemned as unfit for habitation by Philippine authorities, the Japanese used the prison as a central receiving station for the transfer of American prisoners to and from forced-labor camps throughout the Philippines.

Lt. George Ferguson, one of Bilibid's Navy inmates, sketched a portion of the prison's layout in his journal. Dr. Ferguson would later die aboard a Japanese hell ship torpedoed by a U.S. submarine.

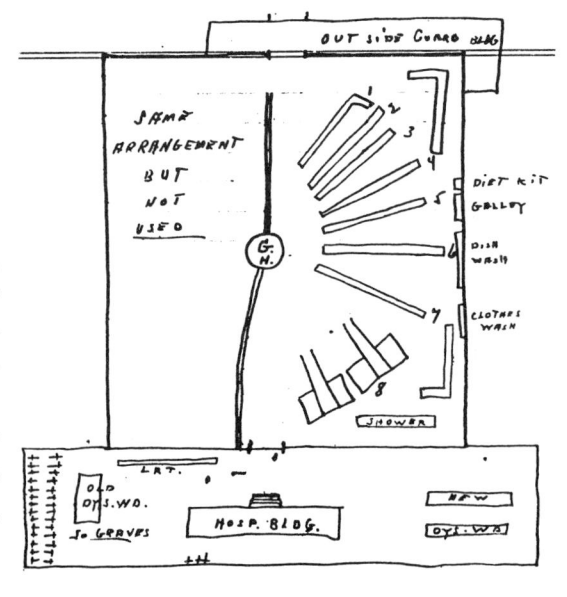

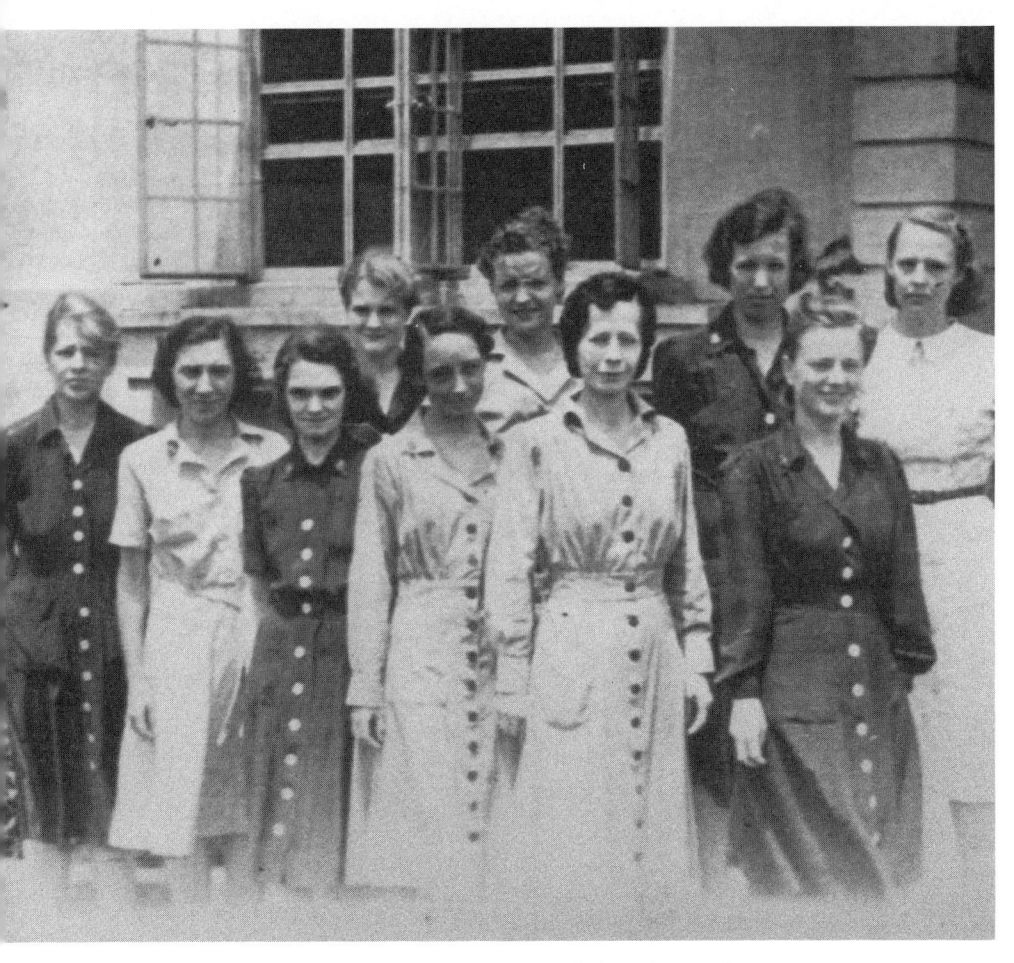

A Japanese guard named Kusimoto snapped this photo of Navy nurses in Manila's Santo Tomas internment camp in September 1942. From left: Susie Pitcher, Helen Gorzelanski, Margaret Nash, Mary Rose Harrington, Eldene Paige, Goldia O'Haver, Laura Cobb, Bertha Evans, Edwina Todd, and Dorothy Still. By the time of their liberation, all were suffering severe malnutrition.

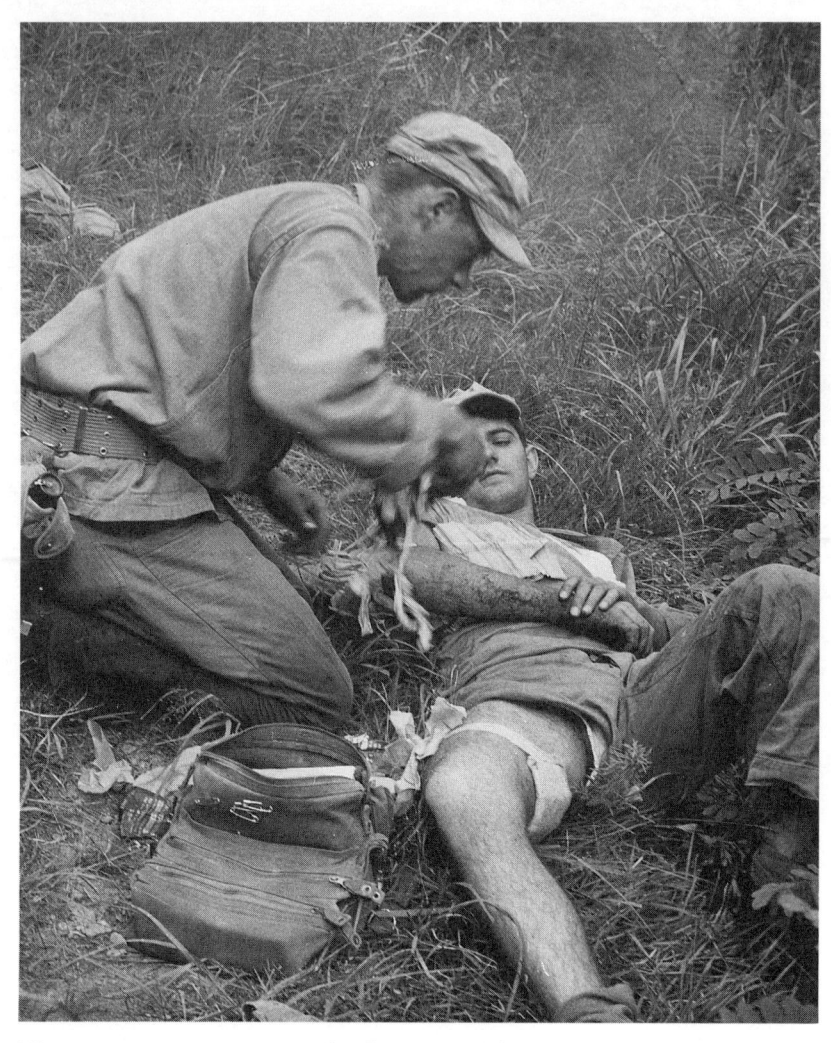

The company corpsman is the first critical link in the evacuation chain. Medical aid bag at his side, PhM3c Don Meloan applies a battle dressing to a wounded Marine at Okinawa.

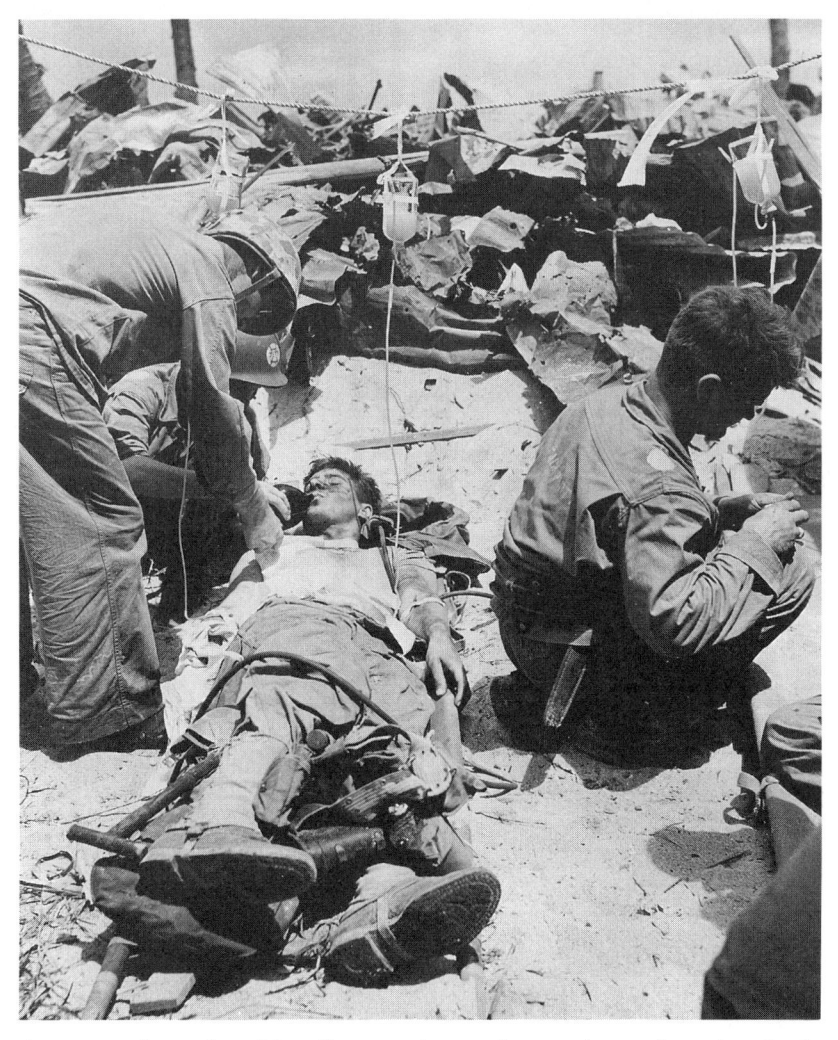

An entrenching shovel handle provides a splint as plasma flows into both arms of this badly injured Marine at an improvised aid station on Eniwetok. Before serum albumin and whole blood were available later in the war, plasma—the liquid portion of blood minus the platelets and red cells—was commonly used as a blood-volume expander for the prevention and treatment of shock.

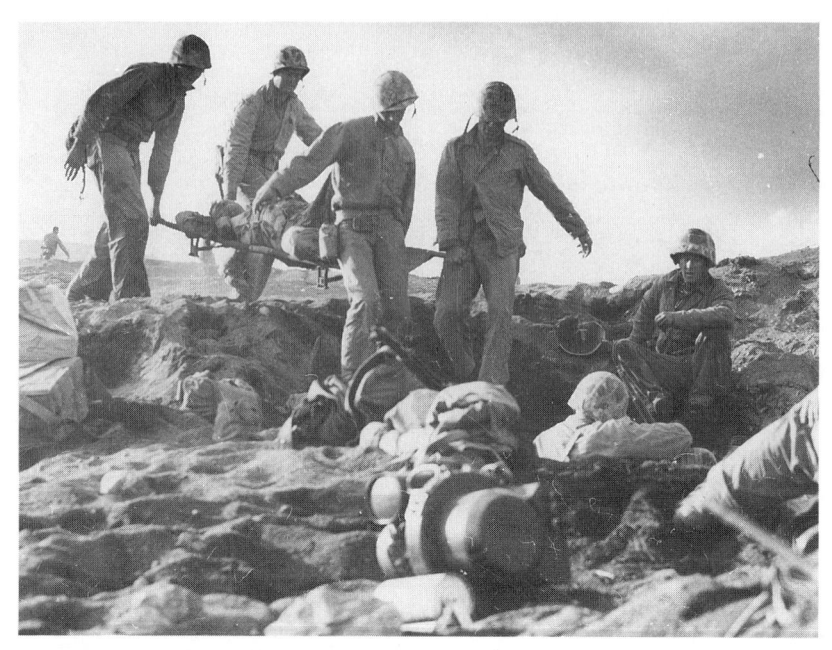

A litter team brings in a casualty under fire. Shell holes gouged from sand or coral often provided the only protection for a frontline aid station.

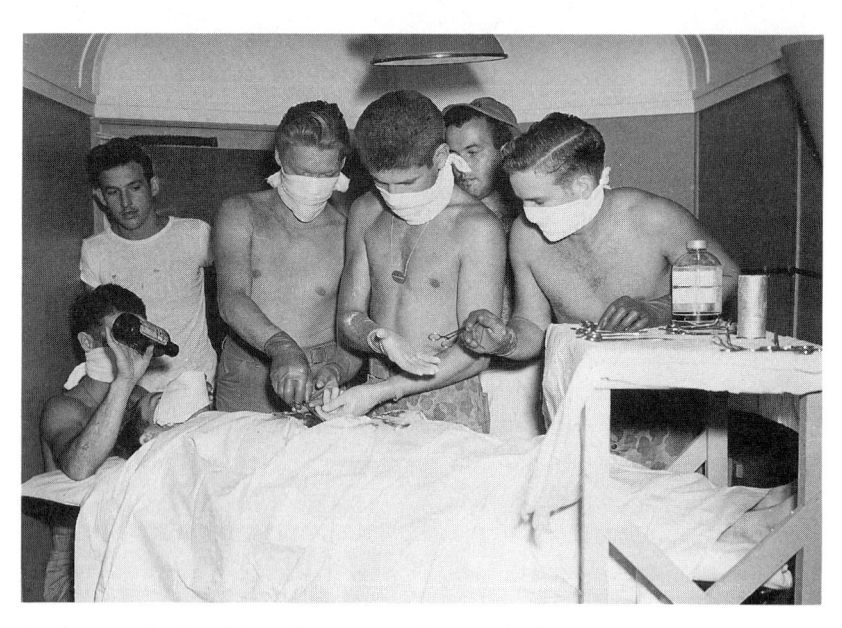

As the anesthetist drips ether into an improvised gauze mask, a young surgeon and his assistants perform emergency surgery somewhere in the South Pacific.

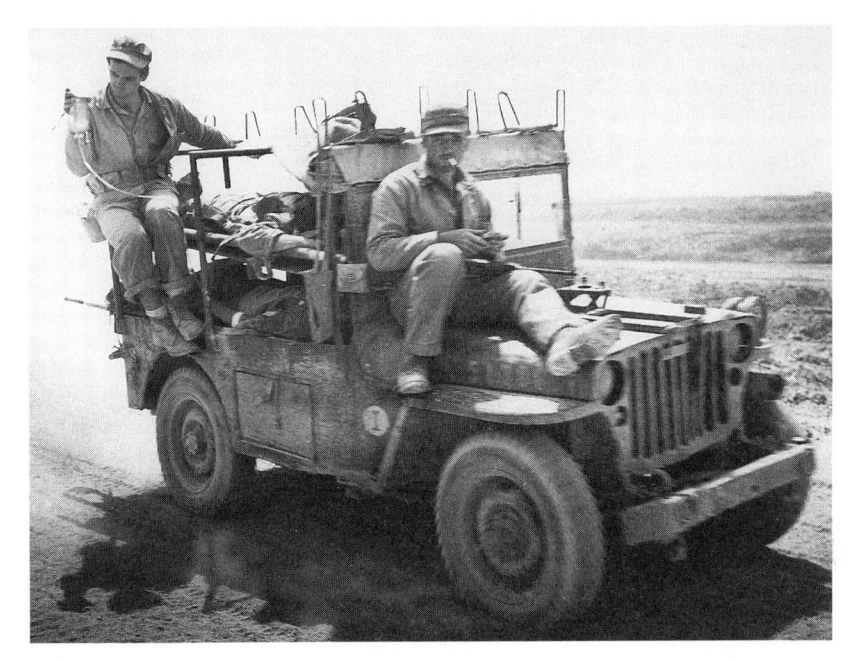

With two patients aboard, a corpsman administering plasma, a driver, and a Marine riding shotgun, jeep ambulances often provided the only quick evacuation to the beach.

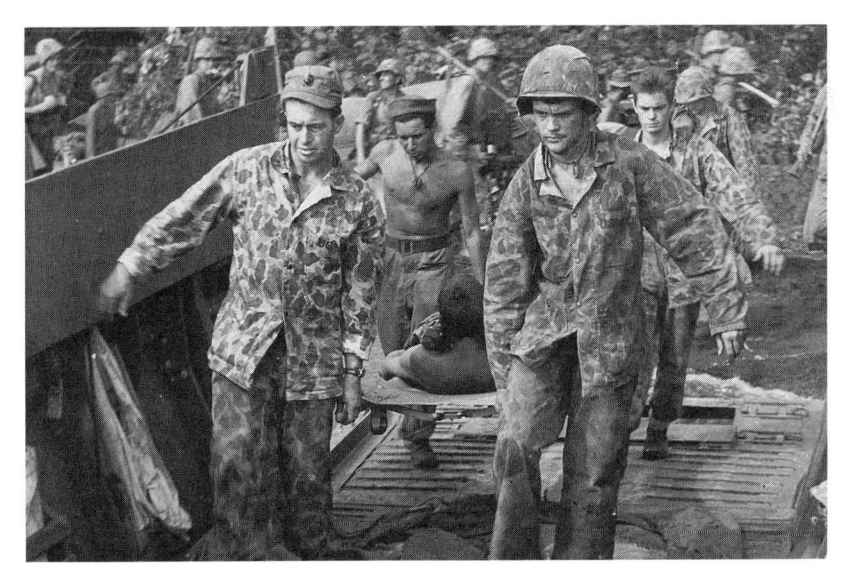

The evacuation chain continues. For a Marine wounded in the battle for Bougainville, the next stop is a landing craft for a trip out to a transport or hospital ship, where he will receive more definitive care.

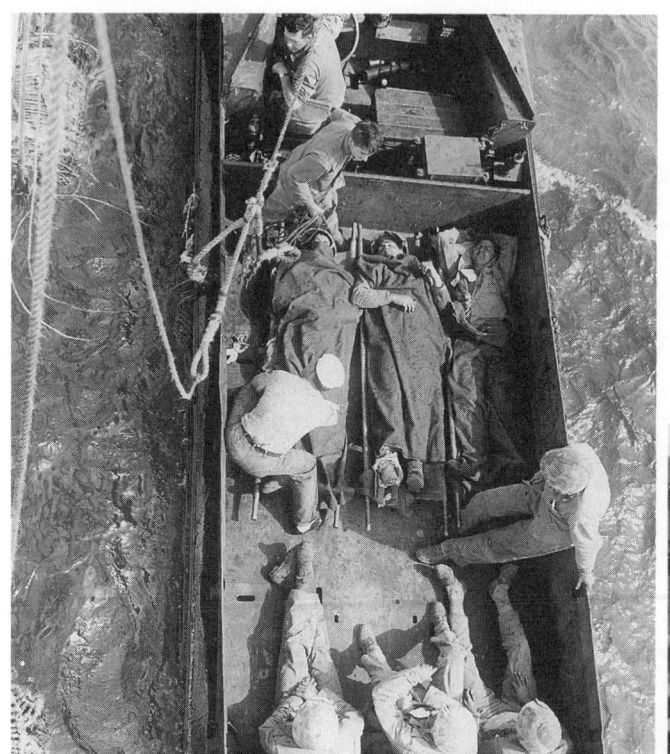

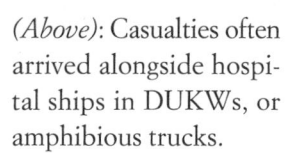

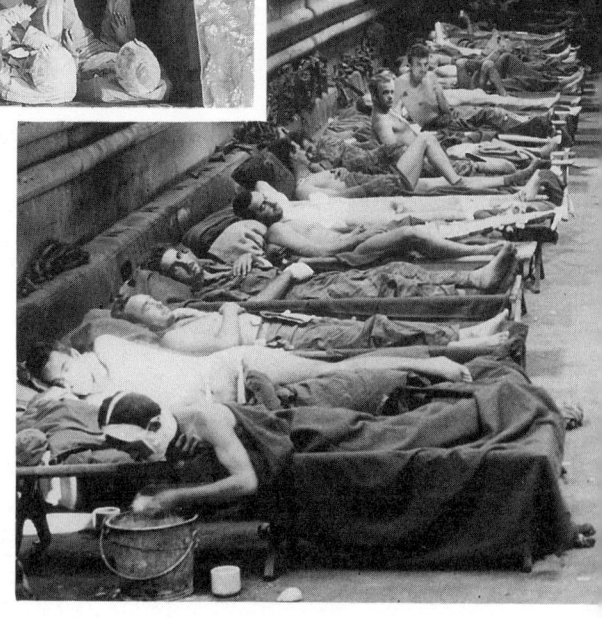

(Above): Casualties often arrived alongside hospital ships in DUKWs, or amphibious trucks.

(Right): Preventive medicine: Corpsmen prepare hypodermic syringes as physicians administer tetanus and yellow-fever shots aboard the USS *Nevada* en route to Iwo Jima. As in previous wars, disease could keep more men off the line than enemy-inflicted injuries.

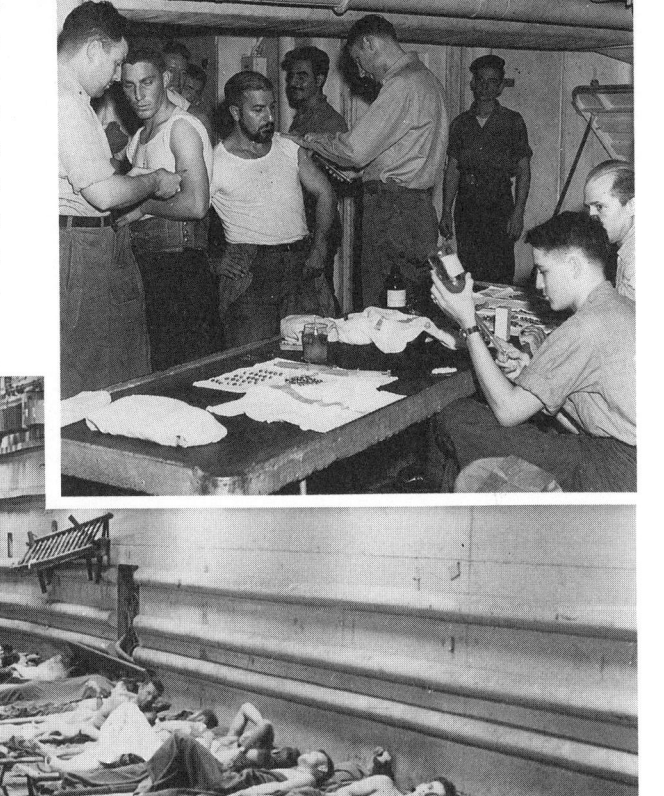

Once it discharged its cargo of troops, tanks, trucks, and supplies on the invasion beach, an LST tank deck offered ample space for casualties. In the early days of the Pacific campaign, there were very few hospital ships in theater, and landing craft and troop transports with negligible medical services offered the only available transportation for the wounded.

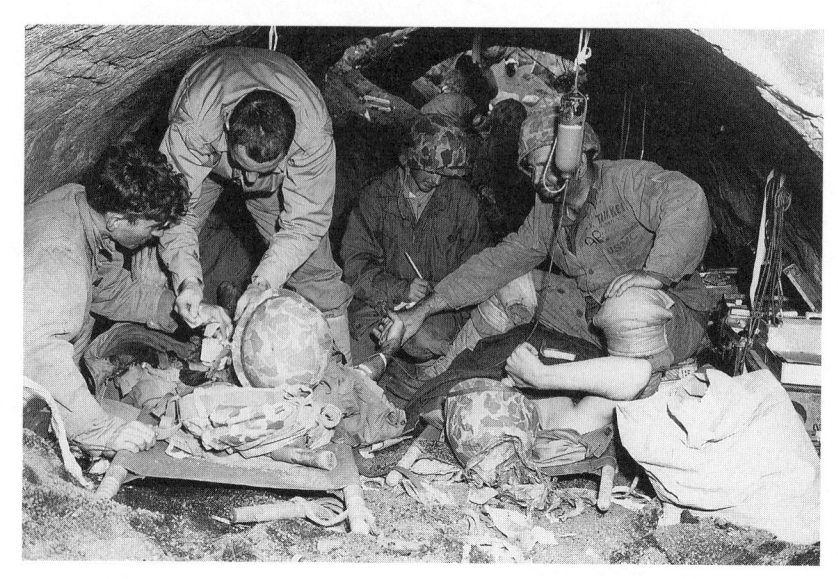

An abandoned concrete Japanese air-raid shelter serves as an aid station on Iwo Jima. Here, a concerned corpsman grips a wounded Marine's hand as he receives plasma and a physician assesses his injuries.

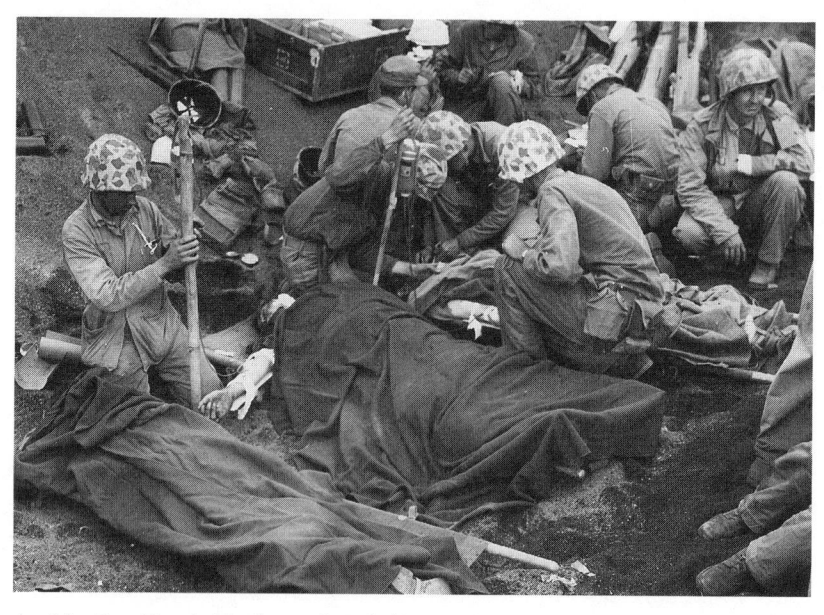

Amidst Iwo Jima's black sand and the wreckage of war, doctors and corpsmen struggle to save wounded Marines shortly after the initial landings. Lifesaving plasma flows into two patients while a deceased comrade lies alongside.

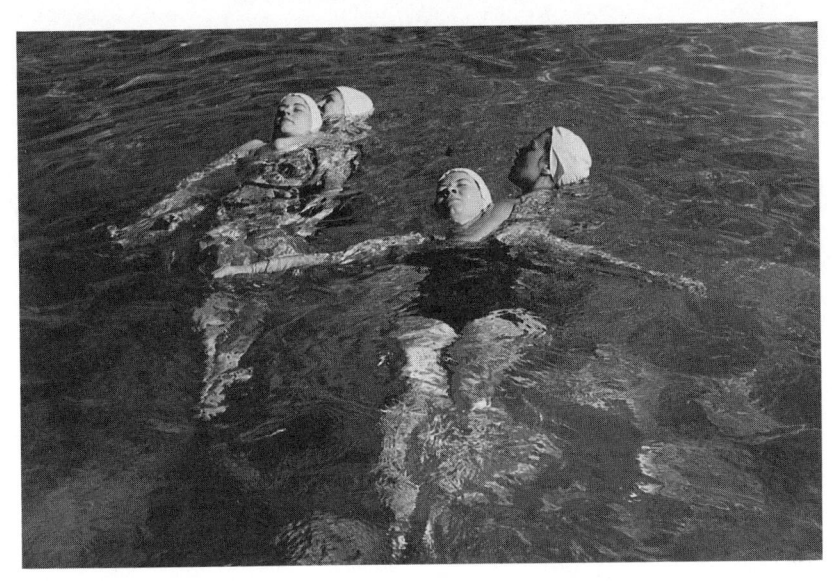

By early 1945, the first class of Navy flight nurses were training at Alameda Naval Air Station for duty in the Pacific. Water-survival instruction was essential.

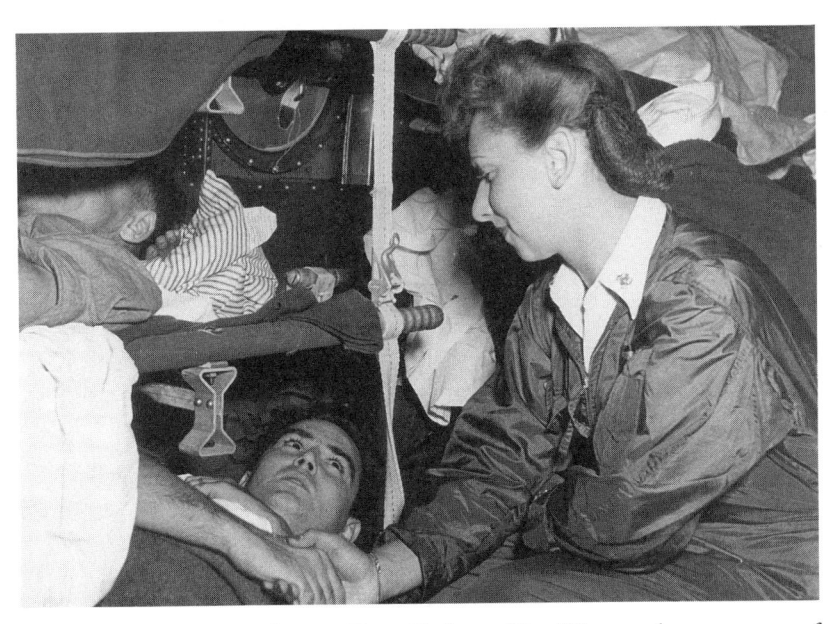

One of Alameda's graduates, Ens. Kathryn Van Wagner, became one of the first American nurses on a foreign battlefield when she accompanied an evacuation flight from Iwo Jima in March 1945. *Courtesy of Kathryn Van Wagner Pribram*

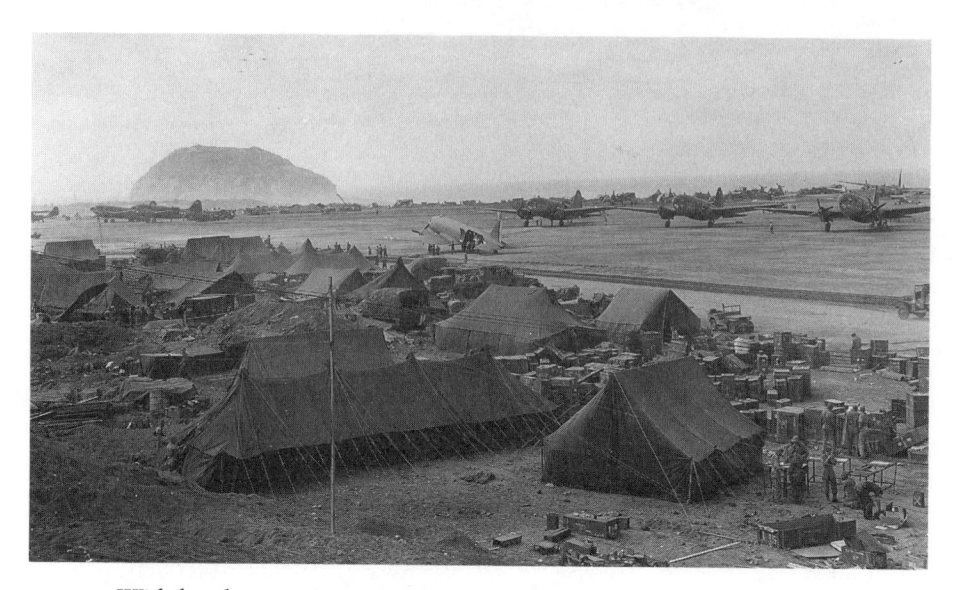

With hard-won Mount Suribachi as a backdrop, Navy R-4Ds (C-47s) line an airstrip on Iwo Jima, waiting to take wounded Marines to a naval hospital on Guam.

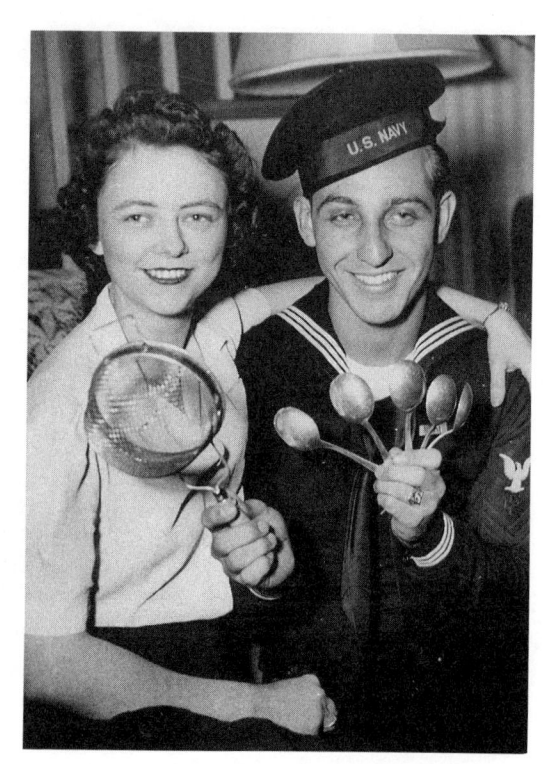

PhM1c Wheeler B. Lipes and wife show off kitchen utensils similar to the ones he used during his historic submarine appendectomy.
Courtesy of Wheeler B. Lipes

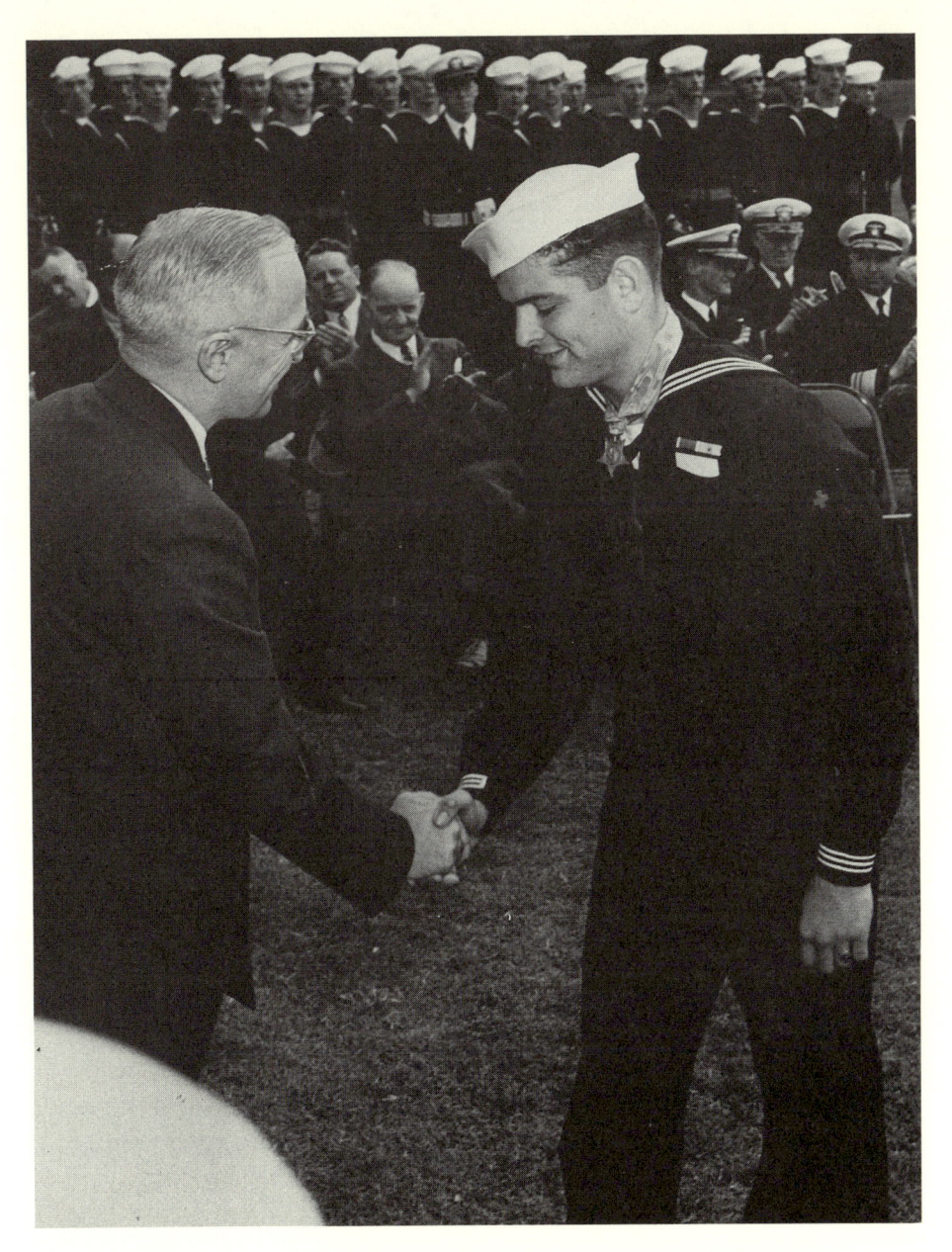

President Harry S. Truman awards the Congressional Medal of Honor to HA1 Robert Bush. During World War II, corpsmen received seven Medals of Honor for their actions at Iwo Jima and Okinawa. A Navy decision not to award the medal to corpsmen in the early campaigns precluded many equally deserving young men from receiving their nation's highest honor.

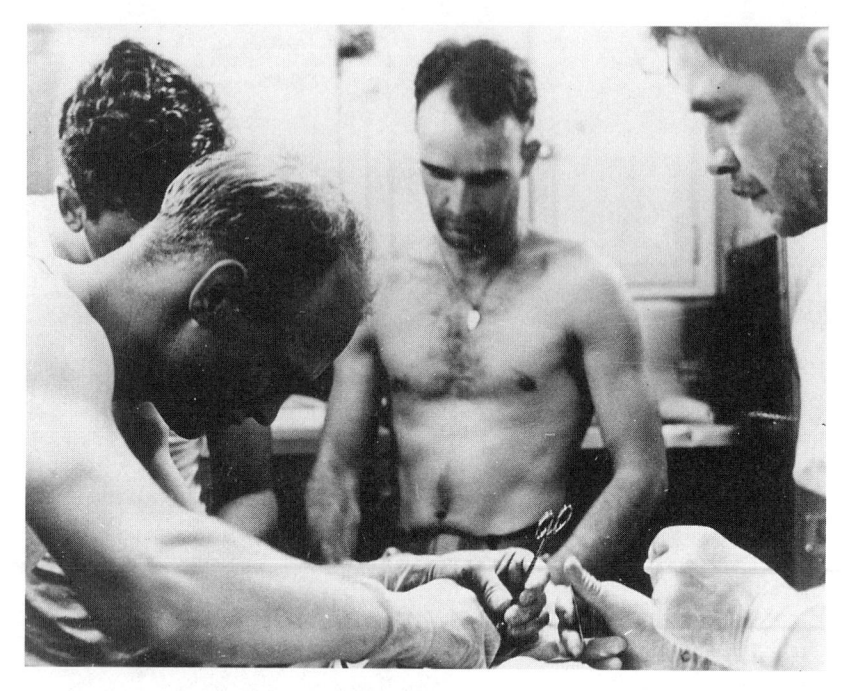

Lt. Robert Worthington, diving officer of the USS *Silversides,* took this photograph of PhM1c Thomas Moore and his team performing an appendectomy on shipmate George Platter. *Courtesy of Thomas Moore*

FIVE

Submarine Surgeons

If corpsmen distinguished themselves supporting the Marines in the island campaigns, they did no less serving the fleet. On many of the smaller combatant vessels, corpsmen provided the only medical care available.

As Japanese forces rolled over the Allies from Wake to Singapore during December 1941 and the early months of 1942, the only offensive weapons the defenders could bring to bear were mostly relics of the Asiatic Fleet—three cruisers, thirteen World War II four-piper destroyers, twenty-nine submarines, a host of small auxiliaries and patrol boats, two gunboats, six motor torpedo (PT) boats, and thirty-six patrol planes (PBYs). Outnumbered and outgunned, the cruisers and destroyers put up a gallant fight, but to little avail. The PTs and submarines, armed with defective torpedoes, did little better.

After the destruction of the Cavite Navy Yard, near Manila, on 10 December 1941, only bases at Pearl Harbor and in Australia served as relatively safe havens for American subs. Even though a well-trained corpsman was always part of the crew, long patrols far from these ports put submariners many days and thousands of miles away from comprehensive medical care. An emergency that could easily be treated in a well-staffed hospital ashore often assumed a very different dimension beneath the sea.

One of the most dramatic stories to come out of World War II was that of an emergency appendectomy performed by a twenty-three-year-old corpsman as his submarine, the USS *Seadragon* (SS-194) cruised submerged in enemy waters. Related in a 1942 article, the story brought a Pulitzer Prize to journalist George Weller and fame to PhM1c Wheeler B. Lipes. It also gave a much-needed dose of inspiration to the home front when good news about the war was hard to come by.

In the last half century the story has been distorted and embellished by its retelling in books, movies, and television. Mythologized by Hollywood and the printed word, that heroic 1942 surgery is firmly established in Navy lore.

Faced with an acute appendicitis, "Johnny" Lipes selected members of his surgical team from the crew and commandeered the wardroom for his operating room. A tea strainer lined with gauze became a makeshift anesthesia mask, and teaspoons from the galley with bent handles served as retractors.

Two other corpsmen performed appendectomies during the war, PhM1c Harry Roby aboard the USS *Grayback* (SS-208) and PhM1c Thomas Moore aboard the USS *Silversides* (SS-236). Lipes and Moore recount their stories and their bizarre repercussions.

It started 11 September 1942, when William E. "Pete" Ferrall, on his fourth combat patrol as commanding officer of the USS *Seadragon,* suddenly faced a perplexing problem. S1c (seaman first class) Darrel Rector had been ill three days with belly pain, nausea, and fever. The sub's corpsman, PhM1c Wheeler B. Lipes, was now confident that the diagnosis was acute appendicitis. Standard therapy was surgical removal of the appendix. But there was no medical officer on board to do the appendectomy, and without it Rector could die.

I was in the after battery section of the submarine—the crew's compartment—when Darrell Rector came back and said, "Doc, I got a pain in my belly. How about giving me a couple of CC pills." These were laxatives. I told him to get in his bunk and rest a bit. His temperature was rising and he had the classic symptoms of appendicitis. The abdominal muscles were getting that washboard rigidity. He then began to flex his right leg up on his abdomen to get some relief.

I said to him, "Does that make you feel better?" and he said yes. I thought for a while he might have something going on in the gall bladder. But he complained less about his back, and his pain began to localize in that right quadrant.

Rector worsened and I went to the skipper and the executive officer and asked them to come back and see him. They asked me what I thought was wrong with him and I told them I thought he had appendicitis. The skipper went back and talked to Rector, explaining that there were no doctors around. Rector then said, "Whatever Lipes wants to do is okay with me."

The CO [commanding officer] and I had a long talk and he asked me what I was going to do. "Nothing," I replied.

He lectured me about the fact that we were there to do the best we could. "I fire torpedoes every day and some of them miss," he reminded me. I told him that I couldn't fire *this* torpedo and miss. He asked me if I could do the surgery and I said, "Yes, sir, I can do it. Everything is against us. Our chances are slim. But if that's what I'm ordered to do, that's what I'll do."

They asked Rector what he thought and he said, "Whatever the doc feels has to be done is okay with me." The skipper then ordered me to do it.

I had no blood-pressure apparatus. I had no access to a laboratory. I couldn't do a blood count. I couldn't do a urinalysis. I didn't have a microscope. I had no intravenous fluid, no nothing. Submarines went to sea without adequate equipment and support and with very few basics.

I couldn't be thinking about his belly without knowing anything about his clotting time, so I did a bleeding and clotting time on him. I nicked his ear, took a drop of blood, inverted a medicine glass, took a stopwatch and a needle, and timed the clotting to be sure I didn't have a hemophiliac on my hands. Then when I got into the belly, the appendix wasn't there. I thought, Oh my God! Is this guy reversed?

You should be able to find the appendix very quickly. The first thing you think about is whether the patient is reversed and is his caecum on the left and not on the right side. There are people like that, with organs opposite where they should be. I slipped my fingers down under the caecum—the blind gut—and I could feel the appendix. It was five inches long, adhered, coiled, and buried down at the distal tip, and the distal tip was turning black. It was gangrenous. What luck, I thought. My first one couldn't be easy.

I detached the appendix, tied it off in two places, and then removed it, after which I cauterized the stump with phenol—carbolic acid. I then neutralized the phenol with torpedo alcohol. We had some sulfa tablets I ground into a powder and then put in the oven to kill any spores. This was all I had. There was no penicillin in those days.

I had given this kid a three-inch incision, yet he healed well and was back on duty in a few days. In fact, the ship's cook said "Doc, you must have sewed him up with rubber bands, the way he eats."

When we got back into port, someone told me I was wanted in the wardroom. I went and there, sitting on the bench behind the table, was Admiral Lockwood [Rear Adm. Charles A. Lockwood, Jr., commander submarines, Southwest Pacific]. I said, "I'm sorry, sir. I thought the captain wanted to see me."

He said, "Are you Lipes?"

"Yes, sir."

He then said, "Well, *I* want to see you." He got up, shook my hand, put his arm around me, and said, "Well, you fellows have had an exciting time." So I stood there and talked to him for four or five minutes before [George] Weller came in. He and I then talked at some length.[1]

I received mail from everywhere, and the majority of the letters that came were from mothers who said, "I didn't want my son to go in the Navy, but when I read this story of how you care for the patient, it makes me feel better."

When I got back, it was not my understanding that I had done anything more than my job, that I certainly wasn't out there to be a surgeon, but was there to do whatever it took to alleviate pain and suffering and save life if I could do so. I wasn't being heroic. And I didn't even write a note to my wife about this incident, not one word.

Her sister saw a little three-line blurb in the Philadelphia paper that said, "Sailor removes shipmate's appendix in submarine." Period. That's all. She remarked, "That sounds like something Johnny would do," and then the next thing she knew, the reporters were beating on the door.

After we submitted our report, there was a great deal of conster-

---

1. For his story "Doc Lipes Commandeers a Submarine Officers' Wardroom," published in the Chicago *Daily News* 14 December 1942, George Weller received the Pulitzer Prize for distinguished reporting.

nation at the Bureau of Medicine and Surgery back in Washington. An old warrant officer I knew was on duty the night the message about the operation came in. He told me later how much trouble I had caused him. There were many doctors back there who were very upset about what I had done. I guess they were afraid that because I had performed an appendectomy, everyone in the fleet would be running around looking for the first opportunity to do one. They forgot there were commanding officers and you had supervisory chains that would preclude this.

The day I retired I got one of those canned retirement letters signed by the surgeon general. It gave me credit for bravery in action during the sinking of the submarine *Sealion*.[2] Yet neither it nor any document I ever received mentioned the appendectomy. However, since the incident had given the Navy good publicity and presented to the public the fact that Navy men were well trained and dedicated, the omission was that much more evident.

In the ensuing years, not a month has gone by that I'm not reminded of that incident. Weller's story has even appeared in high-school literature books. When my grandson was in the seventh grade, he found it in one of his books. In fact, he proudly told the teacher that that was his grandfather. The teacher said something like, "Go away little boy, don't tell stories." It's also been the subject of movies and TV programs. There was a series in the fifties called *The Silent Service,* in which the incident was portrayed in an episode called "Operation Seadragon."

I was on an airplane one time and the man next to me was reading a magazine containing one of those Ripley's Believe It or Nots. It told of a submarine sailor who removed a shipmate's appendix. This guy turned to me and said, "Can you believe that?" I read it, shook my head, and said, "Don't believe a word of it."

Darrell Dean Rector, Lipes's patient, did not survive the war. He died on 24 October 1944 in the tragic sinking of the USS *Tang* (SS-306) by one of its own torpedoes.

A repeat performance of Wheeler Lipes's surgery was not long in coming. On Christmas Eve 1942, during the fifth patrol of the USS

2. See oral history titled "Pigboat Doc," page 45.

Silversides (SS-236), PhM1c Thomas A. Moore informed his skipper, Lt. Comdr. Creed Burlingame, that F3c (fireman third class) George Platter's abdominal pain was indeed a case of acute appendicitis. The situation was remarkably similar to the one Lipes had faced.

A kid named George Platter came to me about three or four in the morning and told me he had a pain in his belly. We had a lot of that around the ship. So I gave him some paregoric and told him to go on back to bed and he'd be all right. I found out years later this was not the best thing to do.

He returned about seven or eight o'clock and again said he had pain in his belly. I told him that I thought he had appendicitis but I wouldn't bet on it, and the paregoric would probably take care of the bellyache. So I gave him another teaspoonful and he went back to his bunk.

About an hour later he sent someone to take me back to his bunk. By then he was tied up like a hairspring. It was getting a little serious. I told the captain that we had a case of appendicitis aboard, and he said we'd just radio for a PBY to come out and take him back to a hospital in Brisbane. We were only four days out of Australia. I then packed Platter's belly with ice. I didn't want to do any damage before he got off the submarine.

After a while, I went to Commander Burlingame and laid it on the line. I was on the code board to send a message to Australia to get that PBY out to us. It was almost midnight and I wondered why the skipper hadn't sent the message. Burlingame told me he had decided not to open our transmitters because we had spent the previous day right off the Rabaul lighthouse, a place he said was as well armed as Pearl Harbor. He also told me he had picked up enemy planes through the periscope all day long, and therefore we were not opening our transmitter that night.

"Well, captain," I said, "you know what's going to happen, don't you? This guy is probably going to rupture his appendix, get infected, and die if you don't get that plane out here."

Of course, I was still holding out for the PBY. I really wanted to get rid of the patient, because he was in dire pain by that time. Our executive officer, Lt. Comdr. Roy Davenport, who was a Christian Scientist, spent part of the day with Platter, as did the captain, who visited him several times. I'm sure he was very concerned.

Davenport was with him about 11:30 when Platter said, "I hate to be disrespectful, but would you get the hell out and get that doc back here?"

After talking with Platter for a few minutes, I went back up to the captain's cabin and told him again I thought the guy needed to go someplace to get some surgery. "In that case," he said, "If worse comes to worst, do you think you can operate?"

I thought about it for about two minutes and said, "I probably can, but I don't know what the outcome would be."

He said, "Doc, if you got to do it, you got to do it. I'll do anything I can. You can have any men you want to help you. The whole ship is at your disposal." He said he would take us down to a hundred feet so there would be no sway or movement. In about five minutes he'd propped me up to where I was convinced I could do that operation. He was a con artist from the word go and an excellent leader of men. There were people on the boat who would have cut their arm off for that old boy.

I then began organizing my team. I got a radioman named [Richard] Stegall who had been around the hospital quite a bit so he knew more than the rest of them, and a guy named Danko. We decided the executive officer could sit at the head of the table.

We used the wardroom for the OR [operating room]. I probably did that because of what Lipes said about his. I didn't have the complete story, just hearsay, and didn't know how much was gossip and how much was true. I'd even heard Lipes had used spoons for retractors. There were no retractors in my medical kit so I had the machinist back in the machine shop make some. We got our other instruments from the galley. We didn't use torpedo alcohol for sterilizing them, we just boiled them in water.

By that time I had enough of a tray draped so we could put out the sterile instruments we had. I had one tube of Novocain and a spinal needle. I'd never paid much attention to general anesthetic because we always had a trained anesthesiologist do that. But I had had a chance to see spinals being administered, because I'd either held the patient or handed the doctor the instruments he used to do it. I'd seen a lot of them and had had plenty of time to observe technique.

We turned Platter over on his side and got a trickling of spinal fluid through the needle until it was good and clear. I had 150 milligrams of Novocain already premeasured in a vial, figuring that would last about an hour and a half, enough time to finish the operation. I let the spinal fluid drip into the vial until it was full, then put the contents back into the syringe and injected it into the spinal cord. It was real simple. Then we turned him over, painted his abdomen with Merthiolate, removed that with alcohol, draped him with towels, and were ready to go.

I had two assistants gloved up and we went in and found the appendix fairly quickly. But this one was actually adhered to the caecum. I have photographs of the appendix. [Lt. Robert] Worthington opened a cubbyhole between the officers' mess and the [operating] table and took five photographs of the operation.[3]

As I worked, I heard someone say, "Is this operation over yet?" It was Platter waking up. And then he began moaning and jumping up and down on the table. I knew we then had to resort to ether. I told Lieutenant Commander Davenport, who was up at the head of the table, to get a can of ether from the sick bay and a tea strainer and gauze. He put a piece of gauze over the tea strainer and I told him how to drip the ether into it. He was pretty excited and got a little bit too liberal with the ether. It got all over the patient and nearly anesthetized all of us.

In the meantime Platter was still raising Cain on the table. I left my place and went to the head of the table and started the ether dripping until we got him under. Then I showed Davenport how to maintain just enough to keep him under till we could get through. I then returned to my position, regloved, and resumed the operation.

I put a tie around the base of the appendix, walled it off with gauze real good, and then cut it off. We then cauterized the stump with phenol and put a little alcohol on it. I then thought I was free on board. "All I've got to do is sew up a few places here."

Up to this point the operation had taken probably thirty minutes, maybe less time than that. But I thought I should be like all the surgeons and check for bleeding down below. I took one of the sponge holders, put a sponge on the end of it, and sponged down in the abdomen. It came out with blood. It was a hell of a mess. There was something down there that was bleeding. I pulled the gut out through the incision and started examining it for a bleeder, wheeling it about twelve inches at a time. I couldn't find anything down there leaking. I must have rolled that gut around for about two and a half hours. I sweated blood until I finally just gave up. After examining every square inch of the intestine, I still couldn't find the darned bleeder.

I finally told myself that I might just as well finish. I closed the peri-

---

3. Robert Worthington, the *Silversides*'s diving officer, recalls that he used a Kodak Medalist 20 camera without a flash, its aperture wide open at f-3.5. His shutter speed was one-fifth of a second. "And our film speed in those days was [ASA] 25, you know. I stuck my head into the forward entrance of the wardroom and just leaned against the bulkhead and took my pictures."

toneum and then closed the fascial area. When we took the skin towels off to get to the subcutaneous layer I found the bleeder and figured out what had happened. A bleeder that had been tied earlier had gotten loose. It was in the subcutaneous tissue, was bleeding, and oozing down behind the skin towels into the wound. So as soon as I found that I was free on board.

We then transferred Platter to a bunk in the forward torpedo room and I gave him a shot of morphine. He lay there for about ten minutes when the Japs started working us over with depth charges. So he spent his first post-surgical night with about three or four hours of depth charging. In fact, he got knocked clear out of his bunk at one point. But Platter was a pretty rough guy. I have to give him credit. He had a lot more nerve than I did.

No big deal was made of the appendectomy when I did it. The big deal came later when we returned to Pearl Harbor. By then Platter had been back to duty for a good thirty-six days, because he had returned to duty about four or five days after he had been operated on. In other words, he had been well for a long time.

After we had tied up, all the admirals and captains came aboard to hear about our mission. We were all up on deck, standing at attention. The old medical officer in charge of the clinic at the submarine base stepped forward and asked me if I'd had any medical problems out at sea. I said, "A guy had a filling drop out of his tooth and I filled that with a little eugenol and zinc oxide. As far as I know he's still got it. We also had a guy that fell down a hatch and cut his arm in the fleshy part just below his elbow. It took twenty-six stitches to close it up."

Then old Captain [Lynn N.] Hart said, "What did you do about the appendicitis?" He wanted to go below and look at the patient. I told him he was topside, standing right over there. He called Platter over and asked him how he was. Platter said, "Fine. The only way I could feel better is if I were twins."

When the doctor asked Platter to show his incision, Platter grabbed his midriff and said, "You know, Captain, I'm charging everybody on this boat five dollars to see my incision and it's going to cost you the same."

After he'd looked at him, he said to me, "Moore, I want to see you, your executive officer, and your patient and his health record in my office at your earliest convenience." I knew I was in trouble then, and I was right.

Burlingame stood up for me and the rest of the crew, but I got a severe chewing out the next day anyway, after which I went to the navy yard, where they had sent Platter's appendix for analysis. Oh yes. I was smart enough to have pickled that appendix and taken it to the lab. On the way into the lab, a lab technician, a chief, was coming out as an officer, a surgeon, was going up the steps. The surgeon said, "I just came over here to see what kind of appendix that damned fool took out at sea. The chief looked at him and said, "Well, to tell you the truth, it was a hell of a lot hotter than most of the ones you've been taking out." I breathed a sigh of relief and it got my chin up off my shoelaces for a bit.

I was then called to Nimitz's office at ComSubPac [Commander Submarines, Pacific]. The first thing Nimitz did was to congratulate me on taking the appendix out. "That was a gutsy thing to do. I just wanted to congratulate you," he said. "Now, we are going to publicize this and I'll tell you why. Our submarines have done nothing but hold the entire Jap fleet at bay ever since we've been out here. We're a silent service and we haven't been able to say a thing. This is one thing we can talk about. It's a human-interest story and we're going to publicize it any way we can." When I got over to Commander Surface Pacific, they had forty-six war correspondents there ready to talk to me.

In the meantime I had made chief and decided to check out the chief's mess. As I sat down with my newspaper, an old chief looked up and said, "Look at this. A damned fool pharmacist's mate took out an appendix at sea. I'm sure glad that son of a gun wasn't working on me."

News of these appendectomies caused an uproar in the Navy medical community. The Medical Corps, including the highest echelons at the Bureau of Medicine and Surgery, strongly disapproved of appendectomies performed by anyone but certified physicians. In fact, a very angry Navy surgeon general, Rear Adm. Ross McIntire, demanded that such appendectomies cease. In 1943 a ComSubPac directive distributed to all subordinate commands explicitly stated that such procedures should end. The Medical Department then issued a guide for nonsurgical care of submariners with appendicitis until a definitive treatment could be performed ashore.

Although submarine appendectomies were now illegal, appendicitis continued to appear. Throughout the war, pharmacists' mates diagnosed 127 cases on 116 submarine war patrols. In eleven instances appendicitis required the ship to leave its area of operation.

SIX

With the Surface Fleet

World War II saw the largest naval expansion in U.S. history. By October 1945 the fleet numbered over seven thousand vessels, from landing craft and auxiliaries to the *Essex*-class carriers and *Iowa*-class battleships.[1] The hundreds of vessels smaller than destroyers had their corpsmen, to be sure, but the larger vessels rated physicians, corpsmen, dentists, fully equipped sick bays, battle dressing stations, and usually an operating room. The standard medical complement for a 7,250-ton escort carrier was one medical officer, a flight surgeon for the embarked air group, a dentist, and about thirteen corpsmen. A much larger 27,100-ton *Essex*-class carrier like the USS *Franklin* (CV-13) boasted four physicians augmented by a flight surgeon, three dentists, and thirty-one corpsmen.

During routine operations, physicians and corpsmen serving aboard vessels in the South Pacific encountered and treated heat- and humidity-related maladies exacerbated by confinement without air-conditioning—heat exhaustion and stroke, fungus infections, heat rash, and breathing disorders.

1. *U.S. Navy Ship Force Levels, 1917–1989.* Unpublished typescript (revised), 8 December 1989. Ship's History Branch, Naval Historical Center, Washington, D.C.

During battle, modern naval warfare posed a host of problems for the medical staffs of these vessels. Armor-piercing shells, aerial bombs, torpedoes, and fuel-laden suicide planes inflicted mass casualties in seconds. Such injuries as penetrating body wounds, blast injuries, burns, inhalation of toxic gases, and asphyxiation were commonplace. Rendering first aid amidst the chaos of battle meant evacuating casualties to safe areas of the ship, arresting bleeding, and treating shock. Doing their best during the worst of the Okinawa campaign, medical personnel often could do no more than offer words of encouragement as they found themselves on the receiving end of the worst a determined and fanatical enemy could dish out.

SERVICE ABOARD THE MIGHTY MONTY

Robert A. Conard was in his junior year at medical school when he realized that the United States was likely to go to war. He took the exams for the Navy Medical Corps, passed them, and, when he graduated from the Medical College of South Carolina in 1941, was commissioned a lieutenant junior grade and ordered to Washington for medical internship at the Washington Naval Hospital.

After Pearl Harbor, "we knew we were in for it," he says, "and all of us young medical officers at the hospital knew that when we finished our internship, we were going to have to go to war. Realizing that, we made the most of the time remaining, with parties and good times and a last fling." Dr. Conard's experiences were very similar to those of other junior medical officers who served aboard U.S. Navy ships of the line.

They assigned me to a light cruiser, the *Montpelier* [CL-57], which was under construction at Camden, New Jersey. I found a place to live and my shipmates joined me as they reported for duty.

I was impressed with the amount of shipbuilding going on at Camden Naval Shipyard. It was not under the Navy but a civilian yard, the New York Shipbuilding Company. You couldn't help but notice the tremendous amount of activity, with workmen on the sides of our new ship, the flare of acetylene torches, the smell of hot metal, and the clanging noises of construction.

We were assigned a place near our ship in one of the large warehouse buildings, and that's where we first congregated as a crew. I was soon joined by the senior medical officer, then a dentist. We carried out inoculations and checked over the men.

First we established the medical facilities (sick bay, pharmacy, dental office, operating room, and battle dressing stations). The sick bay, as I recall, had about twenty bunks. We also had two battle dressing stations, one forward and one aft, and these had to be outfitted throughout the ship. Everything was going on at a rapid pace, because there was a dire need for warships, particularly in the Pacific.

It was not until September that she was finally completed and we were able to board the ship. Then she was towed over to the Philadelphia Navy Yard, where we carried out the commissioning ceremony, which was quite an impressive event for us. We were all in dress whites and everybody was lined up on the deck. The ship was commissioned on 9 September 1942.

We were busy then in getting the ship ready for war, and everything had to be done posthaste; it was quite an active period. A lot of the crewmen were green and had never been to sea, but everybody worked together beautifully, and we were able to get the ship in pretty good shape in record time.

In December we sailed down the Delaware River into the Atlantic in a big snowstorm. When we got there it was very rough, and the submarine danger was extreme at that time. Going down the coast, we were in convoy with several other ships heading south.

I remember being on deck. Most of the crew was seasick because we hit a terrible storm off Cape Hatteras. I was fortunate in that I was just a little squeamish and was able to be out on deck. The captain turned to me and said, "Would you help keep a lookout for submarines?"

I said, "Well, I'll try." But I didn't know how to look out for submarines and, in those huge waves, I don't think I would have seen one anyway.

As the ship got further south into the Caribbean, it became beautiful, with calm blue water and soft breezes. It was a welcome relief from the cold wintry weather we'd just left in Philadelphia. We got to the Panama Canal, and that was an exciting experience, going through the canal and the locks. Then we headed into the Pacific and zigzagged our way southwest.

On our way to the South Pacific a tragic accident occurred. We had two SO3C-1 Seagull Scout Observation seaplanes on the fantail on two catapults, and they were testing how much weight the plane could carry. Unfortunately too much weight was added, and when it was catapulted off and tried to rise, it couldn't. The plane had depth charges on the wings and when it sank they exploded.

I was on the rescue squad, and we went out in our whaleboat. The other man on the plane, the radioman, was fine, but the pilot's chest was crushed. I tried to give him artificial respiration but my hands just went through into his chest and I knew it was hopeless; he was gone. The crew lined the deck when we brought the body aboard. It was a very sad time for us, because we had to get all his personal effects together and notify his family. It was our first burial at sea. We were on the fantail, the bugle played taps, and we were singing the Navy Hymn as the body slid into the water.

Following that incident, we crossed the equator and had a crossing-the-line ceremony in which the traditional hazing went on. I was a pollywog—I had never been across—and was a little bit apprehensive about what was going to happen. Some of us were blindfolded, and we went through a line where they gave us a few licks. Then they made us do some funny things before the Court of King Neptune. Everybody had a good time.

We were first based at Espíritu Santo in the New Hebrides, and from then on we got more and more heavily involved in the war, later being based at Purvis Bay near Guadalcanal. On a typical day aboard ship, we got up at dawn and went to battle stations, where we stayed for a couple of hours, and then we came back, had breakfast, and then held sick call. From then on we took care of any medical cases that needed attention.

Since I was a junior officer, I had several other duties assigned to me. The most onerous was coding and decoding classified messages. This four-hour watch, usually at night, was very tiring and tedious. Another assignment was the censoring of the crew's mail. I was also in charge of the rescue squad, and on a number of occasions we had to leave the ship on specific missions.

My battle station was in the after battle dressing station, between the

6-inch gun turrets in the after part of the ship. It was a very noisy place when the guns went off, and the air would fill with dust and smoke. It was a nerve-racking place to have to sit for long periods at general quarters. We had basic first-aid equipment in there and naturally couldn't expect to do too much in the way of treatment. We assumed that we would take our patients to the main medical facility as soon as the battle was over. Of course, I had Adrenalin, morphine, and so on to inject. We had first-aid material, but we weren't equipped to take care of any very serious casualties in my battle dressing station.

The incessant heat and humidity certainly kept us busy. Taking care of heat rash was very difficult and mainly unsuccessful because the men were always subjected to heat and sweating, and there was not much you could do to help with the situation. We also had a lot of fungus infections. We could take better take care of those with sulfa drugs and antifungal ointments. We had none of the antibiotics presently used. The heat rash in some cases got to be pretty bad, with men developing blistering over the body.

We also had a special rule. Before any possible engagement, we would announce over the loudspeaker system that everybody take a "navy shower" and get into clean clothes to prevent any possibility of infection if wounded. Due to the limited supply of water on the ship, the navy shower consisted of a brief wetting, soaping, and rinsing.

During combat we were below deck, and most of the time didn't know what was going on. Sometimes the situation was announced over the speaking system. I remember one time it was announced, "There's a torpedo heading for the ship." Fortunately it turned out to be a dud, but it was nerve-racking, to say the least. We were very fortunate that our ship was never torpedoed. We were hit with other shells but never torpedoed. However, on one occasion our ship swerved in time to miss a torpedo which unfortunately slammed into our sister ship, the *Denver* [CL-58], which was badly damaged with many casualties.

Our first action was just south of Guadalcanal. Our four cruisers and a number of destroyers were heading for the Rennell Islands, supporting the landings there. I was on the bow of the ship, enjoying the beautiful sunset, with the mountains of Guadalcanal in the distance, when all of a sudden one of the cruisers started firing into the night. I thought, "Well, this is a hell of a time to start practice firing." But then before I could think again, Jap planes started diving and general quarters sounded.

The planes came in and started strafing the deck. Naturally, I was very scared and went frantically aft to get down to my battle station. I found a door I could get into and went down the ladder. A sailor ahead of me fell at my feet. I told him, "This is the real thing. Get to your battle station." I thought he had just slipped and fallen, and then I looked and saw the blood spurting from his chest. Fortunately we were very near the dressing station and we dragged him back in there. There wasn't much I could do, because he had just about bled to death at that point. I tried injecting some Adrenalin into his heart as a last measure, but he died anyway.

The Japanese torpedo planes were diving, trying to hit the ship, and we were turning and twisting to avoid being hit. Our dressing station was in the chiefs' mess quarters. I said, "Let's get under the table," which we did, and it was a very trying experience, with this poor shipmate lying there in a pool of blood and the ship bouncing around.

The attack must have lasted about an hour or so. The next morning I went topside and the *Chicago* [CA-29] was listing in the water.[2] It had been torpedoed, and I think there were about sixty men lost. Then our ships were ordered back. We had no refrigeration for preserving the dead, so we put the sailor in a paint locker. Unfortunately, before we could get back to Espíritu Santo the body began to smell a little bit, and I noted the chow lines were not as long. It was sad. His brother was on the ship.

The sailor was buried ashore; the captain must have felt it was close enough to our base to get back within reasonable time, so we didn't have to bury him at sea. He was the only casualty on our ship during that action.

From this time on, our ship was heavily involved in the war. Our mission, under Admiral Halsey, was mainly to intercept the Tokyo Express, the Japanese ships coming down to reinforce Guadalcanal and later New Georgia and Bougainville. We also participated in a lot of shore bombardment. During that activity, I was in my battle dressing station. The only times I was able to get out was when the firing ceased and we were able to observe what was going on ashore. When we were at our stations below decks, it was pretty difficult in the uproar to distinguish one gun from another.

2. During the attack, two Japanese torpedo bombers scored two hits on the *Chicago,* causing severe flooding and loss of power. The following afternoon while under tow, the disabled vessel drew four more torpedoes, which sank her.

While all this was going on, you resigned yourself to the fact that this is where you've got to be, and you kept your fingers crossed that the ship didn't get hit and that you would come out of it all right. While below, somebody from the galley would sometimes come by and bring us sandwiches and coffee. But many times we went without regular meals.

The heat was a real problem, and, of course, we had no air-conditioning as we know it today. There was a ventilation system on the ship, but that was turned off during battle, so you just had to sweat it out. The dust and smoke that filled the compartment would cause your nose to run and your sweaty skin to itch. It was pretty miserable if you were there for long periods of time. We had to treat a number of cases of heat rash and sometimes heat exhaustion.

How long we would be down there varied a lot with the operation. For instance, at Empress Augusta Bay in November of '43, the battle was preceded by bombardment of the Shortland Islands and other islands near Bougainville the day before. We were at our battle stations a long time for those bombardments, practically all night. Then we got word the next day that the Japanese fleet was coming down, and we had to turn around and head north to try to intercept them. That night the Battle of Empress Augusta Bay took place. It was a long battle—about four or five hours.

It was one of the outstanding battles the *Montpelier* was involved in, with all the cruisers acting in concert. The training that Adm. Tip [Rear Adm. Stanton] Merrill had done really paid off in that battle, because the cruisers would turn together in concerted movements that baffled the Japanese. There were smoke screens and flares lighting the night. This is what made it such an interesting battle. After several hours we got the better of it, and the Japanese fled after we sank a number of their ships.

The next morning as we headed south we had an air attack with about a hundred Japanese planes attacking. A shell from a plane hit the fantail on the catapult, which was only about twenty feet from where I was below deck. Our ships downed a large number of Japanese planes in this attack. One man was injured when some metal pierced his head and lodged in his brain. We had to get him off the ship to a hospital because we couldn't take care of him; it was too complicated.

In about thirty-six hours there, we went through one hell of a lot of battle and manning of battle stations. During that time we were pretty much at our battle dressing station, not coming out except for a break after the big night battle.

The next morning I was able to come on deck to a scene I'll never forget. The deck was littered with shell cases. Everybody was exuberant because of the victory, and we slapped each other on the shoulders in camaraderie. Despite the fact that we were worn out, unshaven, sweaty, and dirty, it was such a wonderful feeling to know that you had won. The comradeship you feel with your fellow sailors at such a time is something you can't appreciate until you've experienced it.

When we headed back down to our base at Purvis Bay in the southern part of the Solomons near Guadalcanal, everybody was just worn out from being involved in such a lengthy combat. As we pulled into the bay, there was a message to the admiral asking, "Is there anything that you need?"

He answered with one word, "Sleep."

One night we headed up the slot to the Kula Gulf area in New Georgia. Our radar had improved considerably by this time, and the Japanese radar was inferior to ours. We surprised them, sinking two of their ships before they even knew we were there. That was great news to us.

Admiral Halsey visited the ship a number of times. He was a character. You could never forget him, because he certainly deserved the name Bull. He was a short, stocky man and swaggered across the deck. Whenever he spoke about the Japanese, it was in very strong terms and he inspired everybody in hatred of the enemy. We gave him his annual physical examination on the ship. We removed a wart from his hand.

In the Marianas campaign, the taking of Saipan was the longest and most difficult. At times I got topside to see the action. It was exciting because we could see the progress of the troops. They had orange markers that were moved forward as the troops progressed. Also we could hear the radio contact between our ship and our scouting plane, which was directing our fire. We could hear the conversations—You need to go so many yards this way or that—and then our ship would fire and there would be an explosion where we hit. When I think of Saipan, I remember the continuous noise of the guns, the flares at night, the ack-ack of antiaircraft fire, the ammunition dump explosions, and the smoldering towns.

And then the terrible time when the terrified civilians were herded to the northern point of the island and told by the Japs that they were going to be tortured if captured. So many of them jumped off the cliff, later named the Suicide Cliff. I remember the horrible sight of bodies floating around the ship—men, women, and children—for several days. It was pretty sad to see the women and particularly the children. But we couldn't do anything about it.

THE FIRST KAMIKAZES

Lt. Walter B. Burwell joined the Navy after the attack on Pearl Harbor. In July 1942 he was assigned to the USS *Suwannee* (CVE-27), then under construction in Newport News, Virginia. CVEs—escort carriers—were converted merchant ships or oilers. Smaller, slower, and cheaper to produce than fleet carriers, they solved the problem of providing continuous airborne support for convoys and amphibious operations. As part of the Philippines invasion at Leyte in October 1944, the *Suwannee* had the unfortunate distinction of being the second Navy ship hit by a Japanese suicide plane. The following is Dr. Burwell's account of that action and its aftermath.

The *Suwannee*'s sick bay had one standard hospital bed and four tiers of three bunks. We also had an operating room and, adjacent to that, a pharmacy and a sick-call area, and a dental office. For the ship's company, we had a senior medical officer; I was the junior medical officer. Each squadron usually brought a surgeon with them. We also had about twelve corpsmen and a chief pharmacist's mate. There was a dentist aboard as part of our ship's company medical division. Of course, he would help out with first aid, health and sanitation inspections, and things like that. But he was kept pretty busy with his dental duties, because in those days the general public had pretty poor dental hygiene. A lot of these boys coming aboard had probably never seen or heard of a dentist before.

We arrived at Nouméa, New Caledonia, in January 1943, and amazed the South Pacific veterans by steaming into the harbor with officers and crew at quarters in whites. We spent the next seven months or so based at Efate Island. From time to time we'd sortie out and run up the Slot to Guadalcanal to support various operations.

We made a quick trip back to San Diego in September 1943 for resupplying, refurbishing, things of that kind. But we made it back in time for the assault on Tarawa. We took part in the shore bombardment for that operation, and then, in succession, supporting landings at Apemama, Kwajalein, Eniwetok, Aitape, Hollandia, Saipan, Tinian, Guam, and Moratai.

On 12 October 1944, we left Seadler Harbor to participate in the Philippines invasion, supporting the landings at Leyte. Our fleet was divided into three groups—Taffy 1, 2, and 3—off the east coast of the Philippines. Our group, Taffy 1, was the southernmost and was to support the landings on Leyte. The Army seemed to have no great trouble with the initial landings on 29 October, and we were able to successfully repulse Japanese aerial attacks on our group.

But, of course, the Japanese navy came down to try to knock us out of our positions. By October 18th we received reports from our search planes that the southern Japanese fleet had put out from Singapore and was heading for the Philippines. By 22 October our submarines had spotted the Japanese center force heading for San Bernardino Strait. The southern force was destroyed at Surigao Strait during the night of 24 October. At the same time, Adm. Takeo Kurita's force came through the San Bernardino Straits to the north expecting to catch us in a pincer maneuver. Even those of us doing mundane jobs were aware that something was going on from all the radio activity and reports.

On 25 October we went to general quarters at dawn. After being released, I had breakfast and went back to my stateroom to take a shower. Our captain announced on the PA system that the whole Japanese fleet was attacking Taffy 3 to the north of us. I looked out on the forecastle and sure enough, it looked like there were a hundred ships on the horizon.

At that point general quarters sounded, and I had to go below to my battle dressing station in the forward part of the ship. It was one deck below the main deck, two or three below the flight deck. We were just about at the waterline.

There was nothing unique about the battle dressing station; it contained twenty-five to thirty bunks, and medical supplies stored in lockers, and was just below and aft of the catapult engine room. There was an open deck one deck above, so you could look out on either side. This was ordinarily used as a barber shop and had a couple of barber chairs there. Many times during general quarters I would sit in one of those chairs, because it was the most comfortable thing I could find.

Shortly thereafter our sister ship, the *Santee* [CVE-29], was hit by the first kamikaze. Nineteen minutes later, another kamikaze managed to get through all the antiaircraft fire and crash into our flight deck about amidships. It penetrated to the main deck. This attack did not do nearly as much damage as the second attack the next day.

On the morning of the 26th, we had maybe twenty-five wounded in the forward battle dressing station from the action of the day before. Things were pretty much under control and we were not even at general quarters. My stateroom was only two decks above our battle dressing station, and I told my corpsman that I was going up there to get a change of clothes and maybe lie down a minute. If he needed me he knew where I was.

For some reason, exhaustion just got the better of me before I even got up there and I crawled into a bunk in an adjoining sleeping compartment just forward of our battle dressing station and fell asleep. I was asleep when the second attack occurred. The thing that woke me was the sound of our antiaircraft guns going off. When I heard the guns, I jumped up and started for the dressing station. Just as I got to the doorway, there was a terrific explosion and we lost our lights. I went into the dressing station and was helping our corpsmen pull some of the wounded out from under wreckage when there was a second explosion. That one shattered all the bulkheads and broke water mains.

After the first explosion my corpsman lit out for my stateroom to get me, thinking that's where I was. But when he got there, he found my stateroom had been demolished and thought I was gone. I will never forget how, after we got working again, he looked up and saw me and said, "My God, you can't be here." Indeed, he thought I was dead. "I'm so glad I'm not here by myself," he continued.

The second explosion forced us to evacuate the battle dressing station. After the first explosion, there was smoke and fire fed by aviation gasoline pouring onto the deck above us. The wreckage in the passageway and ladder to the deck above, caused by bomb and ammunition explosions, prevented entrance or exit to or from our dressing station.

Up to that point we could have remained where we were, at least temporarily. However, the second explosion further wrecked our compartment, buckled our bulkheads, and ruptured water mains above and in our compartment, so that we began to flood. As the water level rose to knee height, the ship was listing uncomfortably and lying dead in the water without steerage because of destruction of the bridge and wheelhouse.

Isolated from the rest of the ship with only the reflection from the gasoline fires above and a few flickering battle lamps for light, I saw my wounded partially covered with wreckage and already awash and knew we had to evacuate. I think there were about thirty of us, including two corpsmen, two stretcher bearers, and perhaps twenty-five wounded resulting from the action of the day before, mostly consisting of extensive burns, blast and fragmentation injuries, traumatic amputations, compound fractures, and multiple severe lacerations. About half the wounded were able to drag themselves about, but the remainder required stretchers.

Though I did not know the extent of damage to the compartments aft of us, I knew they were unoccupied and sealed off during battle conditions. I informed my corpsmen that I would try to find an escape by this route, as it seemed to offer our only hope of evacuation. We opened the hatch to the adjacent compartment, and I was able to get through it and lock it behind me without flooding from our compartment.

Feeling my way with the help of a pocket flashlight, I found the compartment to be intact and dry, though without light or ventilation. Then I worked my way aft through several adjacent unoccupied compartments in the same way, until at last I reached an open space on the main deck. Now, feeling certain that we could make our way out by this route, I returned to my group in the forward battle dressing station.

There, with my corpsmen and stretcher bearers, and with the valiant help of some of the mobile wounded, we moved our stretcher-bound wounded through the hatches from one compartment to the next without leaving or losing a single member of our party. We finally emerged on the open deck and, from there we entered the chief petty officers' mess, where we found two corpsmen tending to about twenty more wounded. So we joined forces to organize an amidships dressing station and began to gather additional wounded in that area.

On the deck above we found about fifteen or twenty wounded, mostly burns and blast injuries, who had made their way into bunks in the chief petty officers' quarters. There was no immediate possibility of moving them to our already overflowing and understaffed amidships station.

One of my corpsmen and I gathered what medical supplies we could carry and made our way up to the chiefs' quarters to treat the wounded there. Just as we arrived at the entrance to the compartment, a sailor, apparently in panic, came running along the passageway screaming, "Everybody's going over the side! The captain's dead! Everyone on the bridge has been killed! Everybody's abandoning ship!"

Now, havoc—contagious panic and cold fear! The wounded who had crawled into the compartment began struggling to get out, screaming hysterically, "Where's my life jacket? Who took my life jacket? Turn that loose! Gimme that! No, it's mine!" Some were shoving toward the entrance, fighting and scrambling over one another. My heart sank as I stepped into the threshold to block the entrance and shout over and over, "Get back into your bunks! There's no order to abandon ship! You don't need your life jackets!"

I could see this was only having limited effect; so, with much inward trepidation but outwardly extravagant bravado, I made myself step into the compartment from the threshold, remove my own life jacket and helmet and hang them in clear view on a coat hook near the entrance. Then I had to force myself to move away from the entrance and the comfort and security of my life jacket and go into the compartment to tend the wounded, fearing that at any moment some panicky sailor might snatch my life jacket and belt, setting off a wild melee. It seemed that time hung in the balance for an eternity, but finally one after another of the men quieted down and crawled back into their bunks, so that gradually things began at last to calm down and sort themselves out.

In the meantime, one of our corpsmen tending the wounded on the flight deck saw the plight of those isolated by fire on the forecastle. He came below to report that medical help was critically needed there. It seemed to me that we would have to try to get through to them. He and I restocked our first-aid bags with morphine Syrettes, tourniquets, sulfa, vaseline, and bandages, commandeered a fire extinguisher, and made our way forward, dodging flames along the main deck.

We were joined by a sailor manning a seawater fire hose with fairly good pressure, and though the seawater would only scatter the gasoline fires away from us, by using the water and foam alternatively as we advanced, we managed to work our way up several decks, through passageways along the wrecked and burning combat information center and decoding area, through officers' country, and finally out on the forecastle.

Many of the men there and the catwalks above had been blown over the side by the explosions. But others trapped below and aft of the forecastle found themselves under a curtain of fire from aviation gasoline pouring down from burning planes on the flight deck above. Their only escape was to leap aflame into the sea, but some were trapped and were incinerated before they could leap.

By the time we arrived on the forecastle, the flow of gasoline had mostly consumed itself, and flames were only erupting and flickering from combustible areas of water and oil. Nonetheless, the decks and bulkheads were still blistering hot and ammunition in the small-arms locker on the deck below was popping from the heat like strings of firecrackers. With each salvo of popping, two or three more panicky crewmen would leap over the side, and we found that our most urgent task was to persuade those poised on the rail not to jump. We used a combination of physical restraint and reassurance that fires were being controlled and that more help was on the way.

Most of the remaining wounded in the forecastle area were severely burned beyond recognition and hope. All we could do for the obviously dying was to give the most rudimentary first aid, consisting of morphine, a few swallows of water, and some words of companionship, leaving them where we found them and moving on to others.

Nonetheless, within an hour or so after being struck in the last attack, power and steerage had been restored, fires were out, ammunition and gasoline explosions had ceased, pumps were working, and ruptured water mains had been shut off. But it was miraculous that we escaped destruction during this period, because we were vulnerable to further air or submarine attack.

By this time we had done what we could for the wounded on the forecastle and I moved back to the amidships dressing station. From there my corpsmen and stretcher bearers were searching out and gathering wounded.

By nightfall we began to run short of medical supplies, and I realized we needed to salvage the supplies left behind in the forward battle dressing station. I was able to recruit a small group of stretcher bearers to help me, and we successfully made our way back there. We found the compartment was still flooded with knee-deep water, but most of our supplies were salvageable in wreckage above this level. We were able to load up our stretchers with plasma, dressings, sulfa, vaseline, and morphine, and haul them out. After two or three trips we had all our supplies safely out and distributed elsewhere.

For the ensuing three days, we still had our hands full, continuing to search for, find, and care for our many wounded scattered throughout the ship, and burying the dead at sea. Then we proceeded to Kossol Roads, Palaus, where we transferred our most seriously wounded to two hospital ships, the *Mercy* and the *Bountiful*. From there we went to Seadler Harbor, Manus Islands, to further lick our wounds for five days. We cared for our less seriously wounded and made temporary repairs so we would be seaworthy enough to proceed to Hawaii.

We arrived at Pearl Harbor on 19 November. As we limped up the channel to the naval base, every Navy ship at anchor or in dock there manned the rail in a salute to the *Suwannee*, and our radio received this message: "Welcome to Pearl! Your successful fight against great odds will live as one of the most striking tales of naval history. The people of our country and those of us in the naval service are gratified and proud of your outstanding performance of duty against the best the enemy could offer. As long as our country has men with your heart, courage, skill, and strength, she need not fear for her future. To each and every one, a well done. Adm. Nimitz."

We stayed in Pearl Harbor only overnight, just long enough to transfer our remaining wounded to the naval hospital and to take on supplies, and then headed for major repairs at the Puget Sound Navy Yard in Bremerton, Washington, where we docked on November 26, 1944. The repairs took about a month. I walked through the ship once more and realized I must have led a charmed life. The bunk I had been lying in at the time of the first explosion had been destroyed by the second explosion. It was absolutely unbelievable.

I departed with great pride in my ship and shipmates and their accomplishments, for I had witnessed innumerable instances of cool courage, bold bravery, and unselfish heroism blended with faith, friendship, and self-sacrifice. But I had gained no fondness for naval warfare, and was thankful to go on to other endeavors.

For his heroic work on the *Suwannee* Dr. Burwell received the Silver Star.

✚

FLIGHT SURGEON ON THE SPOT

In March 1945, as the Pacific war drew closer to the Japanese home islands, the aircraft carrier USS *Franklin* (CV-13) was conducting bombing raids on Japan as part of Task Force 58. Early on the morning of 19 March, as the ship was steaming just fifty miles off the coast, an enemy bomber slipped through the combat-air-patrol screen and dropped two semi–armor piercing bombs on the ship. Both exploded among a number of armed and fueled aircraft. The resulting explosions and fires claimed the lives of over eight hundred Navy and Marine personnel and nearly sank the vessel.

Lt. Comdr. Samuel R. Sherman, MC, USNR, was the flight surgeon aboard the carrier and the only physician on the flight deck after the attack.

I went to Pensacola in April 1943 for my flight-surgeon training and finished in August. I was then sent back to the West Coast in late 1943 to wait for Air Group 5 at Alameda Naval Air Station, California.

Air Group 5 soon arrived, but it took about a year or so of training to get up to snuff. Most of the people were veterans from other carriers that had gone down. Three squadrons formed the nucleus of this air group—a fighter, a bomber, and a torpedo bomber squadron. Later we were given two Marine squadrons, the remnants of Pappy Boyington's group.[3]

Since the Marine pilots had been land based, the toughest part of the training was to get them carrier certified. We used the old *Ranger* [CV-4] for take-off and landing training. We took the *Ranger* up and down the coast, from San Francisco to San Diego, and tried like hell to get these Marines to learn how to make a landing. They had no problem

---

3. Maj. Gregory Boyington, USMC, shot down twenty-eight Japanese aircraft in a four-month period. That achievement and superb leadership of his squadron won him the Congressional Medal of Honor.

taking off, but they had problems with landings. Luckily we were close enough to airports so that if they couldn't get on the ship they'd have a place to land and wouldn't have to go in the drink.

Anyhow, we eventually got them all certified. Some of our other pilots trained at Fallon Air Station in Nevada and other West Coast bases. By the time the *Franklin* came in, we had a very well-trained group of people.

I had two Marine squadrons and three Navy squadrons to take care of. The Marines claimed I was a Marine. The Navy guys claimed I was a Navy man. I used to wear two uniforms. When I would go to the Marine ready rooms, I'd put on a Marine uniform and then I'd quickly change into my Navy uniform and go to the other ready room. We had a lot of fun with that.

As their physician, I was their general practitioner but also their father, mother, spiritual guide, social director, psychiatrist—the whole thing. Of course I was well trained in surgery, so I could take care of various surgical problems. Every once in a while I had to do an appendectomy. I also removed some pilonidal cysts, fixed a few strangulated hernias, and, of course, some occasional fractures incurred during training exercises. I took care of everything for them and they considered me their personal physician, every one of them. They called me Dr. Sam.

Eventually the *Franklin* arrived, in early 1945. It had been in Bremerton being repaired, after being damaged by a kamikaze off Leyte in October 1944. In mid-February of '45 we left the West Coast and went to Pearl first and then to Ulithi. By the first week in March, the fleet was ready to sail. It took us about five or six days to reach the coast of Japan, where we began launching aerial attacks on air bases, ports, and other targets.

Just before dawn on 19 March, thirty-eight bombers took off escorted by about nine of our fighters. The *Franklin*'s crew was getting ready for another strike, so more planes were on the flight deck. All of a sudden, out of nowhere, a Japanese plane slipped through the fighter screen and popped up just in front of the ship. My battle station was right in the middle of the flight deck because, as the flight surgeon, I was supposed to take care of anything that might happen during flight operations. I saw the plane coming in, but there was nothing I could do but stay there and take it. The plane just flew right in and dropped two bombs on our flight deck.

I was blown about fifteen feet into the air and tossed against the steel bulkhead of the island. I got up groggily and saw an enormous fire. All those planes lined up to take off were fully armed and fueled. The dive-bombers were equipped with these new Tiny Tim heavy rockets, and they immediately began to explode. Some of the rockets' motors ignited and took off across the flight deck on their own. A lot of us were just ducking those things.

It was pandemonium and chaos for hours and hours. We had 126 separate explosions. Each explosion seemed to pick the ship up, rock it, and then turn it around a little bit.

Of course, we suffered horrendous casualties from the first moment. I lost my glasses and my shoes. I was wearing a kind of moccasin shoes because I didn't have time that morning to put on my flight-deck shoes. Those moccasins just flew right off immediately. Regardless, there were hundreds and hundreds of crewmen who needed my attention.

Fortunately I was well prepared, from a medical-equipment standpoint. From the time we left San Francisco and then stopped at Pearl, Ulithi and so forth, I had done what we call disaster planning. Because I had worked in emergency hospital service and trauma centers, I knew what was needed. Therefore I had a number of big metal containers, approximately the size of garbage cans, bolted down on the flight and hangar decks. These were full of everything I needed—splints, burn dressings, sterile dressings of all sorts, sterile surgical instruments, medications, plasma, and intravenous solutions other than plasma.

The most important supplies were those used for the treatment of burns, fractures, lacerations, and bleeding. In those days the Navy had a special burn dressing which was very effective. It was a gauze impregnated with vaseline and some chemicals that were almost like local anesthetics. In addition to treating burns, I also had to deal with numerous casualties suffering from severe bleeding; I even performed some amputations.

Furthermore, I had a specially equipped coat with all the little pouches similar to those used by duck hunters, and a couple of extra-sized money belts in which I carried my morphine Syrettes and other small medical items. Due to careful planning, I had no problem whatsoever with supplies.

I immediately looked around to see if I had any corpsmen left. Most of them were already wounded, dead, or had been blown overboard.

Some, I learned later, got panicky and jumped overboard. Therefore I couldn't find any corpsmen, but fortunately I found some members of the musical band, who I had trained in first aid. I had also given first-aid training to my air-group pilots and some of the crew.

The first guy I latched onto was Lt. Comdr. MacGregor Kilpatrick, skipper of the fighter squadron. He was an Annapolis graduate, a veteran of the *Lexington* [CV-2] and the *Yorktown* [CV-5], and had three Navy Crosses. He stayed with me, helping take care of the wounded.

I couldn't find any doctors. There were three ship's doctors assigned to the *Franklin,* Comdr. Francis [Kurt] Smith, Lt. Comdr. James Fuelling, and Lt. Comdr. George Fox. I found out later that Fox was killed in the sick bay by the fires and suffocating smoke. Smith and Fuelling were trapped below in the warrant officers' wardroom. That's where Lt. Donald Gary got his Medal of Honor for finding an escape route for them and three hundred men trapped below. Meanwhile, I had very little medical help.

Finally a couple of corpsmen who were down below in the hangar deck came up, once they recovered from their concussions and shock. I had hundreds and hundreds of patients, obviously more than I could possibly treat. Therefore, the most important thing for me to do was triage—separating the seriously wounded from the not-so-seriously wounded. We'd arranged for evacuation of the serious ones to the cruiser *Santa Fe* [CL-60], which had a very well-equipped sick bay and was standing by alongside.

Lieutenant Commander Kilpatrick was instrumental in the evacuations. He helped me organize all of this, and we got people to carry the really badly wounded. Some of them had their hips and arms blown off and other sorts of tremendous damage. All together, I think we evacuated some eight hundred people to the *Santa Fe.*

Then orders came that all air-group personnel had to go over to the *Santa Fe,* because they were considered nonexpendable and had to live to fight again in their airplanes. Kilpatrick and I began supervising the evacuation between fighting fires, taking care of the wounded, and so forth. Kilpatrick, being an Annapolis graduate, knew he had to obey the order, but I managed to stay.

After the air group evacuated, I looked at the fires, felt the explosions, and thought, Well, I had better say good-bye to my family right now because this ship is never going to survive. We were just fifty miles off the coast of Japan, about fifteen minutes' flying time, and dead in the water. The cruiser *Pittsburgh* [CA-72] was trying to get a tow line to us, but it was a difficult job and took hours to accomplish.

Meanwhile, our engineering officers were trying to get the boilers lit off in the engine room. The smoke was so bad that we had to get the *Santa Fe* to give us a whole batch of gas masks. But since the masks didn't cover the engineers' eyes, their eyes became so inflamed from the smoke they couldn't see to do their work. The XO [executive officer] asked me if I knew whether we had any anesthetic eye drops to put in their eyes so they could tolerate the smoke. I told him we had a whole stash of them down in the sick bay; I used them when I had to take foreign bodies out of the eyes of my pilots and crew members.

He asked if I could go down (about four or five decks below), get the drops, and bring them to the engineering officer. I replied, "Sure, give me a flashlight and a guide, because I may not be able to find my way, even though I used to go down three or four times a day."

I made it down there and got a whole batch of eyedropper bottles. After the men put the drops in their eyes, they could tolerate the smoke immediately and were able to get the boilers going.

It was almost twelve or thirteen hours before the doctors trapped below were rescued. By that time I had the majority of the wounded taken care of. However, injured people were still trapped in various parts of the ship, like the hangar deck, and hadn't been discovered. We spent the next seven days trying to find them all.

Taking care of the dead was terrible. They were all over the ship. The ship's medical officers put the burial functions on my shoulders. I had to declare the men dead, take off their identification, and, with the chaplain's help, remove from them whatever possessions hadn't been destroyed. We then slid them overboard, because we had no way of keeping them. A lot of them were my own air-group people—pilots and aircrew—and I recognized them even though the bodies were busted up and charred. I think we buried about 832 people in the next seven days. It was really terrible to bury that many people.

It took us six days to reach Ulithi. Actually, by the time we got there we were making fourteen knots and had cast off the tow line from the *Pittsburgh*. We had five destroyers assigned to us that kept circling all the time, from the time we left the coast of Japan until we got to Ulithi, because we were under constant attack by Japanese bombers. We also had support from two of the new battlecruisers.

At Ulithi I got word that a lot of my people in the air group, who were taken off or picked up in the water, were on a hospital ship that was also in Ulithi. I visited them and they told me that many of the men killed from the air group had been in their ready rooms waiting to take off when the bombs exploded. The Marine squadrons were particularly hard hit, having few survivors. I have a list of dead Marines which makes your heart sink.

When the survivors of the air group reassembled on Guam, they requested that I be sent back to them. I also wanted to go and pleaded my case with the chaplain, the XO, and the skipper. Although the skipper felt I had earned the right to be part of the ship's company, he was willing to send me where I wanted to go. Luckily, I rejoined my air group just in time to keep the poor derelicts from getting assigned to another carrier. The air-group commander volunteered these boys for another carrier. But most of them were veterans of the *Yorktown* and *Lexington* disasters and had seen quite a lot of action. A fair number had been blown into the water and many were suffering from the shock of the devastating ordeal.

The skipper of the bombing squadron did not think his men were psychologically or physically qualified to go back into combat at that particular time. A hearing was held to determine their combat availability, and they needed a flight surgeon to check them over. After I assembled the pilots and checked them out, I agreed with the bombing-squadron skipper. These men were just not ready to fight yet. Some of them looked like death warmed over.

Admiral Nimitz conducted the hearing. He remembered me because I'd pulled him out of the wreckage of his plane when it had crashed during a landing approach at Alameda in 1942. He simply said, "Unless I hear a medical opinion contrary to Commander Sherman's, I have to agree with Commander Sherman." He decided the air group should be sent back to the States and rehabilitated as much as possible.

In late April 1945 the air group went to Pearl, where we briefly reunited with the *Franklin*. They had to make repairs to the ship so it could make the journey to the Brooklyn Navy Yard. After a short stay, we continued on to Alameda.

The Navy then decided to break up the air group, so everyone was sent their individual way. I was given what I wanted—senior medical officer of a carrier, the *Rendova* [CVE-114], which was still outfitting in Portland, Oregon. But the war ended shortly after we had completed outfitting. I stayed in the Navy until about Christmas and was mustered out in San Francisco, at the same place I'd been commissioned.

Dr. Sherman received a Navy Cross in recognition of his bravery on the *Franklin*. He died in 1994.

SURVIVOR OF THE INDIANAPOLIS

In July 1945 the war in the Pacific neared its climax. The costly battle for Okinawa was over, and planners were fine-tuning strategy for the invasion of the Japanese home islands. In the New Mexico desert near Alamogordo, physicists of the Manhattan Project achieved their goal, detonating a nuclear weapon perched atop a one-hundred-foot-high steel tower. Its use might now make the invasion of Japan unnecessary.

Meanwhile, the USS *Indianapolis* (CA-35) had just undergone extensive repairs at the Mare Island Naval Shipyard in California following a devastating kamikaze attack near Okinawa on 31 March, an incident that cost the heavy cruiser nine dead. The former Fifth Fleet flagship now received a highly classified assignment—to carry to Tinian the essential components for Little Boy, the Hiroshima atomic bomb.

Having delivered its deadly cargo, the *Indianapolis* would be the last U.S. warship to be sunk in World War II. Traveling alone on 29 July, she was torpedoed by a Japanese submarine. Although some 800 members of her 1,199 man crew got into the water, four and a half days passed before rescuers arrived. Only 316 were pulled from the ocean. The pathetic story of the *Indianapolis* and her crew has been told and retold many times, yet the horror of the tragedy that cost the lives of 880 men is no less appalling a half century later. For the precious few fished alive from the shark-infested Philippine Sea, memories are still vivid. So are the enduring nightmares.

Capt. Lewis L. Haynes, MC, USN (Ret.), the *Indianapolis*'s senior medical officer, tells how it was.

After our repairs were completed [following the kamikaze attack], we were supposed to go on our post repair trial run. But instead, on July 15th, we were ordered to San Francisco to take on some cargo. I was amazed to notice that there was a quiet, almost dead navy yard. We tied up at the dock there, and two big trucks came alongside. The big crate on one truck was put in the port hangar.

The other truck had a bunch of men aboard, including two Army officers, Captain [James F.] Nolan and Major [Robert R.] Furman. I found out later that Nolan was a medical officer. I don't know what his job was; probably to monitor radiation. The two men carried a canister about three feet tall and about two feet square, up to Admiral Spruance's cabin, where they welded it to the deck. Later on I found out that this was the nuclear ingredients for the bomb, and the large box in the hangar contained the device for firing the bomb. And I had that thing welded to the deck above my cabin for ten days!

We stayed tied up to the pier until after we got this cargo on board. Then we pulled away from the pier and anchored out off Hunter's Point. This was July 16th. What we were really waiting for, I found out later, was for them to explode the bomb at Alamogordo to see if it worked. And after the bomb was exploded, at four o'clock in the morning, we got dispatch orders to proceed. As we got under way on July 16th, Captain [Charles] McVay told his staff we were on a special mission.

"I can't tell you what the mission is. I don't know myself, but I've been told that every day we take off the trip is a day off the war." Captain McVay told us his orders were that if we had an abandon ship, what was in the admiral's cabin was to be placed in a boat before anybody else. We had all kinds of guesses as to what the cargo was.

After refueling at an eerily quiet Pearl Harbor, we made a straight run to Tinian at as much speed as they could economically go, about twenty-five or twenty-six knots. Everybody was at Condition Able, which was four hours on, four hours off. It was like going into battle the whole way out. The trip from San Francisco to Tinian took a total of ten days.

When we unloaded our special cargo at Tinian, I noticed a couple of general Air Force officers handling these crates like they were a bunch of stevedores. I was even more sure we had something important.

We were then ordered to the Philippines for training exercises preparing for the invasion of Kyushu. Captain McVay asked for an escort but was told we didn't need one, as it was supposedly safe to go to the Philippines. What he wasn't told was that there were Japanese submarines along that way and that Naval Intelligence knew it.

On July 29th I was pretty tired because I had given the whole crew cholera shots all day. I remember walking through the warrant officers' quarters and declining to join a poker game, as I was so tired. I then went to bed.

I awoke. I saw a bright light before I felt the concussion of the explosion that threw me up in the air almost to the overhead. A torpedo had detonated under my room. I hit the edge of the bunk, hit the deck, and stood up. Then the second explosion knocked me down again. As I landed on the deck I thought, I've got to get the hell out of here!

I grabbed my life jacket and started to go out the door. My room was already on fire. I emerged to see my neighbor Ken Stout. He said, "Let's go," and stepped ahead of me into the main passageway. I was very close to him when he yelled, "Look out!" and threw his hands up. I lifted the life jacket in front of my face and stepped back. As I did, a wall of fire went *whoosh!* It burned my hair off, burned my face, and the back of my hands. That's the last I saw of Ken.

I started out trying to go to the forward ladder to go up on the forecastle deck. There was a lot of fire coming up through the deck right in front of the dentist's room. That's when I realized I couldn't go forward and turned to go aft. As I did I slipped and fell, landing on my hands. I got third-degree burns on my hands—my palms and all the tips of my fingers. I still have the scars. I was barefoot and the soles of my feet were burned off.

Then I turned aft to go back through the wardroom. I would have to go through the wardroom and down a long passageway to the quarterdeck, but there was a terrible hazy smoke with a peculiar odor. I couldn't breathe and got lost in the wardroom. I kept bumping into furniture and finally fell into this big easy chair. I felt so comfortable. I knew I was dying but I really didn't care.

Then someone standing over me said, "My God, I'm fainting!" and he fell on me. Evidently that gave me a shot of adrenaline and I forced my way up and out. Somebody was yelling, "Open a porthole!" I can remember someone else yelling "Don't light a match!" All the power was out and it was just a red haze.

The ship was beginning to list, and I moved to that side of the ship. I found a porthole already open. Two other guys had gone out through it. I stuck my head out the porthole, gulping in some air, and found they had left a rope dangling. I looked down to see water rushing into the ship beneath me. I thought about going out the porthole into the ocean but knew I couldn't go in there.

Instead I grabbed the rope which was attached to an overhanging floater net. I pulled myself through the porthole and up to the deck above. I then went to my battle station, which was the port hangar. My chief, [CPhM John A.] Shmueck, and a lot of casualties were back there. I think the moon was going in and out because at times I could see quite clearly, other times not. We were trying to put dressings and give morphine to badly burned men when an officer came up and said, "Doctor, you'd better get life jackets on your patients."

So Shmueck and I went up a ladder to the deck above, where there were some life jackets. We got a whole bunch and went back down and started to put them on the patients. I remember helping a warrant officer. His skin was hanging in shreds and he was yelling "Don't touch me, don't touch me." I kept telling him we had to get the jacket on. I was putting the jacket on when the ship tipped right over. He just slid away from me. The patients and the plane on the catapult all went down in a big, tangling crash to the other side. I grabbed the lifeline and climbed through to avoid falling. And by the time I did, the ship was on its side. Those men probably all died as the plane came down on top of them. All the rescue gear and everything we had out went down, patients and everything together.

I slowly walked down the side of the ship. Another kid came and said he didn't have a jacket. I had an extra jacket and he put it on. We both jumped into the water, which was covered with fuel oil. We weren't alone in the water. The hull was covered with people climbing down.

I didn't want to get sucked down with the ship, so I kicked my feet to get away. And then the ship rose up high. I thought it was going to come down and crush me. The ship kept leaning out away from me, the aft end rising up and leaning over as it stood up on its nose. The ship was still going forward at probably three or four knots. When it finally sank, it was over a hundred yards from me. Most of the survivors were strung out anywhere from a half mile to a mile behind the ship.

Suddenly the ship was gone and it was very quiet. It had only been twelve minutes since the torpedoes had hit. We started to gather together. Being in the water wasn't an unpleasant experience except that the black fuel oil got in your nose and eyes. We all had black oil all over—white eyes and red mouths. Soon everyone had swallowed fuel oil and gotten sick. Then everyone began vomiting.

At that time I could have hidden, but somebody yelled, "Is the doctor there?" And I made myself known. From that point on—and that's probably why I'm here today—I was kept so busy I had to keep going. But without any equipment, from that point on I became a coroner.

A lot of the men were without life jackets, and a lot of them were injured. The kapok life jacket is designed with two large armholes. You could put your arm through one of those armholes and pull an injured shipmate up on your hip and keep him out of the water. And the men were very good about doing this. Furthermore, those with jackets supported men without them. The fellow without one put his arms through the spacious armholes and held on, floating in tandem.

When daylight came, we began to get ourselves organized into a group and the leaders began to come out. When first light came we had between three and four hundred men in our group. I would guess that probably seven or eight hundred men made it out of the ship. I began to find the wounded and the dead. The only way I could tell they were dead was to put my finger in their eye. If their pupils were dilated and they didn't blink I assumed they were dead.

We would then laboriously take off their life jackets and give them to men who didn't have jackets. In the beginning I took off their dog tags, said the Lord's Prayer, and let them go. Eventually I got such an armful of dog tags I couldn't hold them any longer. Even today, when I try to say the Lord's Prayer or hear it, I simply lose it.

Later, when the sun came up, the covering of oil was a help. It kept us from burning. But [the sun] also reflected off the fuel oil and was like a searchlight in your eyes that you couldn't get away from. So I had all the men tie strips of their clothing around their eyes to keep the sun out.

The second night, which was Monday night, we had all the men put their arms through the life jacket of the man in front of him and we made a big mass so we could stay together. We kept the wounded and those who were sickest in the center of the pack, and that was my territory. Some of the men could doze off and sleep for a few minutes. The next day we found a life ring. I could put one very sick man across it to support him. There was nothing I could do but give advice, bury the dead, save the life jackets, and try to keep the men from drinking the saltwater when we drifted out of the fuel oil. When the hot sun came out and we were in this crystal-clear water, you were so thirsty you couldn't believe it wasn't good enough to drink. I had a hard time convincing the men that they shouldn't drink. The real young ones—you take away their hope, you take away their water and food, they would drink saltwater and then would go fast. I can remember striking men who were drinking water to try and stop them. They would get diarrhea, then get more dehydrated, then become very maniacal.

In the beginning, we tried to hold them and support them while they were thrashing around. And then we discovered we were losing a good man to care for one who had been bad and drank. As terrible as it may sound, towards the end when they did this, we shoved them away from the pack because we had to.

The water in that part of the Pacific was warm and good for swimming. But body temperature is over ninety-eight, and when you immerse someone up to their chin in that water for a couple of days, you're going to chill him down. So at night we would tie everyone close together to try to stay warm. But they still had severe chills which led to fever and delirium. On Tuesday night some guy began yelling, "There's a Jap here and he's trying to kill me."

And then everybody started to fight. They were totally out of their minds. A lot of men were killed that night. A lot of men drowned. Overnight everybody untied themselves and got scattered in all directions. But you couldn't blame the men. It was mass hysteria. You became wary of everyone. Till daylight came, you weren't sure. When we got back together the next day, there were a hell of a lot fewer.

There were mass hallucinations. It was amazing how everyone would see the same thing. One would see something, then someone else would see it. One day everyone got in a long line. I said, "What are you doing?" Someone answered, "Doctor, there's an island up here just ahead of us. One of us can go ashore at a time and you can get fifteen minutes' sleep." They all saw the island. You couldn't convince them otherwise. Even I fought hallucinations off and on, but something always brought me back.

I only saw one shark. I remember reaching out trying to grab a hold of him. I thought maybe it would be food. However, when night came, things would bump against you in the dark or brush against your leg and you would wonder what it was. But honestly, in the entire 110 hours I was in the water I did not see a man attacked by a shark. However, the destroyers that picked up the bodies afterward found a large number—in the report I read, fifty-six bodies were mutilated. Maybe the sharks were satisfied with the dead; they didn't have to bite the living.

It was Thursday [2 August] when the plane spotted us. By then we were in very bad shape. The kapok life jacket is good for about forty-eight hours before it becomes waterlogged. We sank lower down and you had to think about keeping your face out of water. I knew we didn't have very long to go. The men were semi-comatose. We were all on the verge of dying when suddenly this plane flew over. I'm here today because someone on that plane had a sore neck. He went to fix the aerial and got a stiff neck and lay down in the blister underneath. While he was rubbing his neck he saw us.

The plane dropped life jackets with canisters of water, but the canisters ruptured. Then a PBY showed up and dropped rubber life rafts. We put the sickest people aboard and the others hung around the side. I found a flask of water with a one-ounce cup. I doled out the water, passing the cup down hand to hand. Not one man cheated and I know how thirsty they were.

Towards the end of the day, just before dark, I found a kit for making freshwater out of saltwater. I tried to read the instructions but couldn't make sense of it or get it to work right. My product tasted like saltwater and I didn't want to take a chance, so I threw it into the ocean. I then went to pieces.

I watched the PBY circle and suddenly make an open-sea landing. This took an awful lot of guts. It hit, went back in the air, and splashed down again. I thought he'd crashed but he came taxiing back. I found out later he was taxiing around picking up the singles. If he hadn't done this, I don't think we would have survived. He stayed on the water during the night and turned his searchlight up into the sky so the *Cecil J. Doyle* [DE-368] could find us. The ship came right over and began picking us up.

The *Cecil J. Doyle* had a big net down over the side. Some of the sailors came down the side of the netting and pulled our rafts up alongside. They put a rope around me; we were too weak to climb up. I remember bouncing off the side of the ship as they hauled me up. When they tried to grab hold of me I remember saying, "I can get up!" But I couldn't. Two sailors dragged me down the passageway. By the wardroom pantry, someone gave me a glass of water with a mark on it and would only give me so much water. I drank it and when I asked for more, he said that was all I could have this time. Then the skipper asked me what ship I was from. I told him we were what was left of the *Indianapolis*. The next thing I knew, I was sitting in a shower. I remember corpsmen or seamen cleaning off my wounds, trying to wash the oil from me and dress my burns. I remember trying to lick the water coming down from the shower. They put me in a bunk and I passed out for about twelve hours. I recall the first bowel movement I had after I was picked up. I passed pure fuel oil. The other fellows found the same thing.

The *Cecil J. Doyle* took us to Peleliu, where we were taken ashore and put into hospital bunks. They came in and got our vital statistics—we had discarded our dog tags because they were heavy. They changed our dressings. Some of the men got IVs, though I didn't. While there I began to eat a little and get some strength back.

After two or three days at Peleliu, someone came in and said I was going to Guam. The next thing I knew, they hauled me out on a stretcher and onto a hospital ship. The commanding officer of the ship, a friend of mine, was Bart [Bartholomew, surgeon general of the Navy from 1955 to 1959] Hogan. Bart came in and said, "I know you don't feel well but you're going to have to go before the inspector general. I'm going to send a corpsman in and I want you to start at the beginning and dictate everything you can remember about what happened, because as time goes on you're going to forget and things are going to change."

So I sat down and dictated off and on for three days on the way to Guam. When I'd get tired I'd fall asleep, and then I'd wake up and the corpsman would come back. When we landed, Bart gave me a copy of what I'd dictated and I took it when I went to the inspector general's office. I told my story, answered their questions, and gave them this report unedited, saying, "Here it is. This is probably as accurate as I can be."

Normally I don't have the nightmares. Last night I didn't sleep well. And I won't sleep well tonight. But eventually my mind will turn off and I'll be all right. It's like when I try to say the Lord's Prayer. I cry, or I sit down and try to talk to somebody about it. As long as I stay away from talking about individuals—my friends . . . I was on that ship over a year and a half and we were all close friends, and we'd been through a lot together, and I knew their wives and their families. As a doctor you get more intimate than normal.

SEVEN

Mercy Ships

The story of Navy medicine concentrates on the details of treating people. Yet we sometimes overlook how the patient reached medical care. Medical facilities in the Pacific theater were especially hard pressed to keep up with the leapfrog island assault on Tokyo. Mobile and base hospitals proved very effective in providing definitive care to many of the casualties, but the concentrated and very intense combat that described such island campaigns as Tarawa, Saipan, Guam, Peleliu, Iwo Jima, and Okinawa required another option—hospital ships.

The concept of floating hospitals was nothing new to the Navy, the *Red Rover* having served during the Civil War. The USS *Solace* (AH-2) saw duty during the Spanish-American War and, in World War I, it shared assignments with the *Comfort* (AH-3) and *Mercy* (AH-4). Although capable of providing medical and some surgical support, these vessels served mainly as ambulance ships, ferrying patients to shore-based hospitals.

When the United States entered World War II, there were but two hospital ships in the Navy's inventory, the second USS *Solace* (AH-5) and the USS *Relief* (AH-1). When launched at the Philadelphia Navy Yard in 1920, the *Relief* represented a colossal leap in hospital ship design, fully capable of performing state-of-the-art medical care. In fact, it was the only American vessel ever designed as a hospital ship from the keel up, and that distinction remains valid today.

During the 1920s and 1930s, the *Relief* either served in Atlantic ports as a naval-base hospital or plied Caribbean or Atlantic waters following the fleet. In peacetime, one hospital ship would suffice for the entire Navy. After Pearl Harbor, everything changed.

The requirement for hospital ships depended upon the theater of operations. In Europe the Army was the predominant service, and circumstances did not require hospital ships. For example, during the Normandy invasion of June 1944, evacuating casualties the short distance back across the English Channel via LSTs and transports was a simple affair. Once the Allies had established a beachhead in France, field hospitals and air evacuation to hospitals in Britain became routine.

The Pacific theater was a different story. Evacuating casualties from remote islands to mobile or base hospitals in already reconquered islands meant covering vast expanses of water. Until air evacuation became routine late in the war, only a fleet of hospital ships could transport large numbers of critically injured men and take care of their medical needs on the way.

In the early days of the Pacific war, that mercy fleet was just a dream. To augment the strategic plan for reconquering the Pacific, a crash program began for bringing more of these special vessels on line. The federal government appropriated civilian merchant ships for conversion to hospital ships, some while still in the yards. Other, older Navy vessels, some dating back to World War I and with many miles on them, took on a new look as yard workers gutted and modified, welded, and riveted, installing the accoutrements of a floating hospital—operating rooms, wards, double-decker patient bunks, ramps, X-ray machines, and refrigerated morgues.

Until the new hospital ships began arriving in the Pacific in the latter half of 1944, only the *Solace* and *Relief* were available. Fleet tactical doctrine dictated that the two white hulls stand well offshore out of harm's way, serving as casualty-receiving centers and ambulances ferrying casualties to far-flung mobile and base hospitals. Specially designated LSTs transported casualties from the beach. Once troops and vehicles were off-loaded, these surgically augmented LSTs, designated LST(H), staffed with four surgeons and twenty-seven corpsmen, could provide rudimentary care to about 350 casualties, albeit under primitive and unsanitary conditions.

By the beginning of 1945, the role of the hospital ships was evolving. At Iwo Jima their primary mission was not to evacuate casualties but to treat them in the combat zone. And by then, six additional mercy ships had arrived in the Pacific to help share the load. Nevertheless, huge numbers of casualties generated by the vicious fighting at Iwo Jima and Okinawa filled these vessels to capacity, again forcing them into an ambulance role ferrying patients back to hospitals far from the fighting.

Operating these vessels was often complicated by restrictions imposed by the Geneva Accords and natural hazards as well. Mixed Army-Navy and male-female crews added another unique perspective. The following accounts capture the essence of life aboard hospital ships.

✚

FOREST FIRES, LIGHTNING, AND THE MOON

Bound by strict international laws, the daily routine of a white-hulled mercy ship was seldom uncomplicated. Open to boarding by any nation, they were not equipped with the still highly guarded radar to help guide their way through treacherous and often poorly charted Pacific waters. At night, skippers like Comdr. Harold F. Fultz, USN, of USS *Comfort* (AH-6), had to rely on expedient and often ancient modes of navigation, aided by illumination from forest fires, lightning, and the moon.

It's a good guess that fifty forest fires are gnawing their way right now through the coastal hardwood forests of New Guinea and the Philippines. It's a safe bet, too, that almost every night vivid heat lightning is flashing there with uncommon frequency, while of course the moon performs on schedule.

No war affected these illuminators. They were nature's footlights on the close-to-shore stages of the drama of conflict. Their light was varying, yet occasionally substantial, and revealed navigational dangers to many a ship just in the nick of time. Perhaps no type of vessel benefited more from these natural lighthouses than a hospital ship. Steaming almost continuously and alone, often with hundreds of helpless patients on board, following tracks that were off the beaten paths, and blinded by her own glaring illumination, she needed every possible clue to check her position.

This is the story of the USS *Comfort*. The Navy commissioned her at San Pedro, California, 5 May 1944. On 21 June 1944, she sailed out of Los Angeles for Brisbane, Australia, brand new and rarin' to go. She was a unique setup, our first hospital ship to be Navy-manned and Army-staffed. The Navy crew was responsible for the ship, while the Army provided the hospital personnel. The complement was 300 Navy and 220 Army, which included twenty-eight Army nurses; 600 patients could be cared for.

It was a voyage of magnificent distances and a lonely one, too. Being illuminated, we could not mix with blacked-out convoys and so had to keep just over the horizon from them. For eighteen days we saw nothing but sky and sea. Many had never been so far offshore before. It may have been imagination, but somehow I detected an uneasiness, a kind of murmuring such as must have occurred on Columbus's first voyage. It drifted up to my cabin about like this: "Nearly three weeks and no ship or land. Do you suppose those ninety-day wonders up there on the bridge know how to use those fancy instruments, and do they understand those big navigation books?"

To allay any such apprehensions, I announced in the ship's paper that barring bad weather, Cape Moreton, Australia, would rise from the sea dead ahead at 0900 the following Wednesday. Thus the Navy had committed itself, and it was a source of considerable relief when old Moreton put in an appearance about 0915 on the day promised, even though not quite dead ahead. All was well. The seamen had won the confidence of the landsmen.

In Brisbane, a hospital unit from Pittsburgh had been scanning the horizon for us for a long time and was ready, bag in hand. By *bag* I mean about one thousand tons of hospital-unit impedimenta. If the congested loading of all this caused them any inconvenience, the attitude of complete surrender that accompanies seasickness took over as we plunged into heavy weather. The long wait in Brisbane had made our new passengers' sea legs a bit shaky.

Full and down though we were, the loading had not been haphazard. Who and what a hospital ship carries is all regulated by international law. Outside her regular Navy complement, only persons of medical status may embark. Thus if you are not a medico of some sort, the only way you may ride is to break a bone, or meet some other misfortune. As for cargo, only regular medical supplies and equipment and regular ship's supplies may be carried. Under no circumstances may ambulances, vehicles of any kind, or mail be transported.

Laws governing services rendered are also very clear. Once a cruiser engineer needed some two-inch pipe desperately. Another time a destroyer skipper had an emergency machine-shop job. Both of these officers were old friends of mine but all I could give them were cups of our excellent coffee. The slightest assistance of this kind to a combatant ship would have made us liable to destruction. And you may rest assured that a full account of the indiscretion would have been on Tokyo Rose's next broadcast.

The names of military hospital ships must be communicated to all belligerents, who must respect these ships and not capture them. The ships and their boats must be painted white with a horizontal band of green and must fly the Geneva flag. At night, funnels, sides, and upper decks must show illuminated red crosses; a vessel darkens at her own risk. The sick, wounded, or shipwrecked of all belligerents, regardless of nationality, must be cared for. Any belligerent may visit them, refuse to help them, and order them to steer a certain course. An extreme emergency might warrant their detaining them. A hospital ship is forbidden any maneuver or stratagem to deceive the enemy. Being liable to boarding by the enemy, we could carry nothing of a confidential or secret nature. We had to be an open book. Thus we were deprived of radar, which would have greatly reduced our navigational worries.

The comparative immunity from rough treatment promised by international law was all very well, but a hospital ship must take care not to be lulled into a false sense of security. Mines, fires, and collisions, for example, are no respecters of such ships. Drills for abandoning ship were especially important. Fuel-oil tanks were filled with saltwater as soon as they became empty. This precaution ensured no list in case a tank was holed and so improved the chances of launching boats.

But to return to our seasick progress out of Brisbane. We had other things to think about besides rough weather and complicated laws. Our destination was Hollandia in New Guinea, and that meant passing through China Strait, Raven Channel, and the Tufi Leads. One glance at the chart and any navigator can see why these names are notorious. They are the passages in the great coral fields off the southeast corner of New Guinea, the "slots" through which a ship must squeeze to reach the northeast coast of that island.

There was a great deal to be studied. We saw how very important timing was going to be in far-Pacific coasting. For example, China Strait (north bound) should be made at daybreak, Raven Channel negotiated with a high sun and never at night, while the Tufi Leads were best run in complete darkness. Clearly our vital problem was to pass major hazards during daylight, and at night to select as safe waters as possible. At sunset we must never find ourselves approaching a stretch whose passage was considered dangerous after dark.

It was a break that at morning twilight on 20 July 1944, below the China Strait, there was that combination which is the dream of a navigator: stars, and a clear horizon under them. A star is no help unless a horizon goes with it, because you are measuring the angle between the two.

A sunken coral reef bars the approach to China Strait as if the place held the Golden Fleece. There's an opening, to be sure, but to find it you must either get help from the sky or spot a distant mountain peak. No peak showed on 20 July, so the clear sky was very welcome. The Strait itself is a series of dizzy turns through tropical loveliness. The big rollers of the Bismarck Sea cannot follow through the reefs, so all hands promptly forgot their seasickness.

By arriving at Raven Channel about 1000 with a good sun shining, we were fortunate again. This channel is a tight squeeze between long coral reefs, and, right in the middle, a sharp pinnacle lurks just below the surface. It's advisable to have the sun high and behind you so you can see this pinnacle. Only one ship at a time passes through, and at night ships keep away altogether.

This left the Tufi Leads. In this area of extensive scattered coral, a ship is guided through a long narrow slot by means of ranges, or leads, on the shore. In daylight these ranges are hard to make out, but at night their powerful lights are easy to follow. Throughout the war such beacons burned brightly in several spots in the far Pacific, where the danger from natural hazards exceeded that from the enemy. Our good luck held. We approached these ranges in inky darkness and picked them up twenty-five miles away. There was little trouble in "getting on," which means keeping the two lights exactly in line, one on the other. In this Tufi channel you finally pass a lighted buoy close aboard, continue exactly 6.2 miles along the range, then turn sharply to the right. It was here that we had our first help from forest fires. We passed the buoy, started on our 6.2-mile run, and had gone only 5.4 miles by clock when a forest fire dead ahead on the shore near the blacked-out town of Tufi warned plainly that we must turn at once to avoid the beach. The current had fooled us.

By midnight all the slots were passed. Good weather and a forest fire had helped us through the worst stretch I'd ever negotiated in my thirty years at sea. Little did I suppose that we would go through these slots so often that they would come to be called our milk run.

At dawn came Mitre Rock. Off this queer little sentinel, the sailing directions told of a flag buoy marking a rock. No such buoy was seen, and we tiptoed by. If a ship hits a rock in these parts, it is named after her, a distinction I preferred to waive. Big, safe Hollandia quickly absorbed our Pittsburgh medical unit, and a fine base hospital sprang up there. Then our shuttling began in earnest. For nearly three months we steamed back and forth between the ports encompassed by Biak, Hollandia, and Brisbane, carrying patients, doctors, nurses, hospital units, and medical supplies. Our milk runs involved ten ports in all. In daylight, usually, a cordial reception awaited us, but after dark we were about as welcome as a skunk at a lawn party. Except for far-south Brisbane, no one wanted an illuminated hospital ship in their midst. I'll never forget the good-natured, yet perfectly clear orders I received from the senior officer afloat at Hollandia the first time I called on him. "Captain," he said, "I have a thousand ships here in this port. Either you will have to get out at night or I'll have to take my thousand ships out."

Always the problem was timing. Our orders gave us as much latitude as possible and insisted only on definite times of arrival. But once we started on a trip, we had to keep going. As most of our runs involved several nights, it often was a Chinese puzzle to plan so that the least hazardous waters would come during darkness. Forest fires, lightning, and the moon were all factors. A place might be a mad risk during the dark of the moon, but perfectly safe with a half moon or better. It made a great difference too where the moon was in relation to the danger. We came to know all the coastal peculiarities. Lightning was more dependable in one place than another. And the fires seemed to loom up where most needed despite the fact that, of course, they are only accidental. It was not uncommon to see several well-separated fires at once.

Current was the factor that required the closest watching. It injected the element of risk into any night run, and especially if such a run contained a turn, as at Tufi. At evening twilight we fixed our position by the stars or by the land, and then the long vigil would commence. The stars could not help again until morning twilight brought a horizon, and it was a gamble how much the other aids would show the way. The hours just before daylight were the worst, and like St. Paul on his voyage to Rome, we prayed for the day.

Occasionally we ran plumb into a convoy at night, but as we were lighted and the ships in a convoy were dark, the solution was simple. We closed our eyes and kept on going in an absolutely straight line. Two men connecting a ship's [fire] hose follow about the same tactics: one man holds and looks away while the other man connects.

Little by little we worked the base hospitals up close to the Philippines. The whole world knew these islands were the next goal. Suddenly our milk runs ended. Fueling to capacity and loading to the gunwales with medical supplies, we hurried to Leyte, arriving on 29 October 1944, on the heels of the invasion.

To reach Leyte you stand in from the Pacific and pass between Homonhon and Dinagat Islands through a passage about six miles wide, then steam another sixty across a big, open bay. Despite the liberal width of this opening, it was the policy at this time to have ships leave Leyte by 1500 to ensure reaching the open sea by dark.

We arrived at Leyte at 1100, went immediately to a prearranged anchorage, and started taking on patients and handing out medical supplies at a frantic rate. The place was "hot." All hands wore helmets, and bombings were frequent. We had loading pretty well systematized by this time. Patients who could do so walked aboard. Stretchers could be snatched up out of boats at six points along our sides. Sometimes a vessel larger than the *Comfort* herself moored right alongside. A patient's diagnosis determined his ward, although, of course, immediate attention was necessary for some.

A series of events now took place that culminated in perhaps the greatest adventure ever experienced by anyone on board. The bulk of our patients were to come from Red Beach, and about 1400 word was received that they would be seriously delayed. We were asked whether we would be willing to postpone sailing beyond the customary 1500 limit, and agreed to do so as the moon was nearly full. It was 1800 before we weighed anchor. As we crossed the bay a very weak moon started up the sky, and things looked ominous.

At exactly 2100 of 29 October, as we reached the opening to the Pacific, the weather suddenly went completely out of control. It wasn't a case of nature's valves being wide open. Valves, reducers, safeties, or any other device the elements use for rendering the earth habitable had disappeared. First on the port quarter and finally on the starboard bow, a mad wind tried to tear us to pieces. Some experiences are indelibly stamped on your mind and you carry them to your grave, yet you cannot describe them. A 120-MPH typhoon is one of these experiences.

What a ship! Well designed and honestly fashioned, not a thing of importance failed, nor did material fatigue show in any vital spot. And what personnel! All hands, especially the twenty-eight nurses, carried on with such courage and such attention to the wounded that no patient ever suspected that the roaring, crashing, pitching, rolling, and wall of torrential rain were not things that the ship expected and took in her stride.

Just as no night was ever so dark as to put out the light of a candle, so no storm was ever violent enough to destroy hope. A little after 2200, the pulsating, fast-falling barometer reached bottom, stood for a bit, then rapidly rose. Confidence returned. By midnight all was well. By giving the ship all the speed she would take we had apparently held our own, and our bright illumination had undoubtedly saved us from collision. Strange to relate, the closest land during the height of the onslaught was a place with the cheery name of Desolation Point.

It's a four-day run from Leyte back to Hollandia. Everything possible was done for the patients. This early care of the wounded is very important, and the *Comfort* was often complimented on the condition in which patients were delivered to base hospitals.

There is no missing the lofty signal hill at Hollandia. We ducked in behind it and a convoy of ambulances whisked our human cargo back behind the mountains. There were more poor fellows, many more, waiting at Leyte, so we changed the hospital linen, shined the decks, and headed back. This time we were ordered to heave to 175 miles southeast of Leyte and await orders. Apparently things up front were a bit too hot for us at the moment.

On the second night of our waiting, three bombs straddled us. This was the first time the opposition had ever honored us with attention. We blacked out at once and began to zigzag at top speed. All hands got dressed and kept undercover. There's no chapter in international law that tells you what to do in such a case. Dawn was very welcome.

Promptly we told the world by radio in plain unmistakable English what had happened. Just before noon, a destroyer came tearing over the horizon to present her squadron commander's compliments and express the hope we were all right. A little later in the day, Tokyo Rose assured the world it was all a big mistake, so sorry. It's a bit disconcerting to be an unarmed, defenseless, highly illuminated target alone on a big ocean, and, incidentally, over the deepest place in the ocean. Two more nights we tarried at the spot, and each night just before sunset all hands were called aft for a general mutual reassurance that Tokyo Rose was sincere.

Plenty of stretchers were waiting at Leyte, and we bulged as we stood back for Hollandia. The Hollandia hospital was apparently bulging too, because orders came to take six hundred of their patients back to the United States.

On the morning of 28 November 1944 the *Comfort* rounded the signal hill at Hollandia bound for Los Angeles. The whole harbor knew our destination, and the ships expressed their cries of envy. It was a time for careful watch for epidemics of shot-off toes, broken ankles, and such things. Once more and for the last time, we ran the slots of Tufi Leads, Raven Channel, and China Strait, then settled back without worry and for three weeks followed the sky to California. It's a long sky from the star over the signal hill at Hollandia to the one over Point Fermin, San Pedro, and just to complicate the measurement, the stars slide over a bit each day.

[In Los Angeles] over eight thousand tons of medical supplies were on the dock labeled "Philippines." Of course, such a cargo would sink the *Comfort,* but we loaded all the old Plimsoll Mark would permit, and on 8 January 1945 sailed for Leyte with orders to lose no time.

Just before sunset fifteen days later, we stood into Eniwetok Atoll for final routing. This atoll is about the two-thirds mark and apparently all-the-way routing was not advisable because the war might end, belligerents change sides, or our cargo be needed at another destination. We hove to and sent an officer to the beach for this routing, requesting it be expedited in order that the atoll might be cleared by dark. Back came the officer with a clear message. We were to anchor in the berth off the officers' club and at 2000, boats would call to take our nurses to the club dance. Everybody understood. The atoll held a large number of aviators on their way to very hot spots. At dawn we nosed out for Leyte and made a good run of it.

We were expected at Leyte, all right. A pilot swung aboard the minute we arrived and took us to the inside dock at Tacloban, where a convoy of trucks was waiting. Everything came through in good order, even our large amount of biologicals. The Army was so kind as to tell us so in writing, and this letter was immediately broadcast to all hands.

There was still considerable patient traffic, but the high tension was gone. We could spend the night now, although with doused lights. Two loads we took down to Hollandia, then Manila was recovered and orders came which sent us into our most serious huddle. Forest fires, lightning, and the moon would have to stand by in earnest. We were to head back for Leyte, but, at the Homonhon-Dinagat opening, swing south through Surigao Strait and proceed up the unlighted west coast of the Philippines to Subic and Lingayen. Getting there would be no risk, as there would be about a half moon in the right direction for silhouetting the shore. But the return trip was another story, for if there were any delays along the route, a very meager moon would be left for us. The huddle was short, the situation clear. A definite night risk had to be accepted on the return trip, and would consist in making a sharp turn off the southwest corner of Negros Island during the second night.

The first night was over a safe stretch, and the next day we passed all the bad spots in Mindoro Strait. We were then in the Sulu Sea, and our real hurdle at the southwest tip off Japanese-held Negros Island was a little over a hundred miles ahead.

At 0200 we took a hitch in our belts and toed the ship in for the coast. Clouds shrouded what little moon there was, but fortunately lightning was not only frequent but in the direction to furnish a silhouette of the shore.

About 0200 a faint outline of the coast was made out and we stood in as close as we dared and then paralleled the shoreline. At night you see only half as far as you think you do. Then the real lookout began. The trip or tangent of Negros must be sighted definitely and positively and the *Comfort* swung close around it into the Mindanao Sea. Overrunning would be disastrous as there are reefs just below Negros, and turning too soon would ground us on an enemy-held beach.

Anxious moments passed. Two forest fires were welcome sights. Although apparently far inland, they gave assurance that the blur we were calling land was actually land and not a fog bank or cloud.

It seemed hours, but we had been on our parallel course about ten minutes when the chief quartermaster, who had two of the best eyes in the U.S. or any other Navy, sang out "Tangent, broad on the bow!" Presently our two navigators saw it, too.

The *Comfort* was swung into the Mindanao Sea. The race against a waning moon had been won.

It was all plain sailing now. Heavy weather, an unlighted convoy, or perchance a stray mine might be on our track to Hollandia, but these were things over which we had no control. Keeping a ship in deep water, however, is and always will be a professional trust, whether it be wartime or peacetime.

About this time the war moved up rapidly. Hovering at Ulithi Atoll for a while, we finally closed in and stood by at Okinawa. For a week we anchored there near the beach during daylight and ran to sea each night. Okinawa will always bring back memories of the visit General [Lt. Gen. Simon B. Jr.] Buckner paid us.[1] Five hundred patients were aboard at the time. He paused by each bunk and greeted each man as if he were his own son.

It all seems a long time ago, yet how the details stand out! We had the best of everything. No captain ever had better backing. All hands knew that with six hundred wounded and sick below, the ship must not only be kept in deep water but any incident must be avoided that would cause apprehension among those helpless men.

Our most vital instrument was the gyrocompass. It received attention that was devotion itself. Every conceivable navigational help was sought and used. But navigation is not an exact science. No two helmsmen steer alike. Deflection due to wind is not a positive thing, and who can be sure that a current will not, during a long night's run, move a ship bodily over onto some coral reef despite the fact that the book says no such current exists! Then too, on an especially important night, there may be no forest fires. Lightning may decide to be absent, and the moon may take that night to hide behind clouds.

So there's luck involved. Yet *luck* is not the word. The word is God. My cabin was right off the bridge. A few steps and I could be in privacy, a space ideal for prayer. There were many prayers. All were answered.

---

1. Lieutenant General Buckner was killed in action on Okinawa on 18 June 1945, the highest-ranking American soldier to die during the war.

Without divine guidance I am certain that the dangers of the Pacific would not have been avoided for 78,000 miles.

On 16 April 1945 Commander Fultz was relieved, due to a medical disability. Just twelve days later, while cruising about thirty miles off Okinawa, a Japanese kamikaze plunged through the *Comfort*'s superstructure, penetrating two decks. The plane struck the surgery room, then filled with patients, nurses, doctors, and crewmen. The blast killed twenty-eight persons, including six nurses, and wounded forty-eight others. All surgical and X-ray equipment were a total loss, and other parts of the vessel were severely damaged. The ship was able to continue on to Guam under her own power and arrived on 3 May, when a mass funeral was held for the victims.

When temporary repairs were completed, the ship sailed for the United States, arriving at Terminal Island, California, on 28 May. After time in the yard, the *Comfort* sailed for Subic Bay carrying five hundred nurses. Upon her arrival she took up duty as a station hospital. The ship was transferred to the Army in April 1946.

THE WOMEN OF THE <u>BOUNTIFUL</u>

Converted from the aging Navy transport *Henderson* (AP-1), the recommissioned USS *Bountiful* (AH-9) began her second career on 23 March 1944. On that date twenty-one Navy nurses reported for duty in time to see their first action at Saipan. Each had her own impressions of the *Bountiful* experience.

Lt. Ethel Himes

The Lady B, sailing majestically over the calm, deep blue Pacific Ocean, was all decked out in her latest dress of white paint, with a green stripe one foot wide encircling her, her red crosses spaced intermittently on both sides and on the smokestack. With the rise and fall of the bow, the *swish, swish* sound over the water was all that seemed to stir the stillness of the air as she drew ever nearer to the island of Saipan.

In the distance was a blue haze outline of an island that didn't look to be any larger than a small group of foothills one might see around the San Francisco Bay area. As the ship drew closer to the harbor, these hills grew ever larger, and in no time at all we could see mango, papaya, and banana trees, and some unidentified trees which resembled mahogany.

As we dropped anchor, Higgins boats, motor launches, motor whale boats, amphibious ducks, and the like, were heading in our direction. Of course, everyone was very anxious as well as tense and excited, wondering what type of casualties we would obtain. "Here they come, all doctors and nurses to their wards and departments," the senior medical officer said.

All acted accordingly, silently wishing that they might be allowed to remain a few minutes longer to watch all the excitement. There was a dogfight going on about a thousand feet in the air a short distance from where we were, a B-24 and a Japanese Zero. The Zero was shot down shortly after work began.

We loaded over 500 patients in six hours; there were only 150 ambulatory patients admitted this trip. The patients we received were the severest kind of casualties one could ever imagine. Many were in shock and hemorrhaging. Some were shot through the head and probably would be blind the rest of their lives. Some were shot through the chest, already a hemothorax had developed and possibly a pneumothorax along with it. Some had badly mangled legs that had caught mortar fire, and it was a question whether the legs could be saved or not. Some had an arm or a leg cut off, or perhaps an arm just hanging which had to be amputated immediately after admission to the ship. Some had blast injuries that had done quite a bit of internal damage. These fellows were covered from head to foot with Saipan red sand and mud. In many instances the clothing had to be cut off in order not to disturb the general condition of the patient.

On one particular ward, after all the patients were settled down—normal saline, plasma, and whole blood started intravenously, penicillin, sulfonamides, and other medications given—the nurse was making her usual check. It was then she noticed that one patient looked as though he was in great agony. Prior to his admission to the ship, he had lost his right arm to the elbow and his left leg had been badly injured and placed in a cast, so he had good reason to have pain.

We shall call him Jackson. He was clean-cut, about six feet tall. He was fairly good looking, with a few freckles sprinkled over his nose, had curly blond hair—and didn't look a day over sixteen years of age.

"Jackson, is your arm or leg paining you? If so, I could give you another hypodermic," suggested the nurse.

"My arm doesn't pain me, nor do I hurt anywhere in particular at present," he replied.

The nurse looked at him in bewilderment.

"Tomorrow is my birthday," he added, "and I usually have a birthday cake to celebrate the occasion, but I guess that's out this particular time."

"How old are you, Jackson?"

"I'm eighteen and will be nineteen tomorrow."

"You certainly don't look a day over sixteen, if you are that."

He smiled. "I even shave—at least once a week."

This got laughs all around. The nurse told him not to worry about a thing, gave him a reassuring smile, and left.

Jackson apparently couldn't see how everything would be all right. He was blue the remainder of the day, taking no notice of his surroundings, not desiring to carry on a conversation with anyone who stopped by. He ignored his chow and couldn't even be enticed to eat the ice cream he'd looked forward to through so many months of battle.

The following morning around ten o'clock, the nurse was excused from her ward. A few minutes later she returned with a fairly good-sized package wrapped in brown paper and tied with white twine, which she handed to Jackson. At first he seemed skeptical, perhaps thinking someone was playing a joke on him. All the other patients were watching him closely, not knowing what was in the package and as anxious as he to get it opened.

Jackson tried with his left hand to untie the twine, to no avail. Finally, no longer able to endure the suspense, the nurse pulled out her scissors and cut the twine. Cautiously, Jackson removed the wrapping paper and there before him was a luscious three-layer white cake with chocolate icing and sixteen birthday candles on top, with Happy Birthday spelled out in colors. The young man couldn't say a word as tears came streaming down his cheeks. Then the whole ward sang happy birthday to him, and Jackson insisted that everybody get a piece of the cake.

After that party, the youthful patient showed a renewed interest in life. Anyone who stopped by his bunk was treated to a detailed description of his birthday surprise.

Ens. Rhea A. Jungferman

After receiving the first casualties, we no longer thought of our reactions but set to work trying to do all we could to relieve the seriously wounded boys. The wounds were hideous and our hearts went out to the boys as they poured out their stories to us. One six-foot-four Marine was brought in clutching a Bible he had received from his sister. He was to have his leg amputated. Although he was seriously ill, the thought of losing his leg was unbearable; he wanted to get back and help his buddies drive out those Japanese.

We witnessed the horror of gas gangrene. Several arms and legs had to be amputated. We used refrigeration on the limbs. They were packed in ice for about six hours before the amputation. It was surprising, the difference this procedure made in the operation. The patient needed very little other anesthesia, and the field of operation was not as bloody and odoriferous. The patients responded remarkably well to plasma, blood, and glucose. In fact, so well that many were eating ice cream by the end of the trip.

This was one of their greatest joys. They were grateful to be able to have a bath, and many forgot their injuries, so great was their joy at being away from the barbarous Japanese. It made us feel like we were at last doing the job we had set out to do when we came into the service.

Ens. Jean Condon

Out there in the battle areas, certain incidents intensified our feelings of mercy, kindness, and sympathy towards our boys. One morning as I passed through the wards on my way to duty, an emaciated, harrowed-looking boy with a large foul-smelling, draining cast on his leg called me to his bunk and said, "Nurse, do you use perfume?"

When I replied in the affirmative he went on, "You know, each morning I lie here and wait for you to walk by. It is the bright spot of the day just to be able to smell that wonderful odor. It reminds me of home and my girl."

Needless to say, he shortly had his own individual bottle of cologne. The cologne had a dual purpose. It not only reminded him of his loved ones but was effective in camouflaging the odor from his cast. On the ensuing mornings we watched him sprinkle a few drops of Blue Grass on the bed sheets and gown and then lie back and inhale contentedly. His buddies teased and called him the Blue Grass Boy, but he paid little heed and continued to enjoy his newly found luxury. This boy and all other boys we had aboard the *Bountiful* requested so few things and were without complaints. They asked so little and we had so much to give. I will always remember their gratitude.

SHARK BAIT AND ANGELS

By early 1945, several new hospital ships were either nearing completion or undergoing sea trials. To an ambitious Navy nurse, duty aboard one of these gleaming white vessels was a dream come true.

Lt. (jg) Madge Crouch received orders to USS *Benevolence* (AH-13) and arrived in Brooklyn, New York, in time "to learn a little about the ship and about ship etiquette," she said. As she would soon discover, the ladies in white would carry a very special status.

We had 30 nurses and two Red Cross women, 58 officers, 238 corpsmen, 24 chief petty officers, and a crew of 230 on the *Benevolence*. The skipper was Capt. Clyde C. Laws, an enlisted man who had come up through the ranks. He and Admiral Halsey were good friends and had done a lot of duty together.

Captain Laws was a fabulous character. He was a short, heavy-set guy and when he semaphored, it always looked like he was going to lose his pants. He was so proud of that hospital ship. If we were unlucky enough to scrape the sides of that beautiful white vessel when we docked, he would get up on the deck and start screaming.

He was a father figure to us and even more protective of us nurses than the chief nurse was. When we were in Eniwetok, he made sure that when we went swimming, we swam one place and everybody else swam somewhere else. When he would make his announcements, he would get on the PA system and say, "Angels!" That's what he called us. "Shark bait!" That was everybody else. "Now hear this!"

In May of '45 he issued an order saying he was arming the nurses aboard with guns and they were instructed to shoot anybody who entered their quarters. I still have that order. It reads:

> The rooms and other spaces assigned for exclusive use of women shall be plainly marked. No male shall enter women's quarters except on duty or upon specific invitation. No male shall enter the room of any woman between 2100 and 0700 except under escort of the chief nurse or an assistant chief nurse.
>
> In order that all women on board the *Benevolence* understand their right to protect themselves, they are hereby ordered to assume that any man who invades their room quarters between 2100 and 0700 except under escort by the chief nurse or an assistant chief nurse, does so with carnal intent and shall shoot to kill the intruder.
>
> C. C. Laws, Captain, USN
Commanding Officer

And he was very serious. He even gave us guns! We had .45s hanging up by our bunks! The crew had a fit with this. "My God, those crazy nurses will start shooting and we'll all be killed by bullets ricochetting off the steel bulkheads!"

Well, the funny part was we didn't have any ammunition, but nobody knew that but the nurses.

A DIFFERENT KIND OF HOSPITAL SHIP

Amphibious operations, which characterized the war in the Pacific, generated large numbers of casualties. At the time of Pearl Harbor, the Navy had but one hospital ship, the USS *Solace* (AH-5), in theater. It soon became clear to war planners that even as new white ships were being commissioned and coming on line, something else was needed.

The answer was a whole new class of vessels, the evacuation transports, or APHs. Like hospital ships, APHs were converted cargo transports. But they had a dual role. Painted gray like other combatants, they carried armament—thirteen single 20-mm mounts, four 3-inch guns, and a 5-inch gun. In this transport role, the ships could ferry 1,200 combat troops to the fighting fronts.

For their medical role, the three-ship class—USS *Tryon* (APH-1), *Pinkney* (APH-2), and *Rixey* (APH-3)—had fully equipped operating rooms, radiological departments, laboratories, and a staff of ten physicians, one to two dentists, and fifty-four hospital corpsmen. However, unlike their white-hulled counterparts, these ships were not protected under the Geneva Accords.

By mid-1944 all three APHs saw their first combat. By the end of the war, the concept of armed transports providing front-line medical care proved completely successful.

> Comdr. Anthony DePalma, an orthopedic surgeon, tells of his service aboard the *Rixey*.

I don't know who thought of the APHs, but they were one of the finest things the Navy came up with. They were quite a novelty. I had never seen anything like them. They looked just like any other transport, except they had guns. When I got aboard the *Rixey*, I was surprised to see the kind of men they had gathered as a medical staff. They had excellent people, ten physicians in all the major specialties, and about fifty-four corpsmen.

I think the strongest friendships I formed were with the corpsmen. When they were working, those kids would be stripped right down to the waist. Down in that sick bay you couldn't carry patients on stretchers. There wasn't room for a stretcher to go by in those passageways. You actually could take a stretcher one way only but couldn't pass another one going the other way. These young corpsmen picked up the patients and carted them up and down those ladders and into and out of the bunks. Those guys were unbelievable.

When I first came aboard the *Rixey*, we got down to work right away, because we began making that trip up and down the Slot, back and forth from Guadalcanal and down to New Zealand, bringing casualties from all those islands—Espíritu Santo, Efate, and the others. Most of the casualties were being given very primitive treatment, mostly first aid. We picked them up, worked on them until we were loaded, and then transferred the casualties to transports that were leaving the area. Those ships would then take them to a base hospital or a hospital ship. We stayed right where we were.

It worked like this. We brought in troops, let's say the 1st Marines or the 3rd Marines, or units of those divisions. We then unloaded them, after which we stayed as close to shore as possible. We were right on the beach, about a half mile offshore. We never anchored but were under way all the time, and we acted like a field hospital. We took aboard all the casualties from the other ships, such as destroyers.

This is what we did at Okinawa, when we took all the casualties from the surrounding ships. We did the same thing at Guam. In fact, at Guam we were nine days off the beach. There were no white ships there because they couldn't come in at that time. We could handle several hundred casualties without any trouble.

On a typical day, we got up at 4:30 and went from the transport area to the beach. The bombardment was already going on and we would go right to work. And then we would stay there until things were over. At the end of the day, all the ships would go out to sea. We went out to sea with the other transports as a matter of safety. That way the ships wouldn't be concentrated and targets for suicide planes. Then we all came back the next morning.

After the Japanese began using kamikazes off the Philippines and Okinawa, we got a tremendous number of burns. Many times a ship behind us, in front of us, or next to us would get hit with kamikazes and go up in flames and we would get all the casualties. The burns were terrible and had to be treated right away.

The most hectic days we had out were off Okinawa in the Kerama Retto area, when our ships began using smoke screens to protect the transports. Well, somebody forgot that a lot of people might be sensitive to smoke and we had a hell of a time with people on our own ship who came down with acute pulmonary edema. As a matter of fact, at Leyte, Captain [Arthur H.] Pierson, the senior medical officer on our ship, had to be taken off. The poor guy was a heavy smoker and a bit elderly, too. He almost died. I suddenly became senior medical officer from then on.

We had quite a few operating rooms on the *Rixey*—an orthopedic operating room; a general-surgery operating room; and an ear, nose, and throat operating room. They were small. And then we had an X-ray department with a very competent X-ray man. We also had a good laboratory. In other words, we had the facilities but didn't have the room. It was very tight.

When we were in combat, we were down in the hold working in terrible conditions. The worst thing was the heat, and they didn't have any facilities like showers or air-conditioning. Sometimes the heat would be 106 in those holds, and so unbearable we used to work in our skivvies in the operating room. Yet even though that sick bay was inadequate, we were taking care of hundreds and hundreds of casualties. And we did a lot of definitive work. We had to. For instance, on Guam I did forty-seven amputations. I've got to say one thing about the Navy. We never lacked supplies. We always had enough plasma, antibiotics, and plaster.

As far as equipment was concerned, we had to improvise a lot. We used a turnbuckle—a very crude method—to make traction. For example, if I wanted to make traction on a leg to keep it straight, I would weld a turnbuckle up against the bulkhead and attach the leg to it. You then could adjust the tension.

We had men on the ship make splints for us that we could use externally to reinforce a cast. Very often we used the ship's facilities to help us out. Those boys were very competent.

These methods we devised were useful in saving both lives and limbs. I devised a plan in which we would transfix a badly fractured leg with pins above and below the fracture site, and then incorporate the pins in the plaster. The patient could then be moved all around, from bunk to bunk or from one ship to another. These methods worked very well. When our patients left our ship, there wasn't very much left to do to them. I'll never forget what the doctors said when we got to Pearl. "Tony, we don't have to do anything to your patients except send them home."

PLASMA, PENICILLIN, AND PLASTER

One of those able corpsmen Doctor DePalma grew to depend upon was PhM1c A. Milton Bell. Young Bell had just been transferred from Base Hospital 107 in New Caledonia and arrived aboard the *Rixey* in December of 1943, just in time to see plenty of action.

I was in charge of the pharmacy. We made up all the prescriptions, all the cough medicines. When soldiers or Marines came on board and got seasick, we gave them pink APCs [aspirin, phenacetin, caffeine]. They were like Anacin but were colored pink. We would take a bottle of a thousand APCs and put a big label on it—Seasick Tablets. You'd be surprised how many guys got better.

We already had penicillin on board when I arrived, but we didn't know how to use it properly. As I recall, it came in powdered form in bottles, and we kept it refrigerated. We added saline to it and then shook it up, and then it was ready for injection. It was an early form of penicillin. In fact, to us the whole war was the three Ps—plasma, penicillin, and plaster. We prepared the penicillin in a 50-cc syringe. Then we would give twenty-five individual shots of 2 cc each. Each cc was the equivalent of 10,000 units. Today, a 250-gram pill equals a quarter of a million units! Each shot we gave was 20,000 units, and we had to give it every four hours around the clock. And the needles got pretty dull, because we didn't have disposables. We had little half-inch needles. We autoclaved them, put them on the syringe, gave the guy a shot, removed the needle from the syringe, dropped it in the pot, and then re-autoclaved them.

We also made plaster bandages, which were coarse six-inch bandages. We took the bandage off one reel and wound it onto another reel, passing it through dry plaster. The plaster would then be picked up in the gauze of the bandage. We made a bandage that would be five or six yards long and rolled into a roll about 2 1/2 inches in diameter. We then wrapped it in plain wax paper and stored it in a box in a dry area. When you needed the bandage, you put it into a stainless-steel tub filled with water.

The plaster bandages were used for broken legs, broken arms, and body casts. Let's say someone got shot in the clavicle. He would need a body cast that would hold the shoulder up to immobilize the clavicle. For burn cases, which we had a lot of, we used finer bandages about 2 1/2 or 3 inches wide. We used tongue depressors to fold the bandage back on itself, back and forth, so it would fit in a one-pound can.

You know how a Simoniz can looks? The Navy bought cans like that filled with petrolatum, but they weren't sterile. We removed the petrolatum and heated it in a little pot on a hot plate. After packing the can with the bandages, we poured the petrolatum over them, sealed the can, and autoclaved it so it was sterile. When burn cases came aboard and the skin just came off, we sprinkled the burns with a little sulfathiazole and covered them with the petrolatum-impregnated bandages. The patients felt better when you covered their burns, but that treatment also caused terrible scarring. It was the wrong treatment, but we didn't know it at the time. Today you treat them differently.

For anesthesia we used sodium pentothal, which was new at that time. I became an anesthetist. When I wasn't in the boat transferring patients from the beach to the ship, I would be aboard assisting in surgery doing anesthesia and helping suture patients.

Another thing we learned to do as corpsmen was to expose the vein on the arm below the elbow with instruments, so we could cut down on it to insert a cannula. We then tied the cannula in place with suture cord so it wouldn't pull out. Then we could administer plasma, serum albumin, and whole blood without having to stick the patient each time. And the cannula remained in the arm until we had to take it out.

If you were giving anesthesia, we used the same cannula for that. We would make up a big batch of sodium pentothal in a 50-cc syringe and then administer a half cc at a time. If the patient was awake you'd have him count backwards, starting from a hundred. By the time he reached eighty he was asleep. We did amputations and all kinds of heavy surgery with sodium pentothal.

Often when we had to administer whole blood, we would find the blood was out of date. We then got the crew to give blood. It was almost like a direct transfusion. If we needed A blood we asked for an A and verified it by the dog tag. This crew member or one of the Marines or soldiers we were carrying would then be placed on the table and we took a pint of blood. Then we'd transfuse it right into the patient. The donors then got two ounces of whiskey, but not immediately. We "owed" it to them. That's what they were entitled to, and the captain would sign off on it. I think they got Canadian Club.

Those of us who were on the shock team carried scissors and a very sharp knife. We also had plasma and needles and I learned how to get into a vein quickly. I was very good at it. You had to be very careful you didn't cut through a vein or artery. We lost a few patients in surgery that way. Once, when we were transferring patients from Guam to Hawaii, one of the doctors elected to remove a bullet from a patient's neck, and we prepared for surgery. About ten minutes into the operation, he accidentally cut the carotid artery. The patient died on the table and we buried him at sea. Things like that happened.

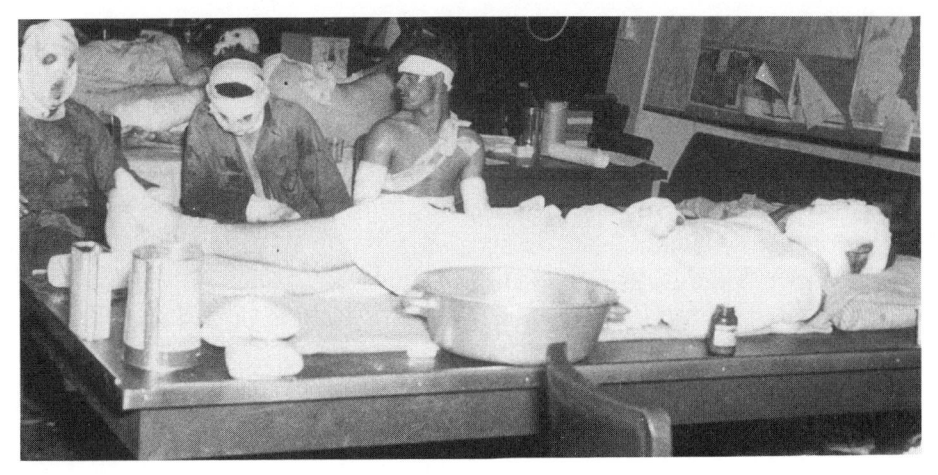

During the Battle of Leyte Gulf, the wardroom of the USS *Suwannee* becomes an impromptu sick bay following the first kamikaze attacks of the war. Because the sick bays of small escort carriers could not handle mass casualties, the medical staff of two physicians, a dentist, and about a dozen corpsmen used whatever space they could. *Courtesy of Walter B. Burwell*

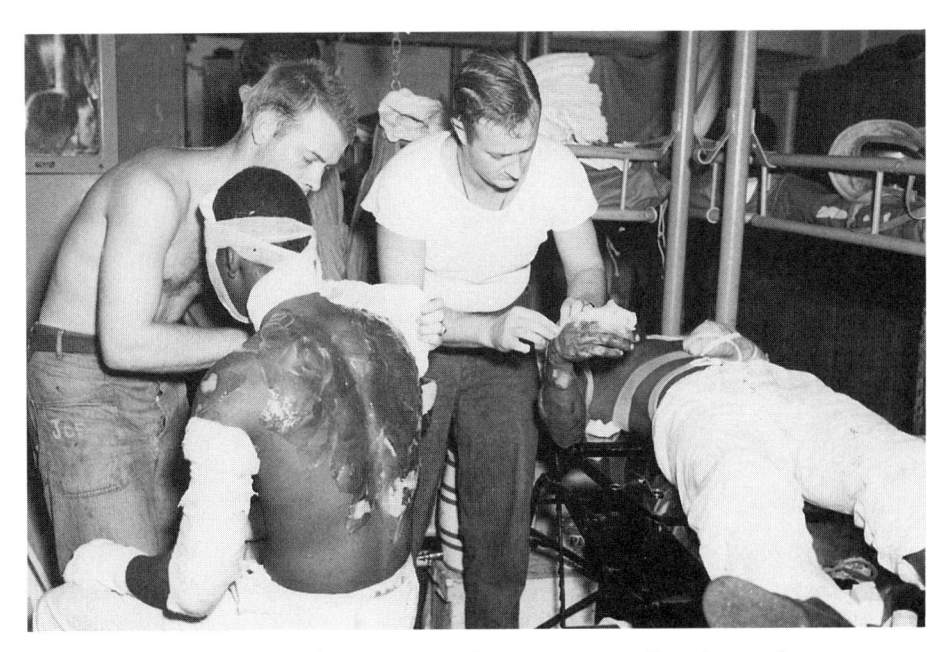

Packed with ordnance and aviation gasoline, carriers suffered most from suicide planes. Here, corpsmen treat burn casualties in the chief petty officers' quarters of the USS *Kalinin Bay* (CVE-68) during the Battle of Leyte Gulf.

(Right): Comdr. Eugene Owens examines Dr. Lewis Haynes's dressings at the naval hospital on Guam following the USS *Indianapolis* disaster. The fatal torpedoes that exploded just beneath Haynes's stateroom inflicted serious burns on his hands and feet. Capt. Charles McVay, the ill-fated cruiser's skipper, stands at right. *Courtesy of Lewis L. Haynes*

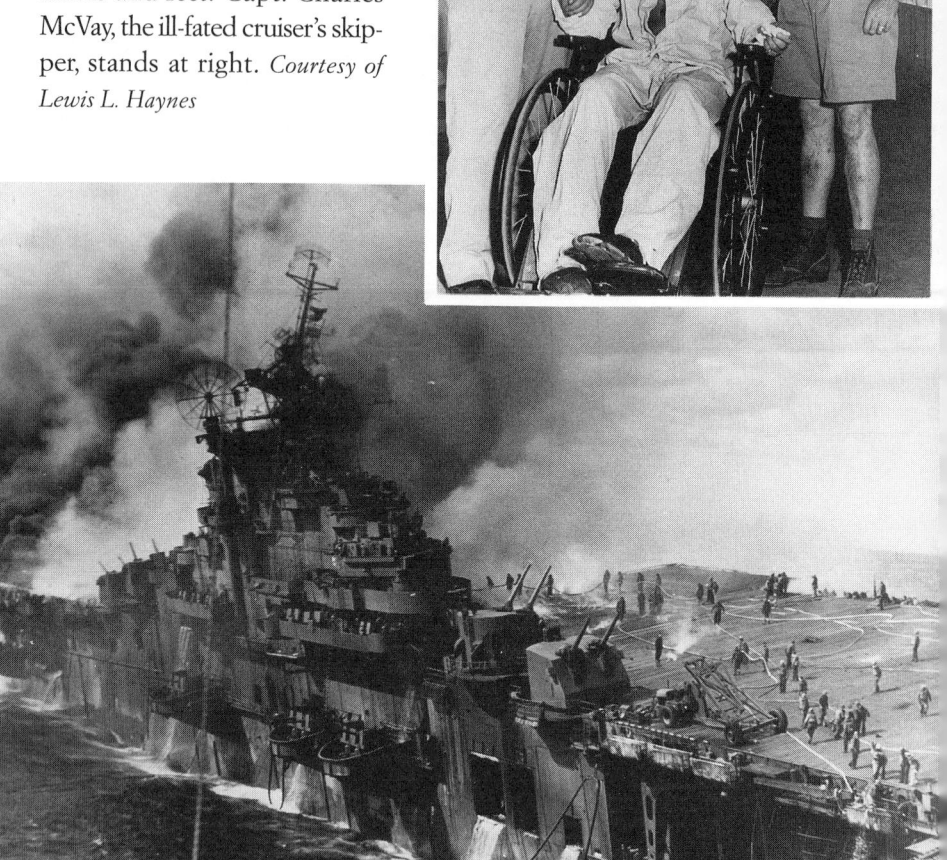

Blazing aviation gas and water pour from the battered USS *Franklin* (CV-13) as firefighters work amidst exploding ordnance to save her. Over eight hundred sailors and Marines lost their lives when the carrier took two direct bomb hits on her flight deck just fifty miles from Japan. The *Franklin* survived the attack and made it back to New York under her own power.

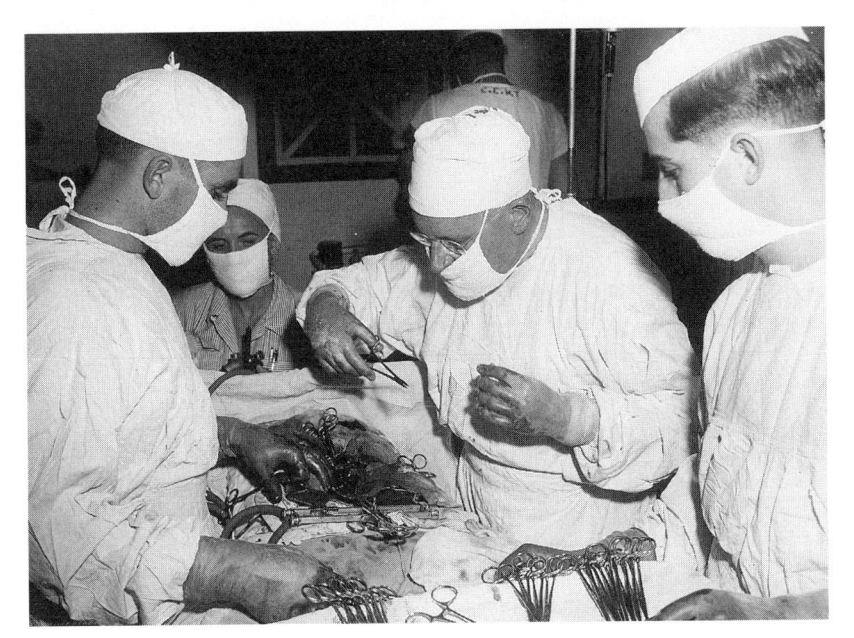

Surgeons repair a shrapnel-inflicted intestinal perforation as the hospital ship USS *Solace* stands off Okinawa during the last and bloodiest campaign of World War II. Clean ships like this offered a brand of medical care parallel to that found in many contemporary stateside hospitals.

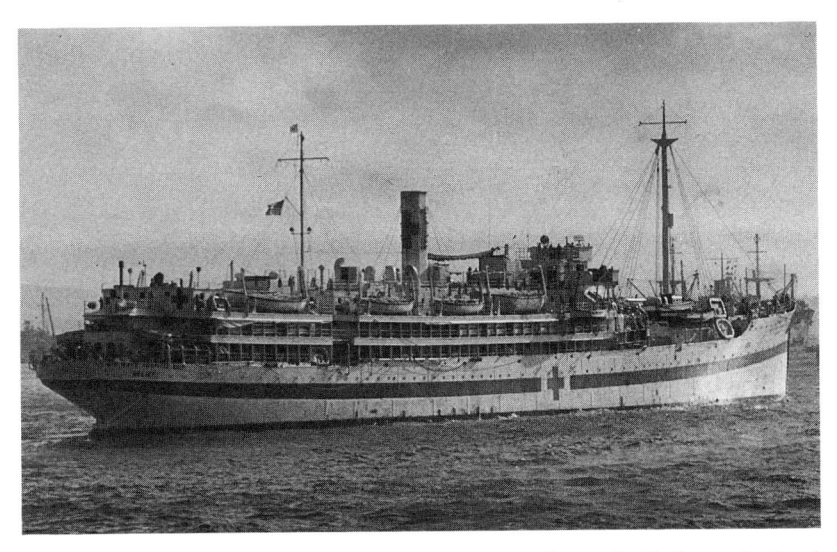

The USS *Relief* (AH-1), the only American vessel ever built from the keel up as a hospital ship, was the oldest mercy ship in the fleet when this photo was taken off the Okinawa beaches in June 1945.

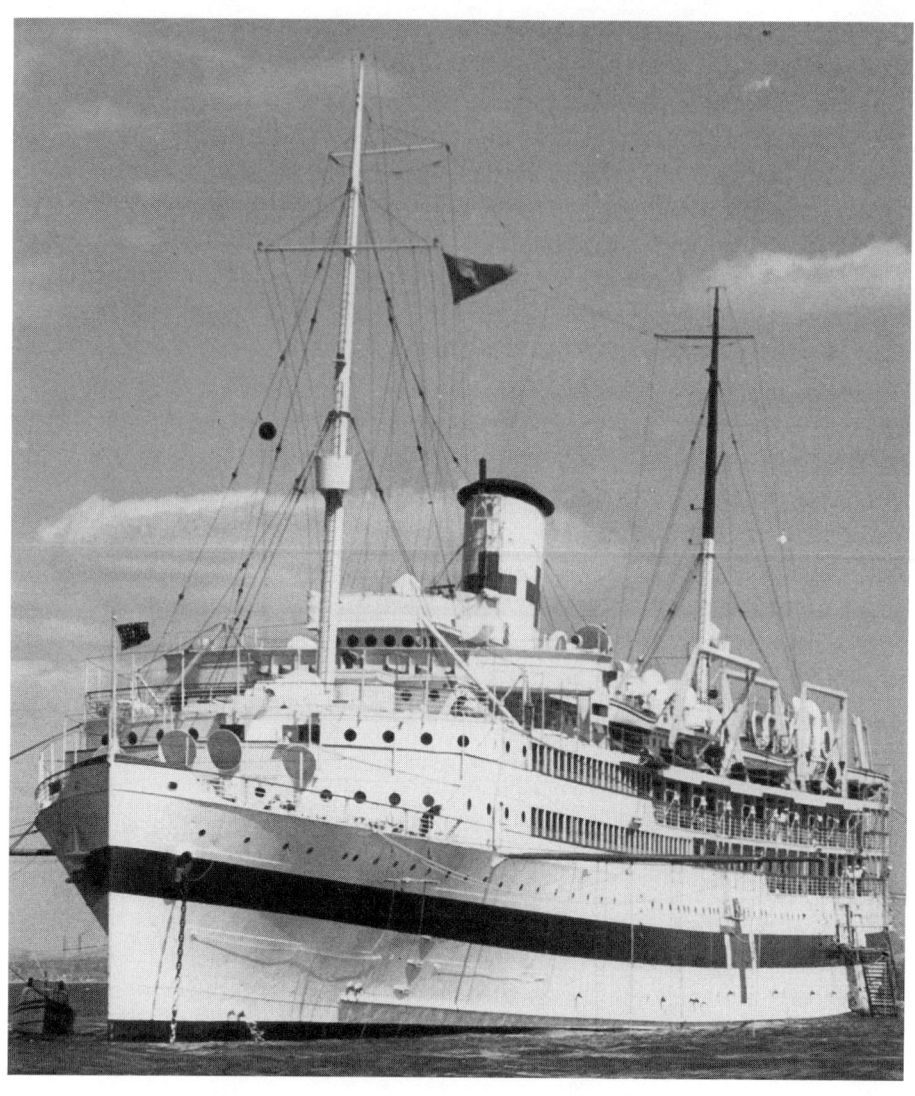

Built in 1927 as the liner SS *Iroquois,* the *Solace* was the only hospital ship in the Pacific on 7 December 1941.

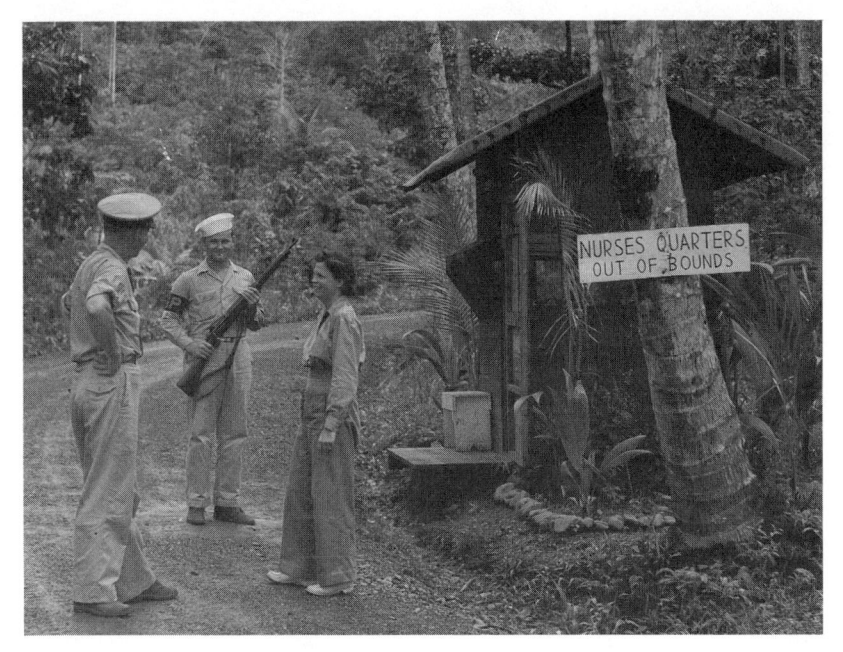

The Navy discouraged fraternization aboard its hospital ships. The situation at fleet and base hospitals ashore was no different.

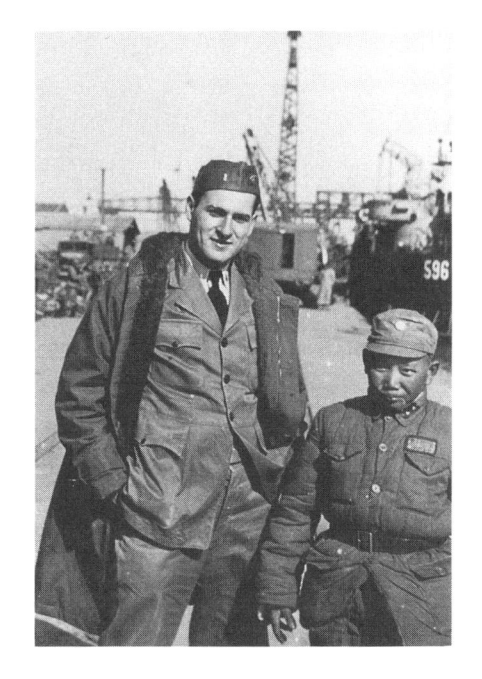

Lt. (jg) Henry Heimlich and a Chinese soldier pose for a snapshot on the Shanghai waterfront. *Courtesy of Henry Heimlich*

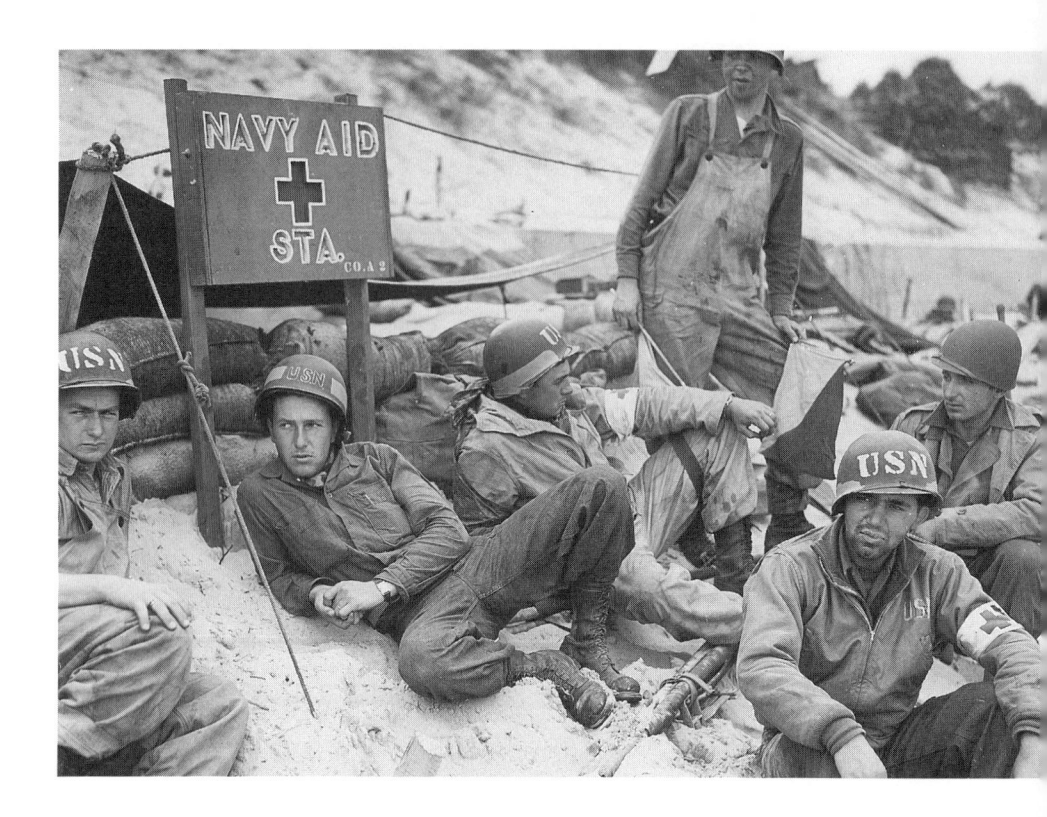

Corpsmen await business on a French invasion beach.

On his fifth trip to Normandy, Lt. (jg) Dale Groom took this photograph of *LST-357* high and dry on Utah Beach. Note the barrage balloons, meant to discourage strafing by low-flying aircraft.
Courtesy of Dale Groom

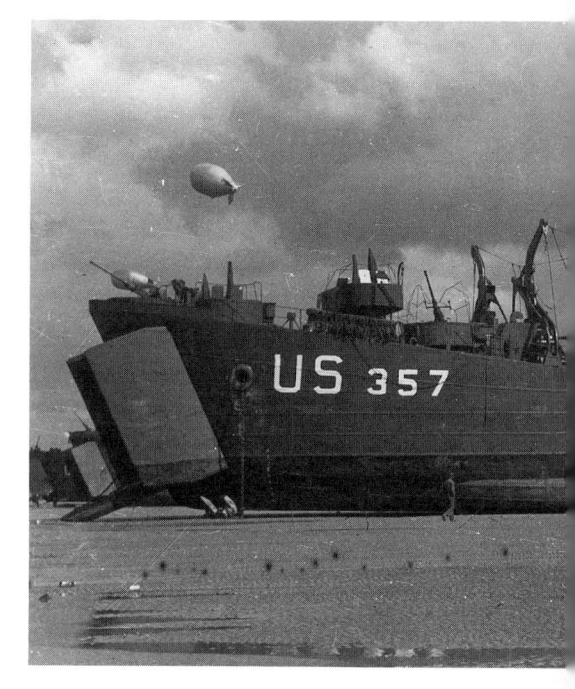

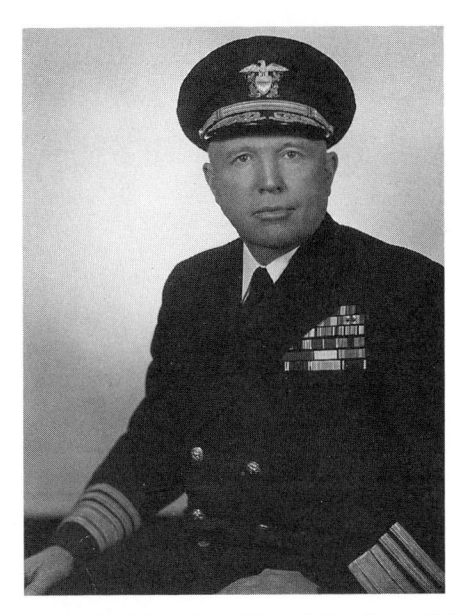

Surgeon General of the Navy Vice Adm. Ross T. McIntire led the Medical Department through World War II and was President Franklin D. Roosevelt's chief physician.

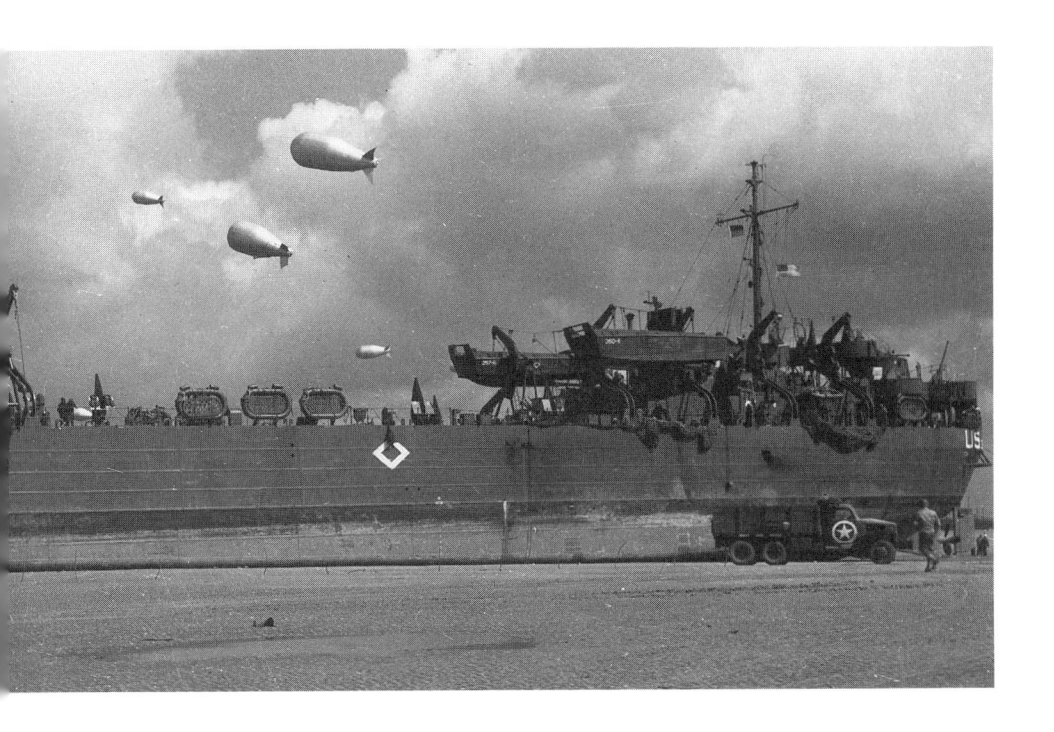

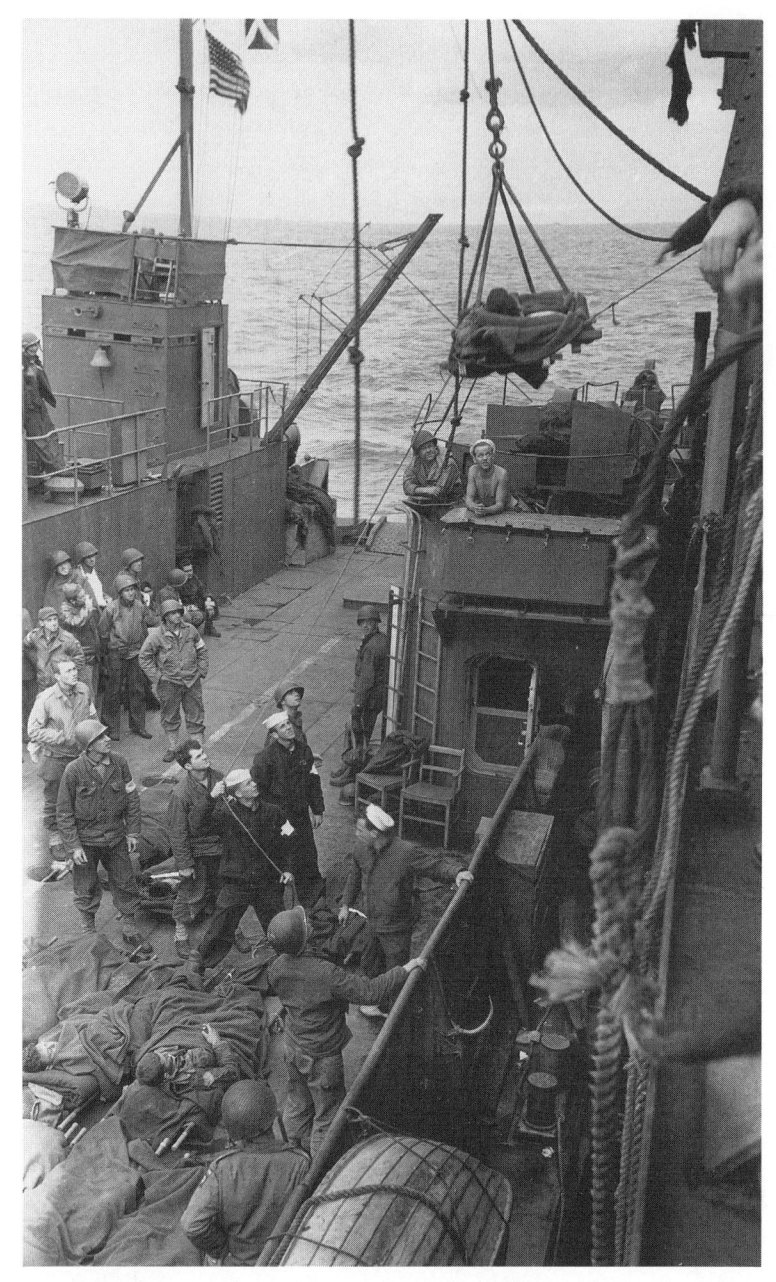

Casualties being brought aboard *LST-357* on D-Day, 6 June 1944. The wounded came out from Omaha Beach in small landing craft and were hoisted aboard by sling. *LST-357* received only about a dozen men before turning back to England that evening for the second load of Army personnel and their equipment. *Courtesy of Dale Groom*

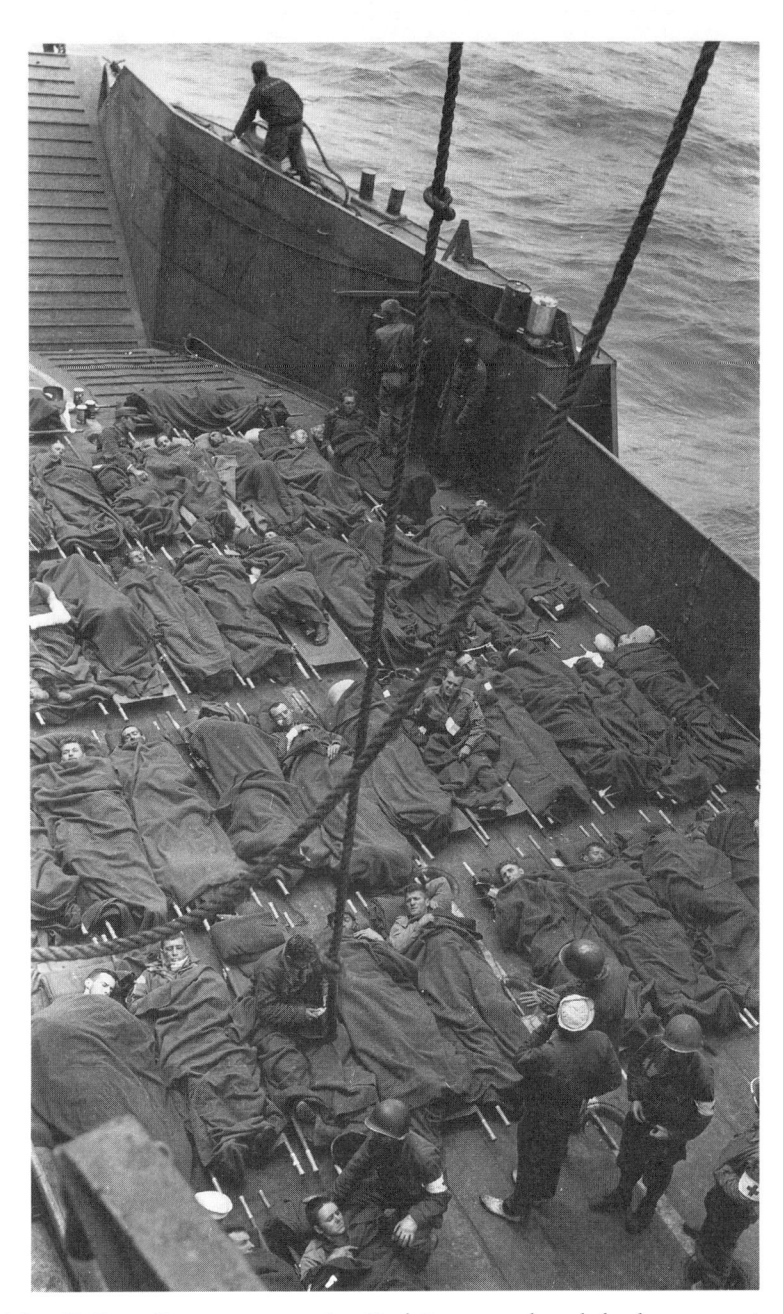

After D-Day: Corpsmen wearing Red Cross armbands look over a mixed load of casualties, Americans and German POWs. The LCT's crewman (top) is about to tie up to *LST-357,* ramp to ramp, so litters can be carried directly aboard. This was a far more expeditious method than the over-the-side slings of D-Day. *Courtesy of Dale Groom*

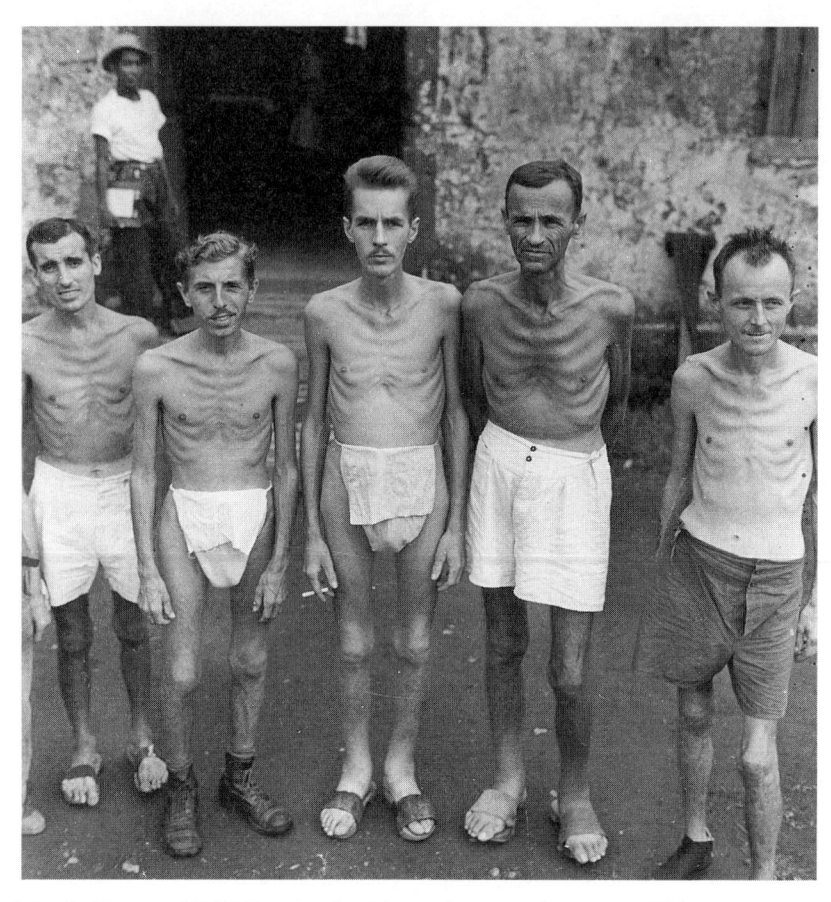

Newly liberated POWs pose for Navy photographers on 8 February 1945, shortly after being freed from Bilibid. These were the lucky ones.

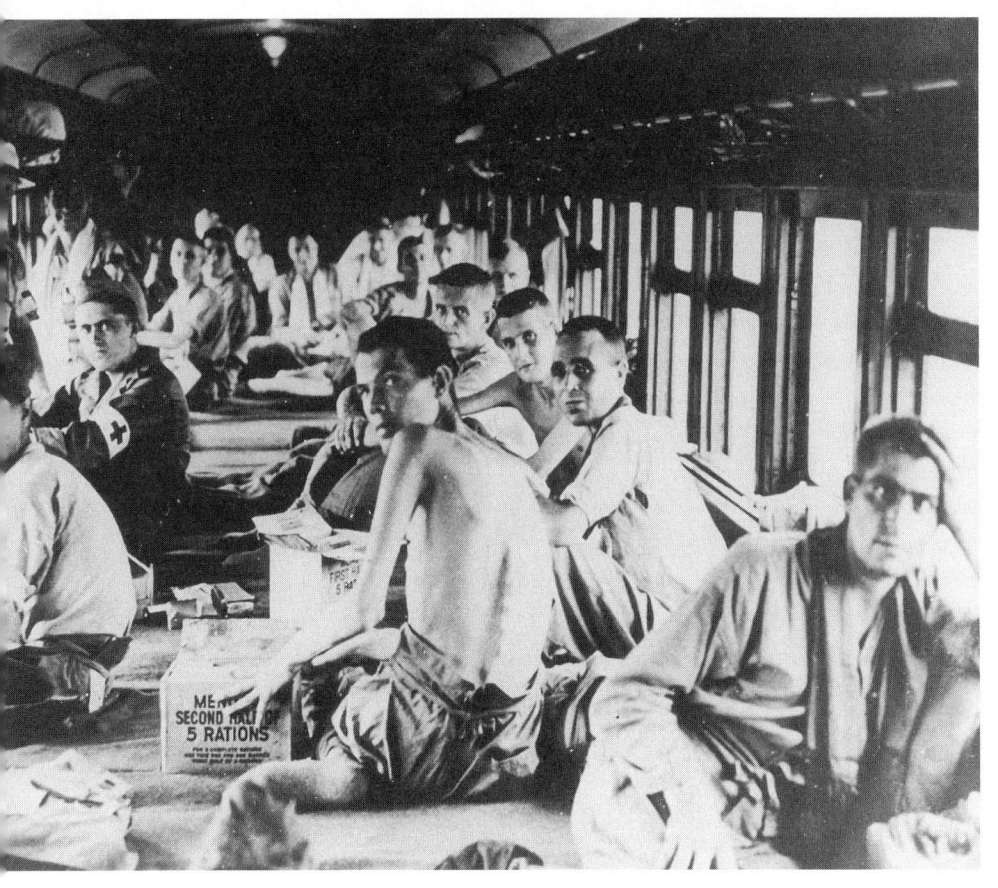

Sick and emaciated POWs occupy a hospital coach on their way to freedom at the port city of Nagasaki. The boxes of K rations would tide them over until they received showers, medical treatment, new clothes, "real food," and passage home aboard a hospital ship.

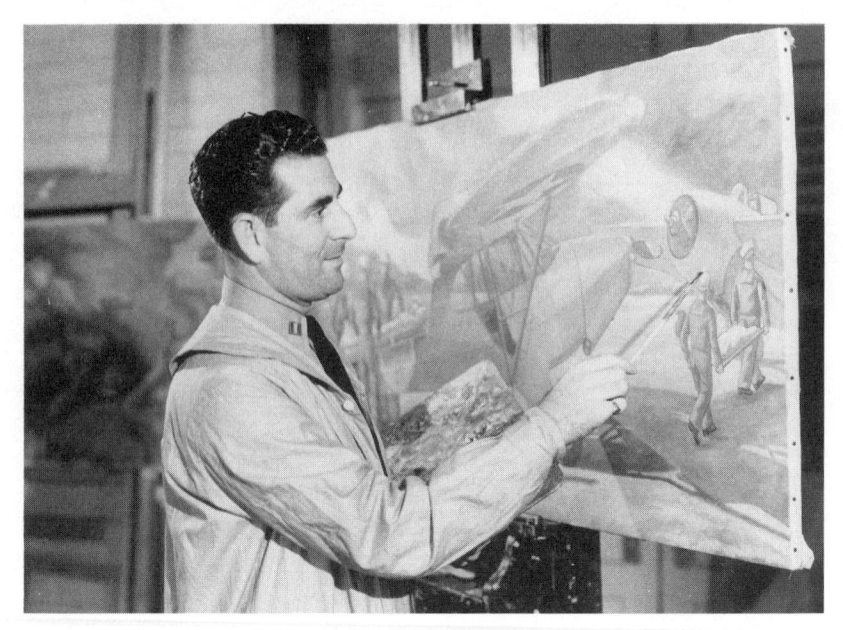

Lt. Samuel Bookatz is shown at work in his studio at the Bureau of Medicine and Surgery. *Courtesy of Samuel Bookatz*

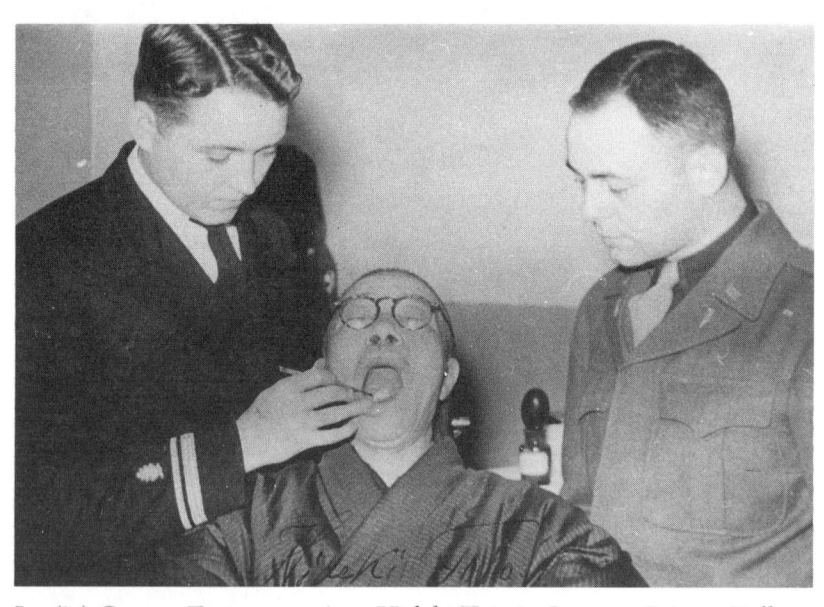

Lt. (jg) George Foster examines Hideki Tojo in Sugamo Prison. Following extraction of the infamous prisoner's remaining upper teeth, Lt. (jg) Jack Mallory would fabricate a new and controversial denture. *Courtesy of National Naval Dental Center*

EIGHT

The Rice Paddy Navy

One of the lesser-known naval activities of World War II took place in the CBI (China-Burma-India) theater. In 1943 the government of Chiang Kai-shek, in cooperation with the U.S. Navy, organized what became known as the Sino-American Cooperative Organization (SACO). Led by Comdr. Milton "Mary" Miles, USN, and Lt. Gen. Tai Li, SACO had several aims.[1] Because weather affecting the Pacific Fleet originated in China, planners desperately needed reliable meteorological information. There was also a pressing need for accurate intelligence regarding Japanese fleet movements. The SACO agreement took care of these needs. Navy personnel flown from India over the Hump into China set up and monitored weather stations in far-western China. In eastern China, a network of coast watchers reported Japanese fleet movements.

A strong Navy presence in central China, where the Chinese government had fled, had another vital benefit—arming and training a Chinese guerrilla army to fight the Japanese invaders.

---

1. Miles had gotten this nickname at the Naval Academy from fellow cadets, whose favorite pinup girl was Mary Miles Minter, a motion-picture actress of silent films.
   Tai Li was Chiang Kai-shek's powerful head of the secret police, known as the Himmler of China. He ruthlessly carried out the generalissimo's instructions, eliminated political opposition, and reserved for himself the fruits of illegal smuggling operations.

GUERRILLA DOCTOR

During the first two years of the war, Lt. Comdr. Cecil Coggins, MC, the former obstetrician turned intelligence officer, had had several assignments, none of them related to medicine. Late in 1943 he received orders as chief field surgeon for U.S. Naval Group China, the American half of SACO, already known as the Rice Paddy Navy.

Even though Coggins again became a practicing physician, he operated behind Japanese lines as Col. Koh Jin Tsuh, wearing the uniform of the Chinese guerrilla army. He also had ample opportunity to indulge in intelligence activities, particularly relating to biological warfare.

First of all, I reported to the chief of SACO, Comdr. Milton E. "Mary" Miles, USN. Dressed in khaki shirt and shorts, he was relaxed and very cordial and made me feel welcome. We sat together and reviewed a rough plan by which medical services could be made available to all guerrilla forces in China, taking into consideration the many supply and personnel difficulties already occurring and which continued throughout the war.

The plan called for a large permanent base hospital, to be located in Tung An in Chekiang province, about forty miles southwest of Shanghai. There were to be two doctors and a dentist, one pharmacist, a chief pharmacist's mate, and about twenty hospital corpsmen. This installation was called "Pact Doc," and it was to constitute the largest and only fixed hospital in all of SACO. My task was to act as field surgeon to accompany mobile hospitals into the field in close support of our guerrilla columns.

While I could accompany only one mobile hospital at a time, I would exercise loose control of personnel in other mobile hospitals. Each one of these was comprised of one MASH (mobile army surgical hospital) unit. During my service with the guerrillas, I built four semi-permanent hospitals with capacities of one hundred beds each and with two doctors and five corpsmen in attendance. Needless to say, each of these hospitals had to be abandoned in succession by the advance of the Japanese army.

I certainly thrived in such an environment. I found out later that Mary Miles had foreseen many of the difficulties of a mixed command, and in an early communication to Washington had written:

> We need good men—better than average men and they should be able to fight . . . in any job assigned to them without fighting their shipmates. No high hat, red-tape clerks allowed. All SACO characters must and will associate without worrying whether they are commissioned, or in what service. Of course, they all ought to know more than one job. Our recruits should not be "Old China hands." The less they know about China, the less they will have to unlearn. We can indoctrinate them all here so that they will meet with Chinese approval.
>
> Our volunteers must be prepared to eat and live in Chinese style and expect nothing else. They must renounce drinking, as this is too dangerous a job to endanger by dissipation. As to women, it's easy to make a law about them because there aren't any here.

On 27 November, Miles sent a memorandum to Tai Li setting up a conference. All I was told was that I was going to meet the man of mystery, Lt. Gen. Tai Li. I wondered what he would be like, and the stories that I had heard passed through my mind.

Mary Miles regarded Tai Li as a sincere, devoted friend of the generalissimo and of himself. This friendship lay at the bottom of all the success achieved by SACO.

I was ushered into the presence of Lt. Gen. Tai Li. We bowed and he politely waved me towards a chair. Eddie Liu [interpreter] was there. Also present was Col. Hsiao Sin-ju, whom I had met in Washington. We sat down and were all served tea. Tai Li was a round, pleasant-faced gentleman with brown, very observant eyes and a soft gentle voice belying his reputation.

When all the political amenities had been observed, and not until then, did Mary get down to business. He mentioned that I had brought some secret weapons to China with me, and I took up the conversation and explained the powerful plastic, disguised as flour and shipped in regular flour sacks.[2]

---

2. The plastic explosive, disguised as flour, was widely used for sabotage throughout China. Chinese guerrillas destroyed railway locomotives, railroad cars, railroad bridges, and tore up large sections of track.

I then described the loud noisemaker to create a diversion in a crowded place; the little squirt guns of skatole to embarrass Japanese officers; the tiny capsules of botulinus toxin, the size of a matchhead, to be concealed under the fingernail and dropped into a drink or serving of food; and finally, and most important, the two soundless and flashless .22-caliber automatic pistols.[3] One was a Colt and the other a High Standard. I had them with me and presented them as gifts to Tai Li. I handed them to him, explaining that the purpose of these pistols was to shoot sentries at night, one at a time, without disturbing the others. I assured him that the pistols were flashless as well as soundless. Tai Li took one of the pistols, stepped to the window, and, with successive shots, rolled a fragment of horse manure down the hilly lawn. I complimented him on his excellent marksmanship, which was obvious to me.

As for the weapons, I felt highly privileged and very happy to strike killing blows at the enemy by whatever means available. The Japanese were advancing in the north, slaughtering, raping, and burning the Chinese peasants indiscriminately and by the thousands in each city. To the Chinese, to fail to use every possible means of stemming such attacks would have been unthinkable! As for me, I had constantly in mind my memories of the treacherous attack at Pearl Harbor on my old ships and thousands of my former shipmates. That awful vision remains.

At war's end Coggins was still with SACO, but from 1947 to 1949 he reverted to his original role as physician aboard the hospital ship USS *Repose* (AH-16). He subsequently served with NATO as chief of atomic, biologic, and chemical warfare. Dr. Coggins retired in 1959 as a rear admiral. He died in 1987 at age eighty-five.

---

3. The tiny noisemaker, which sounded like the approaching shriek and then explosion of an aerial bomb, was supposed to sow panic in a crowd. A miniature syringe containing skatole, a chemical with the odor of feces, could be squirted on Japanese officers in a crowd, resulting, it was hoped, in great loss of face. According to Coggins, the botulin toxin was never used.

DR. HEIMLICH'S FIRST CAREER

Like Dr. Cecil Coggins, the physician-intelligence expert, another medical officer, Lt. (jg) Henry J. Heimlich, took part in the SACO experience after volunteering for "prolonged extra-hazardous overseas duty in China."

After finishing a surgical internship at Boston City Hospital in September 1943, I went on active duty. My first orders were to the Chelsea Naval Hospital on 10 October 1944. In December I was ordered to the chief of naval operations in Washington, and reported in January 1945.

Shortly after arriving, I was taken into a room with two officers. "All we can tell you about this duty is that it is voluntary, and it's prolonged extra-hazardous overseas duty in China." And that's all I knew until I got to China. I remember thinking that if I was going to get it, I'd rather see China than some landing beach. So I took the assignment.

About a month later I received orders to proceed to U.S. Naval Group China. I traveled with the CO of my group, George Basham, and a hundred enlisted men. We took a train to San Pedro, California, where on 26 February we left aboard the USS *Admiral W. S. Benson* [AP-120]. I got sick as a dog for two days right after we left San Pedro.

We traveled alone and not in convoy, because our ship was very fast compared to submarines. On the way out of San Pedro, the ship's crew took antiaircraft practice on a towed target. When we got a direct hit, all of us just yelled with glee.

When we'd been out for a few days, we encountered an unidentified ship and had to go to quarters. As a doctor, I had to go down in the hold and open an emergency medical unit there. It turned out to be an American destroyer.

We arrived in Bombay on 29 March 1945, two days over a month after leaving San Pedro. We then boarded a train for a week, and reported to the commander, India unit of SACO in Calcutta, on 2 April. I didn't know any more about my mission than I had heard in that room back in Washington. I stayed in Calcutta for about two weeks and then received orders to proceed to U.S. Naval Group China via a CNAC [Chinese National Airways Corporation] plane over the Hump.

I never knew what was coming next. On 17 April I was designated an official courier for the purpose of transporting official U.S. Navy communications from Calcutta to commander U.S. Naval Group China in Chungking. Making me a courier allowed them to have me to carry mail and materials on the plane. I wore a half dozen .45 pistols they needed in China. From that point on, I traveled in a gray or khaki uniform without insignia.

The CNAC was flying old C-47s over the Hump. There were holes in the windows to fire through if we were attacked. We had to climb over 17,000 feet to get over the mountains, and when we got to a certain height I began gasping for breath and then passed out, as we all did. Only the pilot and copilot had oxygen. I got to see a little of the Himalayas before I lost consciousness. The next thing I knew my eyes suddenly popped open and there were rice paddies all around on the mountains.

Eventually I reached SACO headquarters in Chungking. The airport where we landed was a small sand island in the middle of the Yangtze River, between the hills. Then I boarded a sedan chair with a guy in front and one in back and climbed many, many stairs to the top, where they dumped me on the street with my bags and my guns. I remember the children laughing at me and coming over and touching the guns. Ultimately I reached SACO headquarters. Again I was taken to a room with two officers, and they explained what SACO was all about.

I learned that I had come to China to replace a doctor at one of the Navy camps in the Gobi Desert, Camp 4 in Inner Mongolia. He had broken a tooth in a basketball game. The Americans and Chinese in these camps would play fierce basketball games. A Nationalist general in our area, Fu Tso Yi, had an army of 100,000. I was to build him a medical corps.

I didn't know what was going on in Mongolia until I got there. I received my orders to go to Naval Unit 4 on 21 April. I caught another CNAC flight from Chungking to Lanchow, in northwest China. While I was in Lanchow, I met a Lt. Angus A. MacInnis. He was a weatherman and was going to a place further west—Penglian—to set up a weather station. We had an old Chinese-owned Dodge truck and a Chinese driver. The truck broke down and the driver took the engine completely apart, put it back together and then it worked.

Before reaching Camp Four we crossed the Ordos Desert. We made it to Mongolia on 4 June and initially visited a Spanish missionary. They cooked marvelous food, had great wine, and danced the fandango.

Camp Four was in the town of Shempa in Suiyan Province, but it has a new name now and is also part of Inner Mongolia. Shempa was a walled town built in adobe style. My group originally had twelve members, thus our code name was the Apostles. But it grew to about twenty people, including a chaplain named LaSor. I reported to the CO, a Marine captain named Hilliard. He sent me to the doctor's room, and then I was assigned a horse.

The doctor I replaced left a two-year supply of equipment. We had sulfa drugs but no penicillin. I also had a steam sterilizer built from a five-gallon oil tin, and a still made to produce distilled water. The local coffin maker built me an operating table out of wood with iron hinges and ratchets, so I could raise and lower the head and feet.

A couple of our people were training the Chinese guerrillas. There were 250 Nationalist Chinese guerrillas under two generals, Chiao and Liu. But they were mostly fighting puppets of the Japanese.

I treated both Americans and some of the locals. One evening shortly after I arrived, an eighteen-year-old girl was carried in with a distended abdomen and severe dehydration. I didn't know whether it was a tumor or an infection. But I knew she needed surgery. As we didn't have electricity, I couldn't start a major surgery so close to nightfall.

If she had died our mission would have been in jeopardy. The Chinese did not really trust western medicine and we would lose face. I told her dad I would operate if she lived through the night. I distilled some water, added salt tablets, and gave the saline solution subcutaneously. The next morning she was somewhat improved.

I sterilized instruments and my corpsman assisted me. I gave her a spinal and gingerly cut into her abdomen. As soon as I hit the peritoneum, green and yellow pus gushed all over us. I screamed with joy since this was the only thing I could handle. She had a pelvic abscess. I cleaned it out, left it open, and put drains in. She recovered.

From then on I was mobbed by hundreds of patients. Everyone came to see me. I saw a lot of syphilis and many other diseases and afflictions that most American doctors would not see. It was one of the last areas of plague, both bubonic and pneumonic.

We heard the war had ended while we were there at Camp Four. There was a report on the Armed Forces Radio that the first atomic bomb had been dropped. We all felt it was very promising. About a week later we got a message, the first ever not in code: "It's Over."

We screamed and yelled, but the Chinese were troubled; their future was in jeopardy. In October a Chinese soldier got shot in the chest accidentally during training. The first night I just put on a bandage, because the light was really bad. Chest surgery was in its infancy and I had surely never opened a chest before. It was a through-and-through wound, and by morning he was near death. Therefore, I decided to operate. I found a huge hole from the entrance wound to exit wound, five to six inches. I also found a three-inch hole in one of his lungs and sutured it up. But closing was basically impossible due to massive amounts of torn tissues. Unfortunately, the patient expired during final closure. I always felt guilty; should I have done anything else?

Dr. Heimlich was discharged from the Navy in 1946. In the early 1960s, still haunted by the Chinese soldier lost on the operating table, he developed the Heimlich chest-drain valve, fabricating the prototype from a Japanese noisemaker—the Bronx Cheer. The valve allowed air, blood, and fluid to drain from the lung but kept air from leaking back in through the wound, preventing the injured lung from collapsing. This simple, inexpensive surgical device saved thousands of wounded soldiers during the Vietnam War and is still in common use.

In the early 1970s Heimlich developed the Heimlich Maneuver to save choking victims.

NINE

D-Day

The Americans who stormed Hitler's Fortress Europe on 6 June 1944 were predominantly troops of the U.S. Army. But D-Day was not solely an Army show. It was Navy ships and personnel that brought the soldiers and their equipment from England, and Navy battleships, cruisers, destroyers, and rocket-firing amphibious assault vessels that pounded German fortifications and cleared the way to the beaches and beyond.

By spring of 1944, preparations for the cross-Channel invasion were in full swing. American forces of "friendly occupation" had swelled to nearly a million and half troops, many in the coastal regions of Devon and Cornwall, with others scattered throughout the British Isles.

Augmented by forces from Britain, Canada, other Commonwealth nations, and by token forces of Free French, Free Poles, and troops from other occupied nations, the Allies prepared for the greatest amphibious landing in history. The flotilla that would take them and their equipment to the Continent numbered more than 1,300 warships, 1,600 merchant vessels, and 4,000 landing ships.

Although Navy medical personnel were not present on the French beaches in large numbers, the Navy Medical Department nevertheless played a key role in providing care to the wounded. Physicians and corpsmen aboard specially equipped LSTs and LCTs gave primary emergency treatment once the casualties had been evacuated from Utah and Omaha. And once safely back in England, Navy medical personnel, including nurses, triaged, conducted emergency surgery, and stabilized the injured until they could be evacuated to other hospitals in Britain or back to the United States for more definitive treatment.

As in North Africa and Italy, the Navy Medical Department's primary role was to provide medical service to all personnel between the British ports of embarkation and the assault beaches. Once the landings were in progress, medical personnel were to evacuate casualties from the beaches and provide hospitalization afloat within the combat zone. Navy medical personnel were also responsible for care in the beach areas while operating jointly with the ground forces.[1]

The final medical plan consisted of three phases: the far-shore phase on the Normandy coast was to deal with the prompt exchange of medical supplies and equipment and evacuation of casualties from shore to ship. Afloat, casualties were to receive emergency medical care to the extent possible. The near-shore phase would deliver casualties to the Army at Channel ports in England.[2]

In February and March, medical personnel designated for LST duty began arriving in England. In April, practical demonstrations in casualty handling were held at the port of Fowey in Cornwall. The final plan included ninety LSTs with three medical officers and twenty corpsmen each, thirteen LSTs with two medical officers and two corpsmen, and three LSTs with one medical officer and two corpsmen. Each LST was equipped with medical supplies and equipment to provide surgical and nursing care for two hundred patients on the return to England.[3]

By the last week in April, training exercises for the D-Day landings had reached a crescendo. In the early morning hours of 28 April 1944, these rehearsals took a catastrophic turn. The following are four eyewitness accounts, one of the Slapton Sands tragedy, the others of D-Day and its aftermath.

---

1. "U.S. Navy Medical Department Administrative History, 1941–1945," 731.
2. Ibid., 732.
3. Ibid., 734.

THE TRAGEDY OF EXERCISE TIGER

Lt. Eugene E. Eckstam was a Navy medical officer who participated in the training exercises leading up to D-Day. One of these rehearsals, Exercise Tiger, ended disastrously when German E-boats (torpedo boats) torpedoed three amphibious ships, killing over 750 soldiers and sailors. In order to maintain security for the upcoming invasion, the Slapton Sands incident was never acknowledged at the time and remained a secret for almost forty years.

More lives were lost in one exercise practicing for D-Day than during the invasion of Utah Beach on 6 June 1944. That rehearsal was called Exercise Tiger. Planning for the greatest amphibious operation in history required many such exercises, each designed to test the readiness of plans for the invasion of Normandy and the efficiency of the troops. Duck, Fox, Muskrat, Beaver, and Trousers preceded Tiger, and Fabius followed. Each was larger than the last, and the later ones used live ammunition.

Because it resembled Utah Beach, Slapton Sands was chosen for these exercises, a beach on the English Channel east of Plymouth in Lyme Bay. Other smaller exercises were held many places in southern England, especially at Woolacomb. Exercise Tiger involved some three hundred ships and thirty thousand men. Thirty of the ships were LSTs, which loaded at Plymouth, Brixham, and Dartmouth. The first units landed at H-hour, the morning of 27 April 1944. H-hour was delayed one hour, causing landings and shelling to coincide. And not all ships got the message.

Convoy T-4 consisted of eight LSTs bringing up the rear, which were due to land at H-hour plus 24. I was on LST-507, which was last in line. The convoy circled Lyme Bay at four knots. Only one British escort vessel accompanied us; another remained in Plymouth with a hole in its bow. Much later a replacement was sent, but too late to affect the tragic outcome of Exercise Tiger. German E-boats plied the Channel and Lyme Bay several times a week, and the night of 27 April was one of them.

I was a brand-new naval reserve medical officer, fresh out of an abbreviated senior year and internship, totally unprepared for what was to follow. I knew only about the role of such physicians on LSTs, and this training was short.

My first assignment, in January 1944, had been Great Lakes Naval Training Station in Illinois. At the recruiting center, Mainside, we examined an average of 1,700 recruits a day. In a week I became an expert in hemorrhoids, hernias, and right ears. Then I, and perhaps fifty other new physicians, reported to Lido Beach, Long Island. A few thousand hospital corpsmen of all ranks were there too. Individual outfits of Foxy 29, the code name for our medical unit, were formed by taking two physicians and an assortment of forty corpsmen. We were supposed to drill and train our "men." After the brass saw hilarious marching formations colliding, the Marines took over.

Our training at Lido Beach was the introduction to the LST and its uses as a medical evacuation ship. We had some exposure to gas warfare and endured unpleasant contacts with several chemical agents. Units shipped out at regular intervals on LSTs. We left on 10 March 1944.

As LST-507 was dropping off cargo and loading supplies in various English ports our medical unit was sent to Fowey for a week of intensive training on chemical warfare and general first aid. This all added up to very little preparation for an invasion that looked like it would produce major casualties.

When our medical unit reported back to LST-507, it was in Brixham and had loaded some 290 Army personnel. The tank deck held twenty-two DUKWs [amphibious trucks] with jeeps and trucks topside, all chained to the deck and fully fueled. Army troops were everywhere.

Loading occurred on 24 April 1944. We and two other LSTs sailed from Brixham on the afternoon of 27 April to join five LSTs coming from Plymouth. Only recently I found that our British escort had been warned about E-boats in the area, but the U.S. forces had not been given the correct radio channel to monitor. We sailed along in fatal ignorance.

General quarters rudely aroused us about 0130. I remember hearing gunfire and saying they had better watch where they were shooting or someone would get hurt. At 0203 I was stupidly trying to go topside to see what was going on and suddenly, *boom!* There was a horrendous noise accompanied by the sound of crunching metal and dust everywhere. The lights went out and I was thrust violently in the air to land on the steel deck on my knees, which became very sore immediately thereafter. Now I knew how getting torpedoed felt. But I'd been lucky.

The torpedo hit amidships starboard in the auxiliary engine room, knocking out all electric and water power. We sat and burned. A few casualties came into the wardroom for care and, since there was ample help, I checked below decks aft to be sure no one required medical attention there. All men in accessible areas had gone topside.

The tank deck was a different matter. As I opened the hatch, I found myself looking into a raging inferno which pushed me back. It was impossible to enter. The screams and cries of those many Army troops in there still haunt me. Navy regulations call for dogging the hatches to preserve the integrity of the ship, and that's what I did.

Until the fire got so hot we were forced to leave the ship at 0230, we watched the most spectacular fireworks ever. Gas cans and ammunition exploding and the enormous fire blazing only a few yards away are sights forever etched in my memory. Ship's company wore life jackets, but the medics and Army personnel had been issued inflatable belts. We were told only to release the snaps and squeeze the handles to inflate.

Climbing down a cargo net, I settled into the forty-four-degree water, gradually getting lower as the life belt rose up to my armpits. The soldiers that jumped or dove in with full packs did not do well. Most were found with their heads in the water and their feet in the air, top heavy from not putting the belts around their chests before inflating them. They had never received instructions in their correct usage.

I recall only brief moments of hearing motors, of putting a knee on a small boat ramp, and then awakening halfway up a Jacob's ladder. I was on the only American ship, LST-515, to rescue survivors. This was at dawn, about 0515. I had been in the water over two hours, fully dressed and insulated. Those that had stripped to swim, only God knows where they died. Drowning and hypothermia were the two major causes of death. I often wonder if many "dead" victims were really in a state of hibernation, and what would have happened had we been able to immerse them in warm tubs. But who ever heard of a tub on an LST in wartime? We couldn't even do a reliable physical exam under the circumstances.

Both dead and alive were taken to Portland. The dead went on to Brookwood Cemetery, near London, where they were buried individually. We got dry clothes courtesy of the American Red Cross, and then an exam at an Army field hospital in Sherborne. An Army physician, Dr. Ralph Greene, was there and later did the first American research on Exercise Tiger.

After a month's leave, all were reassigned and most boarded other LSTs for the invasion of Normandy. Others were given shore assignments. For me, Normandy was a piece of cake. LST-391 made one run carrying Rangers headquarters staff to Omaha Beach.

We took 125 injured from Utah Beach to England. The Army tent dispensary at the beachhead had done an excellent job with these men. Our supplies contained only about six 20-cc syringes with 1 1/2-inch needles. We gave 1 cc (20,000 U) of penicillin every three hours to each of the next twenty men with the same syringe and the same needle, but with no withdrawal of the plunger. After a brief boil, syringes and needles were reloaded. There was no other way to keep the schedule.

✛

CORPSMAN AT D-DAY

PhM3c Frank Feduik joined the Navy at age eighteen in 1943. After boot camp at Sampson, New York, he went for six weeks of training at the Hospital Corps school at Portsmouth, Virginia. He then received his assignment to the Philadelphia Naval Hospital, where he witnessed the tragic cost of war for the first time. Casualties of Guadalcanal filled the psychiatric ward, tied to their bunks and watched over by armed guards. "They were very young guys and they were completely gone. Their eyes seemed to be staring somewhere into space," he said.

Following a memorable Atlantic crossing on the *Queen Mary,* Feduik was assigned to LST-338, which landed on Omaha Beach. For the next twelve months, LST-338 ferried men and supplies back and forth from England to France, making over sixty trips across the English Channel and earning the title Workhorse of the Amphibious Fleet.

After Philadelphia, I went to New York and boarded the *Queen Mary* on Easter morning 1944. Believe it or not, it was so congested that I slept in the big empty swimming pool. Actually, I never got up topside, staying in the swimming pool for five days. They utilized all the space they could. We never even unpacked our seabags. You just laid your head back on it and slept. The *Queen Mary* traveled alone because it was so fast [over thirty knots] no sub could keep up with it.

Once I reached England I was assigned to the LST-338. It had just returned from Italy, where it had been in the invasion of Sicily. When I saw this thing, I said, "Oh, God, what is it? This can't be my ship. It's ugly." There was an old saying that if you were assigned to the amphibious fleet in the Navy, you had to have screwed up somewhere. I hadn't done anything wrong and I wondered why I had been assigned to this LST. I spent the rest of my overseas time on that ship.

LST-338 was the command ship for Flotilla 12, Group 36. Our skipper was an old mustang named [Darrell A.] Stratton. We left England on the fourth of June and the Channel was unbelievably rough. They said it was the worst storm of the century. It was just disaster. Nearly everyone got sick. I was just lucky; I never got seasick. I felt sorry for the troops. I thought, "These guys have to be unloaded into these LCVPs and go into battle? There's no way they can fight in this condition."

However, the invasion was postponed and we returned to port. We left again the following day and the weather was a lot calmer. I was on deck during the crossing. Boy, it was dark! We made sure we always had the English corvettes in sight because they protected us from submarines. Every LST also carried a big balloon to keep German planes from coming in low and strafing us. We thought it was a joke, because it was like announcing to the world, "Here we are under this big dirigible!" When we got close to the beach, the Germans began shooting at these balloons. We had been told that if we had to, we should cut the cable from the winch. So when they started shooting, everybody cut their balloons loose. You should have seen that bunch of balloons taking off from those LSTs.

One of my more distinctive memories was the battleships in action on D-Day, the *Arkansas* [BB-33] and the *Texas* [BB-35]. It was such a din! They were behind us as we were going in and the shells would sing their way right over the ship. Some of the targets, I would say, were eight and ten miles inland. Every once in a while you would hear or see a big explosion way inland and we knew they had hit an ammunition dump or something.

It was such a hectic thing, everybody firing this way, beach fire coming at you. They were firing at us from the pillboxes on the beach. You heard the shells whirring by and when you saw them hit the water . . . well, if you were in the wrong place, forget about it.

We did get hit by shrapnel every once in awhile. I was directly beneath one of the gun mounts trying to set up an aid station under gun number 4. As I was coming up the ladder, I heard a noise and then heard a fellow in the gun mount, say, "Round and round she goes and where she stops nobody knows." Evidently a piece of shrapnel had gotten into the gun mount and wound its way around until it exited. I couldn't imagine how cool he was.

On 8 June we got orders to unload our cargo on Omaha Beach. We didn't actually beach ourselves, instead using smaller LCTs to unload the LST. I was able to hitch a ride on one of the LCTs. On Omaha Beach there was chaos and confusion everywhere. I don't think we hit the right part of the beach. We saw a lot of people completely lost who didn't know where they were. I didn't see any Navy corpsmen or Navy aid stations, but I did see a lot of Army medics. They established their aid stations wherever they could. We saw bodies—some were our troops, some were theirs. I saw people with arms and legs missing, parts of bodies. You just couldn't understand it—guys who had not even made it to the beach, some of them impaled on iron rails that were in the water. It was complete mayhem.

After unloading our cargo, we filled our LST with wounded. We treated them mostly by applying tourniquets and giving morphine, after which we marked them with the time. This way you could tell when they were due for the next shot. I remember one soldier whose leg was missing. He had stepped on a mine on the beach. I gave him a morphine shot and told him he would be okay for a couple of hours. He sat up and looked at the stump. I don't know where he got the strength. He screamed, "I'm a farmer. What am I going to do?" I pushed him back and told him he would be okay. He was only twenty years old.

When we met the other ship we transferred the casualties by hand. If you can imagine two ships bobbing with all this stuff going on and wondering whether this guy is going to slip off the stretcher between the two ships. We went back to England that night. We went up the Thames River, loaded up with British troops, and went to Gold Beach. After that, we headed back to England.

We also made about a dozen runs to bring German prisoners back to England. We would load hundreds in the tank deck. They were well guarded by guys with machine guns standing on a parapet. These prisoners were tough, hardened soldiers. One trip was especially memorable. One of my best friends from home, Andy Banko, had gone into the Army. We had said that when the war was over we would tie on a jag and have a hell of a good time when we got back. After I got in the Navy, I didn't hear from him for about a year. And then I got a letter. He was over in Italy and he said something about going to take some mountain called Monte Cassino. I was elated that I had heard from him. I wrote back reminding him of how we would celebrate once the war was over.

Just after that we picked up a load of German prisoners and got a mail pickup in France. My letter to Andy had been returned, with Deceased stamped on the back. Killed in action.

One of my jobs was to make sure the lister bags had water for these troops, because we still had to treat them humanely. But to me, right then, the Germans weren't human. These prisoners were arrogant, very arrogant. I looked at them and thought, I'm giving you guys water and you just killed my buddy? I had no sympathy for them.

One of our strangest cargoes were railroad cars. We had rails welded onto the tank deck of the ship. We pulled up to the hard cobblestone ramps in English ports, built specifically for LSTs to beach themselves, and railroad engines and cars were wheeled right onto our ship. We also had special landing ramps in Cherbourg and Le Havre which had rails. We would go in and connect to these rails. The cars were then pulled by an engine right off our ship, as if it was part of a rail transportation system.

In December 1944, we loaded up with strange little tanks called Snow Weasels. The Germans had broken through our lines during the Battle of the Bulge and we had to get the Snow Weasels over there. We dashed alone across the Channel at night. There was always a red alert on the beach because you didn't know whether there were any German planes, even though the Luftwaffe was about through. The skipper hollered over the PA system, "Open up the doors and get those tanks off. I've got a bunch of French soldiers getting on and they're going to take them out of here. We gotta get off this beach." The French soldiers didn't know what to do. He kept hollering, "Let's go."

Since they didn't do anything I jumped into one of the first ones. Of course, I didn't know how to run a Snow Weasel. There were some controls, one for the left tread, one for the right tread. I just hit the button, started it, and away I went. I don't think I got a hundred yards up the beach when I ran out of fuel. At least I think I ran out of fuel. Well, everybody thought where I stopped must be the bivouac area where we were supposed to leave them, so everyone else stopped too. We came back to the ship and started laughing. We didn't know if anybody came and picked them up. It was funny things like this that made you laugh later on.

LST DOCTOR

Lt. Dale L. Groom, a native of Cleveland, had recently graduated from medical school and was interning at Northwestern University Hospital in Chicago. Because of the war, Groom's internship, normally a year, lasted only nine months. After reporting for active duty at Great Lakes, Illinois, Groom was ordered to Lido Beach, New York, for a month of training with his unit, Foxy-29. Lido Beach was then a staging base for units being deployed to Europe.

We got to Lido Beach in the dead of winter and it was cold. I didn't even know how to salute. They had two doctors team up and they gave us forty corpsmen. We were to train them on how to do IVs, give plasma, blood, morphine, epinephrine, and those sorts of things. Then they gave us officers Colt .45s and carbines to my enlisted men. Someone told me there were some three thousand personnel in Foxy-29 and the training was going on full blast when we got there.

After five or six weeks we were assigned to LST-293, which was in New York at the Brooklyn Navy Yard. I'd seen pictures of LSTs but had never seen one up close before. They gave me a nice cabin and I felt privileged. I thought I had made a good choice picking the Navy and not the Army.

We sailed right away and stopped at a Navy base in Rhode Island, where we picked up some equipment, and then went on to the Boston Navy Yard. From there we went to Halifax, where we joined a sixty-three-ship convoy, most of which were Liberty Ships and not many LSTs. We had an LCT on our deck.

Every day we watched the Liberty Ship on our port side. It had a dog on it and we used to enjoy watching that dog running around. And then, all of a sudden, in the middle of the North Atlantic, a U-boat came. It was broad daylight. When they saw that big LCT on our deck, they must have intended the torpedo for us. But they didn't realize that an LST has a shallow draft and is flat bottomed. So they didn't set the depth of the fish just right and it hit our propeller before going into the Liberty Ship about three seconds later.

There was a hell of an explosion. We were really aghast. I don't remember where I was except when it hit us, it really jarred things. I went up on deck and saw the Liberty Ship just broken in two. There were no survivors.

We also had quite a storm out there that lasted about three days which broke up quite a bit of Navy furniture. In March the North Atlantic is treacherous. The old salts told me it is the worst month of the year, and we really hit it. Having flat bottoms, LSTs didn't ride well in a storm. We had forty-foot seas that looked like mountains to us. Not having a keel, you would get on top and then slide sideways. And that was rather sickening.

I estimate that 95 percent of our crew were sick and I couldn't do a damn thing for them. Even all the old salts were in their sacks. I think I had something like Dramamine, but it wasn't very effective. I did pretty well. My only trouble was that the galley was closed and I had to scrounge up something to eat.

We went around Northern Ireland and down through the Irish Sea. After going around Lands End and Penzance, we put in at Falmouth in Cornwall. After going up the river and dumping our LCT, our LST then went in for repairs, and I never saw or heard of it after that. Our medical unit left the ship and we were sent to Fowey, where we stayed about a week. It was a beautiful Cornish village with a lovely harbor.

We then went to Weymouth and were assigned to two old LSTs. That's when my friend Dr. [Henry B.] Landaal and I split up. He took half the men and I took the other half. He went to LST-314 and I went to 357. We had been together for years, all through medical school, and were close friends.

We got to Weymouth near the end of April and were there at least five or six weeks in the harbor. Every night about midnight or one o'clock, German aircraft came over and we went to general quarters. They dropped mines in the harbor but never hit us. They did some extensive damage ashore during May and wiped out whole city blocks. But I think most of the planes were going to London or Southampton. I guess they just dropped a few on us on the way. But we were at general quarters every night and this was a very stressful experience. This went on for six weeks there in Weymouth. I had to send two of my men ashore who just couldn't take it. All of us were pretty stressed out.

After being there a month or so and being bombed almost every night, we heard some dignitaries were to visit us. Everyone turned to and scrubbed up this old ship and we were proud of her.

We were surprised when our visitor turned out to be the king. When he came on May 25th, I think we were a hundred yards or so offshore, anchored in the harbor. He came in a little boat, and we piped him over the side with his retinue of palace guards and a few British admirals. He was an affable sort of guy and went through the whole ship—up and down the ladders, the tank deck, and everywhere. But he didn't make a speech. He just said a little thing in parting. On behalf of his countrymen, he thanked us for our contribution in the great cause. I guess kings don't give speeches.

Right after that things really got busy. Army vehicles came aboard and I got three hundred stretchers and all kinds of plasma, blood, and medical supplies. I had my stock of things in a space not large enough to accommodate a patient.

I don't remember where we stored all the stretchers. We couldn't store them on the tank deck because it was filled with Army vehicles, and then all the Army troops came aboard. I don't know how many hundred there were. I was told an LST could accommodate 750 troops and their vehicles. And those guys slept and ate in their vehicles.

The day before we left, we were told the assault troops would have our grub—steaks—for dinner. And they would sleep in our bunks at night. And that was natural, since the whole Navy crew was on watch. After we were loaded, they sealed the ship. You couldn't go ashore; no one could come aboard. We were sealed for several days. This was about June 1st, right after the king's visit. They sent all the ship's papers, logs, and personnel records ashore so they would have them in case anything happened. Everyone knew where we were going.

I was the only physician aboard and had twenty corpsmen. Just before we left, the Army gave me one doctor and two additional corpsmen, and I think they were in a beach unit, but the doctor wasn't part of my company at all.

On June 4th we started out in a whole procession, proceeding east down the coast. The 314 was the first LST. Mine, the 357, was the second, and we had a minesweeper on each side and ahead. It was overcast and drizzly. I guess the order went out that D-Day would be postponed, so we went back.

The next day, the 5th, we started out in the same procession, east along the coast for about an hour or two before turning south. It wasn't anything like what we had been through in the Atlantic, and it wasn't as rough as it had been when we had first started out on the 4th. We knew we weren't turning back again. It was during that time the skipper unsealed his books with the official orders. All of us knew for the first time where we were going to land. It wasn't where everyone assumed, where the Channel was narrowest at Dover, but rather where it was a hundred miles across. I was in the cabin when he opened the orders.

I had a very good relationship with the skipper, James J. MacLeod. Just the two of us looked at this book and it was the most amazing thing I ever saw. It had strip pictures of the beach! I asked the skipper how in hell they could have gotten those pictures. I don't know whether he assumed or actually knew, but he told me that commandos swam in and took pictures of the beach. If one of those books had gotten out, the whole invasion would have been a bust. How that information was collected, printed, and distributed without one break in security . . . It was one of the best-kept secrets in history.

By dusk we were well under way. We had a minesweeper on each side and one or two British destroyers as escorts. We were leading a long procession but didn't know how many were behind us. Some of them came from Portsmouth, some from Southampton, and we all joined somewhere out there in the Channel. It was a hell of a long procession. We were all at general quarters and expecting to be attacked. We thought about submarines and E-boats. We also thought about the Luftwaffe. But we didn't have one bit of interference on the whole trip.

When we arrived off Omaha Beach around midnight, we certainly achieved some element of surprise. It was dark, but you could see that a lot of it was afire. Our bombers were overhead bombing the hell out of it, and you could see for miles.

I don't think anyone got any sleep that night. I don't imagine the Army troops slept much, knowing what was in store for them. When the sun came out the next morning, it looked like a good omen. We could see our bombers and our paratroopers, a few of them. Of course, most of them had gone in way inland.

All during the morning we were aware that the battleship *Texas* (BB-35) and the cruiser *Augusta* (CA-31) were out there with us. They were lobbing shells out of those huge guns and making a hell of a noise. I asked the skipper where they were shooting. He said they operated on a grid and they had someone way back there radioing where the shells were hitting.

And then at 6:00 all the bombing stopped. H-hour was at 6:30. Even before 6:00 we began unloading our DUKWs; some of them foundered. We started loading up our rhino barge and putting our DUKWs out and launching our LCVPs. We had six of them; each could carry about thirty men. All of these were circling our ship and waiting to go in. And then, on some signal, they all headed in.

A couple of our officers went in on our LCVPs, and all of them came back. Four or five of our corpsmen also went in, but most of them were with me, waiting to receive casualties.

We cruised up and down the beach trying to get all we could and got about a dozen casualties that day, brought out in small boats and hoisted over the side in slings. Before evening we were headed back to England with those twelve. And I didn't lose any of them.

When we got back to Weymouth we loaded up again on the evening of June 7th and started out for France again on June 8th. On this second trip, the E-boats were waiting for us. The log says it was about one o'clock in the morning. Our convoy had just five LSTs and one Canadian destroyer escort. Since we had been the first in on the 6th, we now were the first [out] for the second trip. This attack occurred on June 9th. We were all at general quarters but never heard them coming. Later we were told that they were painted black.

There were terrific explosions. The decks were afire and these poor people were jumping off. It was a terrible sight. I was with the skipper and I said, "For God's sake, let's stop and pick them up." They were there in the water screaming. He said no, we couldn't do that. The Navy forbade it. If we stopped then *we* went down, and he was right. But it was the most traumatic experience of my Navy career.

I knew some of my men and my friend Landaal were there. They only had two LCVPs on the 314, having lost the rest. Dr. Landaal gave his place in one of those to the injured and said he would take his chances in his life preserver. He went over the side and doubtless died of hypothermia.

The next morning the Canadian destroyer escort that had escorted us returned and pulled a few survivors from the water and several bodies. Dr. Landaal's body was recovered and sent back to the States. Captain [George J.] Szabo, the executive officer, later told me they'd been able to launch a raft and he'd gotten on it with some of the others. The two LCVPs were mainly loaded with the injured. He said the flaming ship went down in twenty minutes after being hit by three torpedoes. I don't think those Army troops had a chance in hell. If they had any life vests, I never saw them. They must have all died.

We continued on at ten knots and got there the next morning. The crossing took from twelve to fifteen hours. We returned to the transport area but were not permitted to beach. It was still terrible on the beach. Small-arms fire was continuous there for three days. We cruised up and down the beach trying to get all the casualties we could and didn't stay in one place. LCTs, LCIs, and all kinds of small boats brought huge loads of them to us. They married to us, ramp to ramp, and as soon as we took those aboard, we started back to England.

On this second trip I lost 1 out of 220. I remember because one of the ship's line officers' jobs was to count the casualties so it could go into the ship's log. We were so damn busy I couldn't observe much except to triage and treat the casualties. The officers' ward room was my operating room. You have to give credit to the Army and Navy beach units for having done some first aid. They had applied tourniquets and improvised some splints, given morphine injections.

I was both the triage and treatment officer. We went a long time without sleeping or eating, I'll say that. I saw missing limbs but didn't have to do any amputations. And I didn't want to. If you stopped hemorrhage and debrided the wounds, you couldn't say whether an arm or leg couldn't be preserved. I refused to amputate a limb when I thought there might be some chance of saving it.

My treatment role was mainly debridement, suturing, and directing all the life support with plasma and blood. The main thing was to preserve life by preserving blood pressure. The corpsmen had to monitor the wounded day and night, giving them fluids. Without that, I'm sure I would have lost quite a lot of them.

I have often been asked how much of my medical education I got to use, and my answer to that is damned little. I didn't have much equipment. We did have Thomas splints, but I didn't have X-rays. I was just doing glorified first aid.

On this second trip we had some German POWs. I remember them because they were yelling, "*Schmertz, schmertz!*" I didn't know what the hell that was. One of my corpsmen told me it was the German word for *pain.* I don't recall how many of the wounded were German. I was only interested in classifying them according to their injuries.

I got some of the crew to use my camera. I had a gentleman's agreement with the skipper. I told him I had the camera and I knew it was against regulations, but I wanted to get some pictures. The agreement was that if we went down, it wouldn't make any difference, and if we didn't go down and we were captured, the camera and all the pictures would go over the side.

Anyway, we got back to Weymouth with the 220 casualties. We had to load them on an LCT because the dock was so busy. I was just exhausted.

I went back to France for a total of five trips. On the third trip we had fewer than the 220 casualties of the second. And we got hardly any on the fourth. By the fifth trip we may not have had any. By that time C-47s were using the improvised runway they'd built above the cliff [at Omaha]. We could see them. They had the advantage of taking their casualties to hospitals way back in England, whereas we could only get them to hospitals near the coast.

This whole Foxy-29 program was a bridge between battlefield first aid and the definitive care with all the staff and equipment back in the big hospitals. Providing this bridge was an innovation of Navy medicine. The planners knew there would be untold numbers of casualties immediately, and you couldn't handle those with hospital ships. Our role was not to provide definitive care but to sustain life and get the casualties back in the best shape we could. That couldn't be done in every invasion, but with England only a hundred miles away, this type of operation was feasible.

NURSES AT NETLEY

One of the hospitals in southern England designated to care for the casualties of the D-day invasion was Navy Base Hospital Number 12. Staffed by Navy medical personnel, the facility occupied the Royal

Victoria Hospital at Netley, five miles from the major Channel port of Southampton. In the months leading up to D-Day, Base Hospital Number 12 was in the vortex of invasion preparations. As Allied fighters and bombers flew overhead on their way to France, the staff made ready to treat unknown numbers of casualties resulting from the invasion. These are the reminiscences of two Navy nurses, themselves veterans of D-Day.

Helen Pavlovsky [Ramsey] joined the Navy in the spring of 1943 and went to England in February of the following year as part of the medical unit designated SNAG-56.[4]

Sara Marcum [Kelley] was a ward nurse originally from rural Kentucky. After graduating from nursing school in January 1943, she joined the Navy Nurse Corps. She served at the National Naval Medical Center in Bethesda, Maryland, for a year, after which she too went to England.

Helen Ramsey

The Army had been at the Netley Hospital before we arrived. I think they took over from the British, and then we came in and took over from them. I don't think the Army was there for any length of time, because they weren't ready for us. The Royal Victoria Hospital at Netley had been built during the Victorian era, and it was a very cold monstrosity. The wards were huge. I have no idea how many beds there were in a ward. There was a fireplace at either end, which made the place terribly cold and damp and certainly not conducive to treating patients.

The Seabees came over and remodeled the whole thing to make it usable. They converted those wood-burning fireplaces—actually wood was at a premium so they burned a kind of coke—to gas and that kept us warmer.

Sara Kelley

The grounds outside the buildings were beautiful, with wonderful surroundings and the view of the water. Unfortunately, the hospital was not in great condition. The plumbing was atrocious. From the bathtubs and the sinks, the water drained into a trough that went halfway around the

---

4. SNAG stood for Special Naval Advance Group.

room before it finally went into a pipe and out. Each room had about thirty or thirty-five beds, but the rooms weren't connected, which is not very efficient when it comes to nursing, because you would have to go out into the main corridor and then around into the room. Usually you were just assigned to one room, and then you would help out someplace else if you weren't busy.

Luckily, the Seabees came and put in showers. They also did some work on the nurses' quarters, so, unlike the Army nurses, who had to live in tents, we were able to live inside.

Helen Ramsey

We knew the ships were gathering for the invasion. It seems to me it took at least a week for all the ships to gather just outside our hospital in Southampton Water [the harbor]. We could go outside and sit on the waterfront and watch. One day it seemed like the whole area was full of ships, and the next morning there was not a single one. We knew the invasion was beginning. We were on alert; we could not leave and were on duty twenty-four hours a day. We didn't know what we were waiting for.

And then the casualties came. It took about three or four days after the invasion. I was an operating-room supervisor. We had two operating-room theaters, one upstairs and one downstairs. At first we started out with one and then we required two, because we just couldn't handle all the casualties in one theater. When I say theater, I mean several rooms, each with its own surgeon, nurse, and corpsman. It was one big unit. I was in charge of the one downstairs.

The first casualties came into my operating room. I remember how busy we were and how they kept coming and coming and we had no place to put them. We put them out in the halls and everywhere. We were only there as a receiving hospital. We received the casualties, took care of them, removed the bullets and shrapnel, did the debridement, cleaned them up, poured penicillin and sulfa into the wounds, and wrapped them up. Then we sent them inland to the Army or to British hospitals inland, or by air to the United States, especially if they were bad burn patients. So we didn't keep them very long.

The operating-room nurses would pitch in and help the doctors do debridements and remove bullets. I still have the first bullet I removed myself and have managed to keep it for many years.

Anyway, we were busy and we never thought about food or sleep or anything else. The doctors as well as the nurses and corpsmen were taking care of patients. We did not sleep for the first twenty-four hours, and then finally sleep had to be rationed because no one would leave their work. The captain issued an order letting certain ones go and get some sleep. And then when they came back others would go. Our food was brought to us in surgery. We lived on sandwiches and coffee for a long time. When we had a minute, we would grab a bite. As the casualty load lightened, things got back to a decent pace.

I also got to use penicillin for the first time. We had little tin cans that looked like salt shakers. They contained a mixture of penicillin and, I'm sure, sulfathiazole, and we would just use them like salt shakers and sprinkle it into the wounds. And I've read since that it was that mixture of sulfa and penicillin used in those early days that saved many a limb and kept infections down to almost zero. They were both miracle drugs. Of course, we also gave penicillin intravenously.

We received casualties fairly steadily, but not at the rate we did at the beginning. As soon as the troops landed on the beaches and went farther inland, the Army went right in and set up their field hospitals, so they could do a lot of the immediate work that we were having to do at the beginning. And that took a load off of us.

Sara Kelley

All types of ships brought the casualties from Normandy. The ships landed in Southampton because our pier could only handle small boats. They brought them by ambulance from Southampton, which was five miles away.

There was a railroad track right behind the hospital. We kept the patients for twenty-four to forty-eight hours, and as soon as they could be moved, they were put on this hospital train and sent to the north part of England and we got ready for some more. We treated mostly Army personnel, but there were also a few Navy men as well. I remember a lot of the casualties were suffering from shell shock. Some of them didn't know who we were. They thought we were Germans and they wouldn't tell us anything except their names and serial numbers. They were classified as mentally ill. Some of them were just farm boys and the shock of war was just too much for them.

TEN

Uncommon Duty

During World War II, not every member of the Navy Medical Department served overseas, aboard ship, or in the many naval hospitals and clinics scattered throughout the continental United States. A few personnel found themselves in very unusual roles. Dr. Sam Gibson, fresh out of medical school, worked closely with the civilian sector seeking better ways of providing blood and blood substitutes to far-flung battlefields where the need was greatest. Dr. Howard Bruenn joined the Navy as a reservist and, due to peculiar circumstances, became President Roosevelt's personal cardiologist. Samuel Bookatz, a young artist from Cleveland, put on a Navy uniform to document on canvas the Navy Medical Department's contributions to the war effort. His duty station was the White House.

SHOCK KILLERS

One of the lingering images of the World War II battlefield is that of a corpsman or medic crouched beside his wounded patient, his outstretched hand gripping a glass bottle. From the bottle flowed a liquid that brought many a soldier or Marine back from the threshold of death. During the early days of the war, that fluid was plasma. Later it was serum albumin.

In the 1930s researchers had perfected the centrifuge technique to separate blood into its components, discovering in the process that plasma, blood's liquid component minus the red cells, could restore blood volume and counteract shock. They had found that freeze-dried plasma could be stored for up to three years, then reconstituted with sterile water and infused into a shock victim with very positive results.

As the U.S. entered World War II, plasma became the treatment of choice on the battlefield, even though it had its limitations. A frontline corpsman loaded down with all his gear could not carry the fragile bottles into combat. Something else was needed and, even before Pearl Harbor, Dr. Edwin Cohn, a gifted Harvard biochemist, began a program to develop a more effective blood substitute.

> In the summer of 1940, Dr. Sam T. Gibson began an internship at the prestigious Peter Bent Brigham Hospital in Boston. As the nation readied itself for war, he obtained a commission as a lieutenant (jg) in the Navy Medical Corps. He spent the war years working with Dr. Cohn on serum albumin, first as a researcher in its development, later in ensuring its purity.

I went on active duty in October of '41. Dr. Edwin Cohn had been working on his plasma fractionation program and wanted to test it on patients. I think he asked the Navy for two jaygees to be assigned to his lab at Harvard. They picked Dr. Lorande Woodruff and me. Dr. Woodruff, who also became my roommate, was a surgical intern from Yale.

Dr. Cohn's program was premised on his idea that albumin would be more desirable than plasma. Albumin was responsible for the osmotic effect of plasma and was the protein that drew most of the fluid from surrounding tissues into the bloodstream when it was administered for shock.

When an individual lost a large volume of blood and went into shock, the blood vessels collapsed. The infusion of plasma to increase blood volume counteracted this. Albumin did the same thing, because the osmotic effect drew fluid from the surrounding tissues and kept the blood vessels open.

To process a unit of albumin, Dr. Cohn took a batch of plasma and added 5 percent ethanol. That precipitated, or separated out, Fraction I. He then adjusted the chemical milieu by adding more alcohol and separated Fractions II, III, IV, and V. Albumin was the fifth fraction.

He prepared the albumin in a 25-percent solution so that 100 ml [milliliters] of 25-percent albumin—one unit—produced the same effect as a 500-ml bottle of plasma. A corpsman then could carry a lot more albumin and get the same effect as a larger volume of plasma—in fact, five times more. The albumin was also in solution, whereas the plasma was a powder and required a bottle of sterile water to reconstitute it. Therefore, a bottle of albumin occupied less space than plasma.

Albumin was really called normal serum albumin human, because they were also working on normal serum albumin bovine. The aim of the latter was to have the bovine source and eliminate the need for human donors.

As I said, Dr. Woodruff and I started in October. We contacted the emergency rooms at Boston City Hospital, Massachusetts General, Beth Israel, and Peter Bent Brigham. We got an apartment and left our phone numbers with the emergency rooms so we would be called whenever they had a patient in shock. When they called us we took some albumin to the hospital, and, after administering it, we'd measure blood pressure and hemoglobin response.

The night of December 6th, 1941, Dr. Woodruff and I had gone to a party and got terrific hangovers. The next morning we went to Dr. Cohn's house for Sunday brunch, the last thing in the world we wanted to do. For an hour I sipped a small glass of vermouth. Neither one of us ate very much that day.

I then took Lorrie back to the apartment so he could go to bed. After I had left him, I turned on the radio in the car, and that was my introduction to Pearl Harbor. This was about three or four o'clock in the afternoon. I stopped at the corner drugstore, called Lorrie, and said, "Wake up. We're at war!" Then I went out on a previously planned date.

Right after Pearl Harbor the professor of surgery at the University of Pennsylvania, Dr. Isidor Ravdin, took a bag full of albumin units and flew to Hawaii to treat the survivors of the attack. When he came back he gave a very glowing report of albumin's benefits to the burn victims.

It was on the basis of this report and on the basis of eighty cases we had tested, from October to January, that the National Research Council approved albumin in January 1942.

Then there was a question of getting contracts for commercial preparation. There were about seven companies that expressed an interest in it and were eventually approved. They had to set up their labs under Cohn's supervision, then accumulate the plasma, fractionate it, and run it through all the tests. As the commercial fractionators—Armour, Sharpe and Dohme, Hyland, Cutter, and three more companies—activated the contracts, we tested a sample from every lot. All this took time, so there wasn't a lot of serum albumin all during '42, and that's why it wasn't used until '43. All the commercial fractionators had to come to Cohn's lab to be trained. Cohn kept a hand in the testing at the chemical end for consistency and so forth.

My role in all this began as one of the original experimenters with serum albumin but then changed. I helped ensure that each lot produced came up to Dr. Cohn's standards. Dr. Lloyd Newhouser was doing the same thing at the Naval Medical School in Bethesda. In August of '43 Newhouser needed someone else, and so I transferred from Boston to his lab. At Bethesda, Comdr. Mary Sproul and I did the testing.

The albumin was packaged in double-ended bottles with stoppers at either end. A tin can about four inches high and about an inch and a half in diameter enclosed each bottle and the apparatus for the albumin's administration. You opened the can with the attached metal key, removed the bottle of albumin, and then inserted the air-filter needle through the top rubber stopper to provide an airway. Then you inserted the needle of the intravenous set—which included rubber tubing, a filter, and an intravenous needle—through the rubber stopper at the opposite end. Then you were ready to insert the needle into the patient's vein and begin administering the albumin.

By November of 1944 whole blood began appearing at the front, in time for the Leyte campaign. Donated just hours before, it was packed in ice and shipped by air from San Francisco to Hawaii. After the ice was replenished, Navy transport planes rushed cases of the blood to Guam, where it was re-iced and sent on to the battlefield. As corpsmen and doctors administered the precious fluid, they found patient response to whole blood even more dramatic than with plasma or albumin, neither of which contained oxygen-carrying red cells. At Iwo Jima, corpsman Stanley Dabrowski noted the difference: "You would get color, pink lips again rather than purple."

Although whole blood augmented plasma and albumin for the war's last campaigns, it never wholly replaced the bottles of those miracle fluids better suited for front-line conditions.

FDR'S CARDIOLOGIST

In March 1944, the Allies had already seized the offensive both in the Pacific and in Europe. The opening days of the month saw U.S. troops hitting the beaches of the Admiralty Islands as they drew ever closer to Japan.

On 3 March American B-17s commenced daytime bombing of Berlin, picking up where the Royal Air Force had left off pummeling the German capital by night. On the eastern front, American-supplied Soviet troops had not merely blunted the Nazi invasion of the motherland; they were now annihilating entire German armies.

In Washington, President Franklin D. Roosevelt neared the end of an unprecedented third term in office. As pundits speculated on whether he might make a bid for a fourth term, it became increasingly evident that the stresses of nearly twelve years in that office had taken their toll. The president's repeated bouts with "flu" and "bronchitis" were newsworthy, yet White House physician and surgeon general of the Navy Vice Adm. Ross T. McIntire reassured the public that their president was basically in sound health for a man his age. Those close to Roosevelt—family and White House intimates—knew better.

On 27 March, McIntire was concerned enough to send the president to the National Naval Medical Center in Bethesda, Maryland, for a thorough examination. There, Lt. Comdr. Howard G. Bruenn, a naval reservist on active duty as cardiology consultant, found the chief executive suffering from hypertension, hypertensive cardiac disease, and acute bronchitis.

The following day Bruenn, under McIntire's orders not to discuss Roosevelt's health with anyone, reported the shocking facts to the admiral. From that day until the president's death some thirteen months later, it was Lieutenant Commander Bruenn, not Vice Admiral McIntire, who literally had his finger on the pulse.

Bruenn traveled everywhere with the president—to Hawaii for a meeting with Pacific commanders Gen. Douglas MacArthur and Adm. Chester Nimitz; to Quebec for a strategy session with British prime minister Winston Churchill; through yet another grueling presidential campaign; to Yalta for a fateful conference with Churchill and Stalin, and finally to Warm Springs, Georgia.

In 1970, following a twenty-five-year self-imposed silence, Howard Bruenn wrote his clinical recollections of Roosevelt's last year, based on personal notes.[1] FDR's medical history had mysteriously disappeared. Bruenn was convinced, as was the Roosevelt family, that the time had come to end years of speculation and rumor and set the record straight. Twenty years after that article appeared, Dr. Bruenn had additional memories of the most unforgettable year of his life.

My new job was something I had been trained for. I had my own office at Bethesda and saw people only by appointment, referred from various areas in the naval district. Officers who were eligible for promotion were seen in the Naval Dispensary in Washington. If there was a cardiac or vascular problem they were sent to me. I was on my own. I had my own staff—technicians, secretaries, and so forth.

I found Dr. McIntire very pleasant and friendly. When he first called me about the president, he said, "I'd like to have you take a look at him."

The initial thing that brought me into the picture was Anna [Anna Roosevelt Boettiger, FDR's daughter]. She put the pressure on McIntire to find out what was going on because the president was not himself. I was very shocked by the president's condition. He was thought to have had an upper respiratory infection and had not quite regained his strength.

When I went over him and I found that he was in acute congestive

---

1. Bruenn, "Clinical Notes on the Illness and Death of President Franklin D. Roosevelt," 579.

heart failure, that put a different aspect on the whole situation. Dr. McIntire asked me to write out what I thought should be done, which I did. When I gave him my recommendations for bed rest, diet, and so on, he said, "You can't do that. This is the president of the United States!"

He summoned the honorary Navy medical consultants. Among them were [Dr. James E.] Paullin, who was the president of the AMA [American Medical Association] at the time, and Dr. [Frank H.] Lahey from Boston. We sat around a table and I showed the assembled doctors the X-rays, electrocardiograms, blood-pressure readings, and results of the physical exam. They asked me what I thought we should do. I said that we had to digitalize him and follow the above procedures. They thought that was all too drastic and extensive.

They went to see the president the next morning and examined him. When they came back they agreed that I could go ahead with the digitalization. I digitalized the president, and in about a week or ten days the results were spectacular. His lungs, which initially had been congested and with a small amount of fluid, were now clear. His heart, which was enlarged, had diminished in size. His coughing had stopped and he was sleeping soundly at night. Dr. McIntire said, "If you have rapport with the president, this is now your problem." And that's how the whole thing got started.

Obviously enough, I was very much impressed and a little apprehensive about my new responsibility. But the president was such a nice person that we had no problem. He became another patient. They gave me a car, and I would go and see him four or five times a week at the White House in the morning and then go back to work at the hospital. Taking care of the president was so-called temporary additional duty. And, of course, I went with him on his trips.

The question of what happened to the president's medical records is one of the strangest things. When I'd come back from seeing him at the White House, I would go to Dr. [John] Harper's or [Robert] Duncan's office and they would give me the chart and I would write a note for that day concerning what I'd found, return it to the administrative office, and then it would go back in the safe.[2] After I wrote the final note, I never saw it again, never saw it.

---

2. Capt. John Harper was commanding officer of the National Naval Medical Center during World War II. Capt. Robert Duncan was the executive officer.

Thank goodness the president did very well, although the pressures were tremendous. You see, the president *was* the government. He was his own secretary of the treasury, his own secretary of state. He was running the works, including the war. On the other hand, he would sleep like a baby on a train, on a ship, on a plane. He had the ability to push problems in the background and really get an adequate night's rest. And that was very helpful.

To reduce his hypertension, we tried to cut down on his weight, and to reduce stress, be sure he got a good night's sleep, cut down on salt— the usual things. But there were no medications for hypertension; there was nothing directly available to control it. In his diet, the main thing we eliminated was quantity and calories.

Dr. McIntire was a nose and throat doctor, and he concerned himself with the president's voice. He wanted to be sure he had a good speaking voice. He did that using sprays.

The president had had some significant medical problems in the past. He had developed a profound anemia about 1938 or 1939. And the polio was an extraordinary thing. He was essentially paralyzed from the hips down and could only support himself with braces. But there was an understanding even before I came. No picture was ever taken of him standing. He was always behind a desk. But it left him with very poor development of the leg muscles. They had just wasted away. But he did have tremendous shoulders and chest. In fact, he weighed something like 185 to 190 pounds.

Taking weight off made it easier on his heart, easier on the blood pressure, easier on everything. Unfortunately some of it came off his face, and he began to look haggard. And then we had a job trying to get him to eat again. He was so pleased with his weight loss, we were forced to tempt him to eat.

Interestingly, he never asked me a question about the medications I was giving him, what his blood pressure was, nothing. He was not interested. He had a job to do and the hell with everything else. I remember when the pressure was put on him to run for the fourth term. All those people around him depended on the president exclusively for their jobs, for their reputations, everything. I'm not only talking about the secretaries, but such people as Steve Early, the press secretary, everybody. The president was the center pole, no question about it. [Robert E.] Hannigan, who was then chairman of the Democratic National Committee, wanted him to run. They all wanted him to run. And he wasn't particularly anxious to do so. It took a certain amount of persuasion to convince him. It wasn't an "I want to be president for another four years" sort of thing.

The state of heart failure I found him in in March 1944 was mainly due to the high blood pressure. From what I remember from his chart, it had first been detected at least several years before I saw him. And then the cardiograms showed that he had underlying coronary disease.

He never complained of any chest pain except on one occasion, when he gave a speech at Bremerton, Washington, on the fantail of a destroyer.[3] He kept on with the speech and came below and said, "I had a severe pain!" We stripped him down in the cabin of the ship, took a cardiogram, some blood and so forth, and fortunately it was a transient episode, a so-called angina, not a myocardial infarction. But that was really a very disturbing situation. That was the first time under my observation that he had something like this. He had denied any pain before. But this was proof positive that he had coronary disease.

One of the first trips the president took for rest and recuperation after I came on was the one he took to Hobcaw, Bernard Baruch's estate in South Carolina. All his trips followed the same type of pattern. We would all be told to appear in the basement of the Bureau of Printing and Engraving, where a special train came in. We were assigned our cars, berths, and so forth. We would leave in the middle of the night about half past twelve or one o'clock. Once we got where we were going, we were assigned bedrooms. I would see the president every morning, examine him, and then I might go down to the pool if we were at Warm Springs. But I was always on call. The Secret Service knew where I was all the time.

Life went on very casually. Guests would sometimes drop in for dinner. The president was really a master of the situation at the table. He smoked his Camel cigarettes, had his martini before dinner. He would go for boat rides, sleep late in the morning, perhaps take a nap in the afternoon. Every day a bag would come in from the White House with the mail and all the papers would be signed. That took about half an hour or so and that was all the business that was done.

---

3. FDR made this speech on 12 August 1944 at the Bremerton Navy Yard, Washington, returning from his Hawaii consultations with Nimitz and MacArthur.

It was on his trip to Hawaii to confer with MacArthur and Nimitz that he was nominated for his fourth term. He was nominated while the train was in the yards in Chicago and accepted the nomination in a railroad car. Anna and the photographers were taking pictures. He was up at one end of the car and we were sitting in the back. As one of the naval photographers took a picture of the president, they also caught me. I was leaning over. That's the first picture in which I appeared. It was this picture that was published in *Life* magazine. The doctors at my hospital—Presbyterian—recognized me and were aware of what was going on. This was the first they knew of my role. I had been warned to keep my mouth shut because wherever I might be, the president might be there too and they didn't want any unnecessary knowledge being spread around.

Should he or should he not have run for the fourth term? I must say, in all honesty, if I had been asked what my opinion or judgment was, I would have been greatly swayed by the circumstances. Here we were in the middle of a great war which had been conducted, fortunately or unfortunately, on an almost personal basis between Stalin, Churchill, and Roosevelt. Roosevelt had a personal relationship with Churchill and Stalin and I thought that was damn important.

I made very little preparation for the trip to Yalta, because I was just a passenger. I was told to appear at the train site. We went down to Norfolk, boarded the ship [USS *Quincy* (CA-71)]; it was a very pleasant journey. We got to Malta and then had a succession of people coming in to see the president, including all the commanding officers of the British Admiralty who were in the Mediterranean. It was quite a party. We took off at night from Malta to fly to Russia—the Crimea.

The president's bed was perpendicular to the plane's axis. It was a big, wide bed. But he refused to have a safety belt. We were afraid that if there was a sudden stop or something, he would be tossed right out of the bed. [Michael F.] Reilly, chief of the White House Secret Service detail, and the rest of us talked it over before we took off and decided that when all the lights were out, I would creep in and position myself on one side of the bed so that if he fell out of bed he'd fall on me. We took off without any problems. The next morning the president said, "It's lucky I recognized you as you came in."

It was quite a hair-raising flight. We had a lot of people going to Yalta—from the State Department, from the chiefs of staff. We must have had a hundred or more. The president's plane took only twelve people. Anna Roosevelt, Admiral [William D.] Leahy, Rear Adm. Wilson Brown, the president's naval aid, and Maj. Gen. Edwin M. Watson were aboard. So were [James F.] Byrnes, Secretary of State [Edward R., Jr.] Stettinius, and the chiefs of staff. We had to fly over Greece, which was then occupied by the Nazis. Everyone was anxious to get on that plane because it was the only one with a fighter escort.

It was not a very nice day when we landed in the Crimea. It was cold and rainy. But they had a guard of honor. [Soviet foreign minister] Vyacheslav Molotov was there; Stalin wasn't, but a couple of other fairly high dignitaries were. They had a few refreshments for us. Yalta was about a five- or six-hour ride by car, and the roads weren't magnificent. The Germans had been there, and it was pretty desolate. It was in February, too, and there was a wintry landscape with devastated houses.

Churchill had written a note to the effect that if you had looked far and wide, you couldn't have chosen a worse climatic place than Yalta. They found that their palace had a lot of vermin. Lavadia Palace, where we stayed, had already been cleaned up by a party of our naval personnel, who'd made it habitable. The Germans had taken all the metal—all the brass knobs had been taken off—it was pretty bare, but clean.

They took good care of us. They would bring the food to us from God knows where. There certainly wasn't much around that place.

When Stalin came to Lavadia Palace for the conference, that was a performance. He and his party were staying a couple of miles away. Soviet troops lined the route. When he got to our place, he got out of the car, and four husky Russians surrounded him as they marched in. There were machine guns all around; he wasn't taking any chances. Stalin was relatively short and broad and a bit brusque. But he was impressive.

Yalta was very stressful for the president. The British were whipsawing him. [Foreign secretary Anthony] Eden would see him in the morning, Churchill in the afternoon. And then there was the conference at night. There was no rest for the poor man.

Roosevelt acted almost as a mediator between Churchill and Stalin. Those two just couldn't get along. He maintained good relationships with both men, until we got back home and the Russians began monkeying around with Poland. Then the president got very upset and wrote a letter to Stalin protesting that this was not what had been agreed upon. But then he never saw Stalin again.

Roosevelt was a very stubborn man, in his own way. He saw the possibilities, and they were not satisfactory—fighting over Berlin or over Poland. It had been agreed that Poland was going to be a democratic nation with the government in exile included. The Russians just turned it around and put their own people in. The president tried the best he could to get the Polish government in exile in London back into Poland, but it was no go.

Prior to the Yalta trip, there was no great change in the president's health. There were a few times when I really got worried about him. He had an attack of gallbladder colic down at Baruch's place. I'm no surgeon, but with a few simple things the episode subsided, and that was that. When we got back, we took an X-ray that showed stones in his gallbladder.

But there were one or two situations that were of some concern. He had seen a movie about Woodrow Wilson and the League of Nations, in which Wilson really got pummeled. The president said, "By God, that's not going to happen to me!" And his blood pressure was very high that night. Then it came down the next morning.

Another time in Yalta, they were having a set-to, particularly about Poland. That night, after the meeting, he had something we call pulsus alternans, which means that every alternate beat was less strong than the previous one. That's a very bad sign, a combination of heart and blood pressure. We certainly put the clamps on him by cutting down his activities for the next twenty-four hours, and the condition subsided. And on the way back he was fine. But he was disturbed about Pa Watson's death.[4] He didn't show any outward signs of upset, but he felt very sorry and reminisced a bit about their past.

What happened at Warm Springs was so dramatic, so unexpected. Actually, the president was having a very pleasant time down there. He loved that place and spent a good deal of time there. He had his two cousins with him, Daisy [Margaret] Suckley and Laura Delano. He was really having a ball. He took the car out driving around the countryside, and so forth. Of course, they bent over backwards for him in Warm Springs because he had been an old patient.

I had seen him that morning [12 April 1945], and he was all right, nothing unusual. He enjoyed his breakfast and I went down to the pool,

---

4. General Watson died of a cerebral hemorrhage aboard the USS *Quincy* on the way home.

not that I liked swimming particularly, but it was a pleasant place to go. And then the Secret Service came down and said that something had happened to the president. They took me right up to the cottage and he was unconscious.

The president's valet [Arthur Prettyman] and I carried him into the bedroom, put him in bed, and I did what I could, which wasn't much. He had all the usual signs of a cerebral hemorrhage—the rigid neck, what they call a subarachnoid hemorrhage, I'm sure. A good deal of his brain had been damaged. I then got in touch with Ross McIntire in Washington. He notified Mrs. Roosevelt and Dr. Paullin, who originated in Atlanta. Paullin jumped in his car and came over, but by the time he got there, which was perhaps an hour or so, I was on the bed giving the president artificial respiration. And then his heart stopped. His breathing stopped first and as I was pumping his chest, Dr. Paullin came in. We put a shot of Adrenalin into his heart—sometimes that starts the heart up again—but nothing worked. And that was it.

We were concerned about his heart all the time. That was the weak spot, but he had a significant blood pressure. We had brought it down somewhat, but under certain periods of stress, it would just shoot up. But there was no stress at that time. He was having his portrait painted by Mme. [Elizabeth] Shoumatoff. And he was perfectly relaxed, going over papers from the White House. But it was a combination of arterial change and the blood pressure, which was a constant strain on the arteries. For some reason, one popped.

Unquestionably, the modern drugs we now have to control hypertension would have had a beneficial effect on his blood pressure, which presumably was the initiating factor in his final illness. In the last ten to fifteen years we have been able to bring down that pressure in practically everybody.

As you know, President Roosevelt was the personification of a father to so many people in this country. I will never forget the train after he died in Warm Springs. The last car had lights, not spotlights, but lights. And there were four servicemen standing at each corner of his casket—Navy, Army, Air Force, and Marine. Almost unbroken, even at that time of night, lining the rails from Georgia up to Washington, people were standing and crying, to say nothing of the stations we went through. It reminded me of the same type of thing that happened when Lincoln died. It was an extraordinary, moving situation. I will never forget it.

Dr. Bruenn died in 1995 at age ninety. A discreet gentleman to the end, he never mentioned the president's special friend Lucy Rutherford during our talk. It is now known, however, that she also was present when the president was stricken.

ARTIST FOR THE PRESIDENT

As a youth in Cleveland, Ohio, Samuel Bookatz aspired to be an artist. After graduating from art school, he learned anatomy at Harvard Medical School, not to practice the healing art but to comprehend what lay hidden beneath the veneer of human skin.

He then won the prestigious William Page Award and received a Prix de Rome mention, enabling him to study and travel abroad. As the Germans marched into France in 1940, Bookatz fled Europe to face an uncertain future at home as the United States prepared for war.

Back in Cleveland, Bookatz continued painting. Luck, timing, and an influential friend landed him a commission in the Navy Hospital Corps with a most prestigious duty station—the White House. His assignment was to document on canvas the Medical Department's contribution to the war effort.

How I ended up in the Navy is an interesting story. I came back to Cleveland from Europe and, after getting resettled, began doing a portrait of David Dietz, one of President Roosevelt's advisers.[5] At that time, 1941, I knew I was about to be inducted. Dietz told me he was going to Washington the next day to see the president. "How would you like to be in the Navy?" he asked. I said that would be great. He returned a few days later and said, "Sam, you're in the Navy, and you'll get to paint."

It might have seemed strange to be joining the Navy as a painter, but it wasn't. Roosevelt had once been assistant secretary of the Navy, and

---

5. Dietz, famous author and science editor, was then serving on the National Research Council as a consultant to the surgeon general of the Army. He was also adviser to the president.

it was his favorite service. As it turned out, he was looking for a good artist to record Navy medical history. One day I was a civilian, the next day I was a lieutenant (jg). Dietz then asked me to come to Washington to meet my new boss, the surgeon general [Vice Adm. Ross T. McIntire], which I did. McIntire was also the president's personal physician.

I reported to the surgeon general's office at 23d and E Streets. They gave me space for a studio there in the old Washington Naval Hospital, where I did a lot of my paintings. When I arrived in Washington in 1942, it was a little town with perhaps two hundred thousand people. With the influx of military, you just couldn't get a room. I finally moved into a little room at a boarding house at 21st and P Streets.

Because I wasn't too clear as to what corps I was in, the uniform shop had sewn the physician's oak leaves on my sleeves. When the surgeon general saw my uniform, he exploded. "Take those oak leaves off; you're not a doctor." So I went back to my room, cut them off, and laid them on the dresser. The old lady who ran the boarding house used to make up my room. One day she saw my insignia on the dresser, called the FBI, and told them she had a spy living in her house. Two agents showed up and began questioning me as to where I worked. I was under orders not to tell anyone where I worked. I told them to call the surgeon general and he would explain everything, which he did. He then told me to get out of that house immediately.

My other studio was at the White House in the Lincoln Bedroom. It was the most fabulous thing you can imagine. I had to paint in the corner of the room to get the best light while Mrs. Roosevelt wrote her newspaper column, "My Day," right next door. Often I would hear her old typewriter clacking away and it would disturb me, but of course I couldn't say anything. When I was through for the day, I'd wash my brushes in the White House sinks, right near where the president's meals were being prepared. I also sketched the president and began a portrait of Dr. McIntire. I still have sketches of Eleanor and the president. Can you imagine that while I painted in their midst, Roosevelt and his advisers were making the decisions and planning the grand strategy for winning the war?

I worked at the White House until 1945, when I was assigned to plastic surgery at Oak Knoll Naval Hospital in Oakland. They needed all the help they could get there, with all those badly wounded boys coming in from the Pacific.

I worked with some of the greatest surgeons in the world cutting cartilage for facial reconstruction right in the operating room. Sometimes the surgeons were so busy, they would ask me to cut a piece of cartilage for a nose or other portion of the face. An artist knows proportions. And I certainly knew anatomy, having studied both at Harvard and in London.

Besides assisting in surgery, I would do sketches of the patients as the operation proceeded. In those days, photographic equipment was big and bulky. And you needed large lamps. When photographers tried to bring it all into the operating room, the surgeons would scream, "Get those damn things out of here, they're not sterile." We didn't have small cameras fifty years ago. I could get up very close and make detailed sketches. The drawing, made on the spot, could then be photographed and projected on a screen. The surgeons would have their conference and then go out and perhaps save the next badly injured patient.

The doctors would allow me to help in other ways. I'd talk with the wounded boys and try to cheer them up. I remember one kid very well. He had half his face blown away and didn't want to see anyone. I'd sit and talk with him. He would show me pictures of what he'd looked like before. After each operation to rebuild his face, I would redraw him. I went to his wedding at the chapel and it was the happiest event you can imagine.

After the war Lieutenant Bookatz remained in the Naval Reserve, retired as a commander, and still paints every day. His work is exhibited in noted galleries and public buildings throughout the nation, including the Corcoran Gallery of Art, the Phillips Collection, the Joseph H. Hirshhorn Museum, the Smithsonian Institution, the Cleveland Museum of Art, the Rochester Museum of Art, and the Library of Congress.

ELEVEN

Ecstatic to Be Free

By February 1945 the battle to liberate the Philippines was reaching its climax as American troops fought their way into Manila. After ferocious street fighting, advanced units of the U.S. Army reached the infamous Bilibid prison and found the pitiful survivors of nearly thirty-four months of Japanese brutality, sickness, and starvation. Many, too weak to lift their heads from their bunks, welcomed their liberators with vacant stares.

YANKS AND TANKS

Ill and bedridden almost the entire time he was in captivity at Bilibid, Dr. Alfred Smith was almost at the end of his rope when liberation finally came.

I don't remember the date I learned the Americans were back in the Philippines, but it was sometime in '44. It was a bright sunshiny day. Two

Japanese planes were practicing dogfighting, and right out of the blue, they turned tail and headed north in a hurry. Within five minutes bombs were hitting the port area. We figured our boys weren't too far away. This was right about the time the Japanese began sending our men on convoys north to Japan.

On the night of February 4th, 1945, about eight o'clock in the evening, half-tracks and tanks suddenly roared past the prison. You could hear machine-gun bullets bouncing off the walls. The tanks never stopped but kept on going. I remember the very first American I saw. He was knocking the boards off the windows with his rifle butt. He looked in and said, "What are you guys doing in here?" He was very fit looking, dark skinned, and wearing a funny kind of helmet we'd never seen before. We were accustomed to the old, flat variety.

Someone answered him. "We've been in here for a long time. Who are you?"

"I'm from Ohio with the First Cavalry," he replied.

"You mean you're an American?"

He said yes, and then someone shouted, "Well then, damn it, give me a Lucky Strike!" He didn't have a Lucky but he did give the guy a Camel. We knew right then that the Yanks and tanks were back and we were free.

Dr. Smith and the Bilibid survivors had their first American chow in many years that day. Shortly thereafter, he began the long trip back from the Philippines by way of Leyte, Peleliu, Honolulu, and San Francisco, arriving home on 17 March 1945. He was hospitalized at the National Naval Medical Center, Bethesda, Maryland, for sixteen months and, declared unfit for further service, retired from the Navy in 1946 with the Bronze Star and a purple heart. He died in 1994.

A NURSE'S STORY

With the fall of Manila in January 1942, Dorothy Still and eleven of her comrades became prisoners of the Japanese, spending the next three years in captivity at Santo Tomas and Los Baños.[1] Liberation for these prisoners came suddenly and quite unexpectedly.

On January 9th, 1945, Americans troops landed at Lingayen Gulf. The Japanese awakened us in the middle of the night and told us they were leaving. They turned the camp over to the administrative committee and advised us not to go outside.

The administrative committee then called us to attention: "Today at this time we're announcing you are free. This is Camp Freedom." An American flag was sent up the flagpole and we sang the national anthem. Tears were running down everyone's face. It was a very emotional moment.

Unfortunately, our freedom only lasted a week. Then the Japanese came back. However, MacArthur's troops came down toward Manila and on February 3d liberated Santo Tomas. After learning about Los Baños, MacArthur assigned the 11th Airborne Division to rescue us.[2]

The raiders already had a map of the camp, given to them by an escapee, Pete Miles. Miles and the Filipino guerrillas would act as scouts and guides for the troops. The plan was to sneak up behind all the guardhouses in the camp, and at a specific moment everything would happen at once.

We didn't know the rescue was going to happen, so we were all feeling pretty low. I was on duty that night. There was a newborn baby and I was trying to feed her with what little powdered milk was left. The mother could hardly nurse the baby. She hadn't had enough nourishment herself. It was just about seven in the morning [23 February 1945]. I had the baby in my arms when I noticed smoke signals going up. Nobody paid any attention to them. Then, all of a sudden, we saw a formation of aircraft coming over.

As the paratroopers started jumping out, the guerrillas and soldiers around the guardhouses began killing the Japanese there. Then the amtracs came in, crashing through the sawali-covered fence near the front gate. I was holding the baby and covering her ears so that the noise

---

1. Ann Bernatitus was not captured.
2. In retaliation for the raid, the Japanese murdered 1,500 inhabitants of the nearby town of Los Baños. For this and other crimes, the prison commandant was later tried as a war criminal and executed.

wouldn't affect her. An amtrac pulled up in front of the hospital, and the American troops jumped out. Oh, we'd never seen anything so handsome in our lives. These fellows were in camouflage uniforms wearing a new kind of helmet, not those little tin-pan things we were used to seeing. And they looked so healthy and so lively.

They were to take the internees out, and any that could walk were to go back with troops in the trucks that came overland with the diversionary force. The internees were not military minded, and they just went in all directions. They didn't want to leave anything. The firing was mostly over in about fifteen minutes, but it took a while to evacuate the internees. In fact, the American troops actually had to set fire to the barracks to get them moving.

Eventually, the troops were able to get about 1,500 people on the amtracs and the rest overland. I left on an amtrac in the second wave. Remarkably, I think there were only two soldiers killed and one internee injured. This whole thing went off with just the most amazing precision that you could imagine.[3]

After our liberation, we were flown to Leyte. We were taken to Admiral Kinkaid's headquarters, where we ate dinner with the admiral.[4] They served us beautiful steaks, which of course we couldn't eat because our stomachs had shrunk so much.

It was surprising to see how much publicity we got. On Leyte we began to see the flashbulbs going off, and then as we got closer to home, more flashbulbs. When we landed in Oakland there was quite a reception for us, including a lot of photographers and media. Then they gave dinners for us, and Mrs. Nimitz was there. It was quite an affair.

We also had a very thorough examination in Oakland, and we went on ninety-day recuperative leave. My health had been good, but while in Los Baños I'd developed the dry type of beri-beri, as had many others. It was very uncomfortable—I ached all over and my knees buckled. There was nothing I could do for it; it was caused by malnutrition. But I quickly recovered once I was able to eat good food again.

3. MacArthur had good evidence the Japanese would soon execute the Los Baños prisoners. In the rescue plan, paratroopers were to drop over Los Baños and attack in conjunction with infantry, who would come ashore in amtracs (amphibious vehicles) from a nearby lake, Laguna de Bay. These vehicles would then evacuate many of the civilians.
4. Vice Adm. Thomas C. Kinkaid was commander, Seventh Fleet and Southwest Pacific Force.

Following her recuperation, Lieutenant Still was temporarily assigned to the Treasury Department on behalf of several bond drives. She also traveled in support of Navy public-relations activities. Toward the close of 1945, she was transferred to Panama. Upon returning home in 1946, she left the Navy and married.

ZOMBIES

Flight nurse Kathryn Van Wagner was at her home base in Guam, fresh out of training, when she flew to the Philippines to pick up survivors of Bataan and Corregidor.

I remember my first evacuation flight of POWs. It was an absolute horror. They were all Americans from Bilibid and were brought to the plane wearing something like pajamas. I spoke to them: "Glad to see you." They looked right through me. They were zombies. Some of them had lost their teeth, and they had lost clumps of hair. They had cigarette burns on their ears, in their nostrils. They looked like they had a disease endemic in Africa—Kwashiorkor. It's severe malnutrition, where people look like stick figures with huge abdomens. They were still able to walk, or rather shuffle, with help. I didn't put them in litters. They wanted to sit up, so we arranged for the bucket seats. They didn't address me. They didn't answer me. I thought to myself, I can't feed these people, it would kill them. I can't give them any food. I can only give them liquids.

We had some bouillon cubes so I made bouillon, handed it to them hot, and I'd hold their hand and say, "Wait a minute. Blow on it. It's too hot." And they would sit there and do exactly what I told them to do.

They had lost their identities. They didn't recognize me as a female. They didn't seem to realize that I was speaking English. They just did what I told them to do. "Sit, stand, come."

I learned later that they had been subsisting on fish head and cabbage soup, sometimes with uncooked rice. None of these patients spoke to me at all, not one word. We took them to Guam, where they began renourishing them. And then I took them from Oahu to Oakland on another flight, after they had been strengthened. Some had schistosomiasis and other parasitic infections, which had caused a tremendous amount of diarrhea.

Once they had been renourished, there was a big change. They were far more alert, but still not talkative. I'd ask them their names and they'd say, "Jim." One-word answers. But they did respond and they did things voluntarily. They were so much better.

During the long years of captivity, news from the outside was scarce. Early on, rumors often wafted through the camps that Germany was on the ropes and that the Axis's days were numbered. Could freedom then not be far behind? But the months turned into years. The Japanese withheld letters from home, and only with the arrival of new drafts of prisoners into camp did shreds of news reach the men regarding the American advance through the Pacific.

The return of U.S. airpower to the Philippines and Japan itself in late 1944 and early 1945 was graphic evidence even to the prisoners that the war was going badly for Japan.

Yet for many POWs scattered throughout Japan and Manchuria, the end of the war came suddenly and without warning. Beatings and work details abruptly stopped. Guards became overly friendly and solicitous, offering food and favors. In some camps the Japanese told the inmates to paint PW on the roofs of prominent buildings.[5]

At Tsuruga Camp in west central Honshu, where American heavy bombers had been hammering the industrial heartland for months, B-29s returned. But this time, bundles slung beneath brightly colored parachutes were dropped from their bomb bays, not bombs. Men rushed headlong into rice paddies where the packages had landed and fell upon them with relish. Some containers broke open, spilling the contents in the mud. No one seemed to mind. There were steaks, candy, cigarettes, canned meat, sugar, newspapers, and medical supplies.

---

5. With the cessation of hostilities and even before the formal surrender documents had been signed, Allied instructions were very strict regarding relief for the POWs. Camps were to be marked to allow the supply of critically needed food and medicine from the air.

Near Kobe, at a camp called Maruyama, Lt. Ferdinand Berley feared that help would not arrive soon enough to save his sick and starving patients. He and two of his comrades took matters into their own hands.

✚
MISSION OF MERCY

We heard the fleet was coming in on the 27th of August to meet for the surrender. Murray Glusman, Stan Smith, and I then got the bright idea that we would go to Yokohama or Tokyo to meet the fleet. We thought our own people would never know where we were. So we got a list of all the patients, their addresses and so on, and one afternoon we just took off.

We didn't have much in the way of clothes. I borrowed a hat from John Bookman and I had a khaki shirt with a Marine Corps insignia on it. We had our wallets, we had money, and we went down to the Kobe station and bought tickets to Tokyo. We went up to the platform, and every time a train came by I'd ask if that train was going to Tokyo or Yokohama, and the answer was no. Kids came up to us and said "baseball" and things like that. It was very friendly.

But we were getting nowhere until finally a very nice gentleman with a briefcase came to us and spoke English. He introduced himself and asked us what we were trying to do. We explained that we were on a mission of mercy. We were from a hospital that had been burned out. We had no medicine and we were trying to get to Tokyo to report our plight. He told us to come with him on the next train and he would show us how to get where we wanted to go.

The next train came along and we sat down together. He took a peach for each of us from his briefcase and told us how glad he was that the war was over and that we could be friends again. When we got to Osaka he went to the train-station master, explained who we were and where we were headed. The trainmaster told us to get up on the platform above, and he would let us know when the train came in.

The station was full of Japanese soldiers and marines, all heading home. When a train came in they climbed over one another through the windows and doors to get a seat. They just mobbed the train. And then the train would take off. Another would come and the same action would be repeated. Finally, after we waited an hour or two, the train master told us the next train coming in would be the one to take us to Yokohama, and then from Yokohama we should take the electric to go to Tokyo.

When the train came in we shouldered our way in there just like the Japs. I found myself sitting next to a Japanese marine. He was as happy as all get out because the war was finished. This fellow had a few hard biscuits, which he shared with me.

As we traveled along through the night you couldn't see very much, but as the morning came on there was destruction in every town we went through. When we got to the bay just before Yokohama, I could see our fleet out there. And that's when I almost broke down and started crying. Goodness, what a beautiful sight that was!

When we got to Yokohama, we got off the train. I remember how the people stared at us, their mouths open. We followed the directions and took the electric to Tokyo. I had been there before the war and the only place I knew was the Imperial Hotel. When we got off the electric, we started walking. Then a Japanese army truck came by and we bummed a ride. We told them we wanted to go to the Imperial Hotel and so they took us there. It's almost unbelievable when I stop and think about it.

Part of the hotel was burned. But the destruction in the area of Tokyo we were in was nowhere near what we had seen in Kobe, Nagoya, Osaka, and all those places. They were just rubble, whereas Tokyo was not. A lot of buildings were still standing.

We went into the hotel men's room down below to clean up a bit. Then we went to the desk. I'll never forget that guy's face when we said we wanted a room. He asked us who we were, and we said we were doctors from Kobe International POW Hospital. He directed us up to the mezzanine to sit. While we were sitting there a Japanese major came by who spoke English, and he asked us what we were doing there. I told him we were on a mission of mercy, because we had 120 sick patients in a place called Maruyama with no food and no medicine, and they were dying one after another. We had come to meet the fleet and tell them of our plight.

They gave us two rooms in the basement and put a guard over us. He was a young Japanese who spoke perfect English and had been studying to be a teacher. During the few days we were there, we learned a lot from him about what would have happened had the landings taken place. He told us they had stashed away many planes for kamikazes. They had ten thousand volunteers who were going to act as human torpedoes and blow themselves up against the landing craft. Nobody had ever invaded Japan and we were not going to do it. Every Japanese would fight to the death. And that meant that all of us would have been killed too. He was very happy the war was over and he could go to visit America one day.

We had beds, we had sheets, we had meals, we had knives and forks and napkins. We had showers, we had soap. And they sent the Kempe [Kempetai, secret police] to interrogate us. The Kempe wanted to know how we'd gotten there and how we'd been able to get there without being killed. And we refused to go back until we could meet someone who represented the American government.

Our interrogator was very, very haughty. As a matter of fact, Murray Glusman got up and pointed to him and said, "Look, you are no longer the victor, you are the defeated. You do not talk to us in that tone of voice anymore. We will have you shot." And the guy turned white and walked out. Outside, Navy planes were flying over almost at treetop level.

Finally the foreign office took over from the Army and the Kempe, and they agreed to take us to the Swiss embassy. We walked there and met with the Swiss delegates and turned over the list I had of all the patients. They promised they would turn it over to the proper authorities. The fleet had been delayed in coming in for the surrender signing because of a typhoon, and so we didn't get a chance to go out to the fleet. And I'm sure the Japanese didn't want us to meet anybody from the fleet.

We then agreed to go back to Maruyama. The next day, with a young Kempe as our escort, we boarded a train back. He got on and kicked people out of their seats so we could sit.

When we got back to Osaka, the place was bustling! There was so much activity, such excitement, I just couldn't sleep. They now had *Life* magazines, food, all sorts of things. Stan, Murray, and I were in such a state of mind, we just couldn't settle down. We tried to rest up on the roof and perhaps catch a little sleep up there.

While we were there we met a young Russian fellow who could speak very good English. I told him I wanted to get back to the hospital at Maruyama to see what had happened there. He was able to commandeer a car taken from some Japanese civilian and drove us to Maruyama. The camp was deserted but for a few cooks, as I recall. Where were the patients, we asked. They told us ambulances had taken them to the Osaka Red Cross Hospital, which was still standing.

About the 27th or 30th of August, we got to the Osaka Red Cross Hospital. All the patients were in beds with sheets and mattresses. They had Japanese nurses taking care of them. Our planes had located where we were and were dropping supplies. Soon we were taken to the train station and sure enough, they had several sleeper cars with berths. All the patients were then loaded in these bunks and we took off for Yokohama. I said good-bye to the others, wondering if I would ever see them again.

On the train to Yokohama, we were so excited we couldn't sleep. There was a reporter who got hold of me and started asking me a lot of questions. Did I know who Frank Sinatra was? Did I know about this and that? Of course, I didn't. I didn't know half the things that had happened the last four years.

When we pulled into the station at Yokohama, I looked out the window and lo and behold, there was Admiral [Richard E.] Byrd standing on the platform![6] Of all people! And I recognized him. I rushed out and introduced myself to him and said, "Admiral, I've got all these sick POWs. Would you mind coming on the train and just walking through. I know they'd just love to see you." He came aboard and shook hands with every one of those hundred or so men.

All the POWs were taken to various hospital ships, but we [Dr. John Bookman and four corpsmen] were directed to an LST. We got some clean clothes, a khaki shirt, underwear, trousers, socks and shoes, shaving gear, and things like that. Then they gave us bunks down below decks someplace. We weren't in the mood to talk to anyone because it was a very, very emotional feeling we had. I remember when they had movies, I would be off crying by myself in a corner someplace. And I'm not the kind of person who cries very much.

Our LST wound up going to Guam, and when we got there they drove us to the hospital. We passed a Jap POW camp and I saw these chaps sitting there looking about as healthy as all get out. I was ready to climb over the fence. You should have seen how well they were being treated!

---

6. The famed polar explorer was also on hand for the surrender ceremonies aboard the USS *Missouri* (BB-63) on 2 September 1945.

When we got to the hospital, they gave us a cursory examination. Then I learned that Murray Glusman and the rest of the staff from the Kobe International Hospital had flown back to the States. They were already home and here we were on this LST! Back to the ship we went and it was a long trip back home. It took us about a month. When I look back on it, that was probably a godsend. It gave me time to get my feet back on the ground, even though they were not back on the ground by a long shot by the end of the voyage. I had such a big chip on my shoulder. I even got angry in the wardroom because they served us rice. Rice, of all things!

I vowed I would not turn down any speaking requests to tell people what had happened. But after a while, I found that you just couldn't dwell on all that stuff. But it took me a long time to get over it.

With the war now over, one of Dr. Berley's trusted corpsmen, PhM2c Ernest Irvin, reveled in his newfound freedom.

THE WAR IS NOW OVER

About six days before we were liberated, the Japs moved us to a Japanese Red Cross hospital in Osaka where we had beds, sheets, and three to a room. I guess they were putting on a show for the people coming to repatriate us.

The Americans started dropping barrels of food. Some would break loose from their parachutes and come crashing down, some on houses. There was fruit cocktail splashed all over the place. About two days after the surrender, Dr. Ohashi [the prison doctor] called us out—that is, those who could walk—and told us the war was over. He said: "There are three reasons. The emperor has ordered everyone to cease fighting." We chuckled at that. "The Americans have invented some kind of atomic bomb. And number three: we have no more navy." We roared when we heard that.

They stacked their rifles, and we were then free to come and go as we pleased. Oh, we did have to log in and out, but no one used their own name. We wrote things like URA Bastard, Go T. Hell, and many others too dirty to print. Before the war, in Shanghai, Tsingtao, and Chefoo, sailors used to write these things in Chinese hotel registers.

We were liberated on the 9th of September. They put us on a train for Yokohama and from there we took a C-47 and refueled in Kwajalein, stopped in Guam for a day or so, then on to Pearl Harbor. From Hawaii we took a flying boat to Alameda.

There were no parades. By then the novelty was over. We just blended in with everybody. We'd go to a restaurant and hear people complain that they hadn't had any butter or sugar. We'd tell them, "You should have been where we were," or we'd simply walk out.

Just days after two nuclear bombs vaporized Hiroshima and then Nagasaki, and the Soviet Union belatedly declared war, Japan sued for peace. Yet even before the victors and the vanquished signed the surrender documents on 2 September 1945, arrangements had been made to liberate and evacuate POWs from the squalid camps scattered throughout Japan and Manchuria. Allied occupation authorities ordered the Japanese to transport the POWs via rail to ports where they could be processed and then evacuated.

✚
THE FIRST WOMEN

Even as the Japanese accepted the Potsdam Declaration on 14 August 1945, the hospital ship *Benevolence* (AH-13) was proceeding toward Japan as part of the Third Fleet. Her function was to care for the casualties the now-canceled invasion of Japan was to have produced. But then the *Benevolence* suddenly changed course for Tokyo Bay: her mission had changed overnight. Thousands of POWs would soon crowd her decks, taxing her facilities and subjecting the crew to a role they were not prepared for. Nurse Madge Crouch remembers.

On the morning of August 29th, they told us we were going into Tokyo Bay. About mid-morning a Japanese pilot came aboard to take us in, because the bay was so heavily mined. We all watched this little Japanese come aboard. He must have been petrified. He took the ship into Tokyo Bay early in the afternoon, and we anchored about 3:00 P.M.

By that time the POWs had already received word the war was over, and planes had begun dropping food, medicine, and dungarees to the guys in the camps they knew about. Personnel had begun to go ashore to locate the prison camps which were close to the Tokyo area. A lot of POWs just walked out of their camps and began making their way to where the fleet was.

We finally got word we were going to embark POWs and were as surprised as anyone. We certainly had had no briefings on how to take care of POWs. Suddenly, without any warning, about five hundred of them somehow got out to our ship.

These men were right from the camps, and it was a psychological shock to suddenly be safe on this beautiful, immaculate hospital ship. They just couldn't believe what had happened to them. Here were these poor, emaciated, filthy dirty, horrible-smelling men crawling with lice in a state of disbelief and ecstatic euphoria. They had had no showers, no delousing, and were starving. Some were carrying small tattered cloths, perhaps containing a picture of a wife and a few precious things they had been able to hold onto all those years. Many were wearing stiff, unwashed dungarees that had recently been dropped by our planes. I will always remember those unwashed dungarees on those poor dirty bodies. They had to put their little possessions into an autoclave on the fantail, because everything was so contaminated.

I remember one officer, either a Marine or a pilot. He had been beaten and tortured. We got him aboard and he died some hours afterward. It was so sad we couldn't save him.

The captain said, "Give these men anything they want to eat," which, of course, was the worst thing he could have done. We had an automatic ice-cream-making machine and most of the men wanted ice cream. They were all so ravenous.

They got sick! The captain had just been overwhelmed and was trying so hard to respond to them. Finally the doctors got to him and told him that he just couldn't do this kind of thing. The POWs couldn't handle it. What they needed was a limited diet in small amounts.

We began sorting them—some had TB, some rotten teeth; some had fractures that hadn't been corrected; some were psychological cases. Nowadays, it's common knowledge how to deal with people who have suffered such trauma. But then we had no idea how to deal with them. We were the first women they had seen in years. And so after they got through those first few days of getting oriented, what they wanted to do most was to talk to you. They wanted to tell you what they had been through. I guess it was a catharsis for them. And they wanted to talk to us because they thought we, as women, would be more sympathetic. We represented their wives, their girlfriends, their mothers.

And when your stint of duty was over for the day, you'd come off exhausted. The torture they described was so awful! We were just doing the best we could with the training we had as nurses. We really weren't equipped psychologically to deal with this.

The men would go through stages you could identify. At first everything was wonderful—like a miracle. And then after a while, nothing was right. At first they couldn't believe having sheets on the bunks and things like that. Then they would hoard food because they weren't sure they would get any more. When you made up their bunks you'd find bread stuffed under the pillows, as though they figured there might not be any food tomorrow.

The big thing for the men, of course, was to get home. They became impatient because they had to wait for transportation, even though we processed them as fast as we could.

And then a very interesting thing occurred. These men were very shaky in terms of their own feelings and psychological welfare. As the time neared for them to leave, many said they were scared to go home. How would the wives or girlfriends left behind accept them? The day before they were to be discharged, they would ask: "How do I look? How do you think she's going to feel when she sees me?"

And we'd talk to them and reassure them. "Oh, she's going to be so happy to see you. She'll understand what you've been through." But you'd think to yourself, "Oh, God, I hope these guys go home to somebody who really understands what they've been through."

TWELVE

Peace

On 2 September 1945, World War II ended dramatically on the deck of the USS *Missouri* in Tokyo Bay. Three years, eight months, and twenty-six days had elapsed since Japanese planes had roared out of a clear Pacific sky on a peaceful Sunday morning.

American troops would now become the occupiers of a thoroughly prostrate and devastated Japan. Every city, almost without exception, had been turned into an ash heap, with Hiroshima and Nagasaki bearing the dubious distinction of having been brought to that condition with but two bombs. Heretofore, American warriors had seen Japan only through their periscopes and bombsights, never up close, and never as victors.

NAGASAKI UP CLOSE

When the war ended, PhM1c Freeman P. Fountain was with the 6th Marines, 2d Marine Division, on Saipan. His unit was soon to be part of the occupation forces in Japan. Seven weeks after the atomic bombing of Nagasaki, Fountain and his comrades entered what was left of the city.

Before we left Saipan they issued us occupational currency, but on board ship it was exchanged for Japanese yen. We also got a small, orange-colored booklet of Japanese words and phrases to use while in Japan.

We landed outside Nagasaki Harbor on 23 September 1945. Since our units were still virtually on a wartime footing, we all went ashore with combat gear and loaded rifles. I was with the scouts and snipers of the 6th Regiment. While in the landing boats, we saw bodies floating in the water. Even though they were bloated and floating face up, we clearly recognized them as being Oriental.

Upon landing we lined up and marched to the staging area, near the site of the Mitsubishi Shipyard on the western side of the harbor. There were several Japanese civilian onlookers, standing motionless with no facial expression.

The bomb had destroyed the shipyard. Steel girders were standing but bent toward the sea. They resembled cornstalks after a windstorm. We camped there for several days and had to set up chlorinated drinking water and latrine facilities, as in the field. Because there was no plumbing, we erected temporary latrines along the wharfs. Excreta would drop into the water below. Later, during the occupation, we used Japanese toilets—oval bowls recessed into the floor with a flushing mechanism at one end. Some of the Marines knocked out the bottoms of chairs, enabling them to sit rather than squat over the toilet.

In the early days of the occupation we lived on a bivouac status. We ate with our mess gear and dipped it into hot soapy water, followed by boiling clear water. We dumped our scraps into a GI can prior to the cleaning. Frequently there were young Japanese boys and girls standing near the GI can holding out an empty container, begging for scraps of food. The sight of hungry youths evoked sadness in all of us. I remember Marines tossing chocolate candy to the children. The Japanese pronounced chocolate as "chocoletto" and said "ah-re-got-o" [thank you].

Early in the occupation we revaccinated all our troops, because there was smallpox among the Japanese civilians. Our vaccination program was successful, as there were no cases of smallpox in the 2d Marine Division. I worked in the regimental surgeon's office (6th Marines) and called in the daily sick reports to the division surgeon's office.

Prostitution was legalized in a small section of the city early in the occupation which incurred the protest of both regimental chaplains. Although condoms were available for Marines going on liberty, we frequently checked the men for VD, the so-called short-arm inspections. There were occasional cases of gonorrhea, which we treated successfully with penicillin.

We were soon granted liberty into the city. We could either walk around the bay or take a small boat across the harbor. I took the boat across and walked home. About half of Nagasaki had not been harmed by the bomb. Apparently, the high bluffs or hills had deflected the blast and offered some protection.

The absence of hostility and the friendliness of the Japanese people came as a total surprise to me. Gifts were exchanged frequently. An elderly man gave me an unusual souvenir, a medal he had picked up in the atomic rubble. It was later identified as a good-conduct medal and was probably worn by a Japanese soldier who hadn't survived the blast. Portions of it had been fused by the heat. I had no way of checking its radioactivity, but years later the activity level was about the same as the dial of a luminous wristwatch. I have that medal in a frame today.

A DENTURE FOR TOJO

Soon after the war, those who bore responsibility for the slaughter of millions faced Allied justice. First at Nuremberg, then at Tokyo, tribunals represented by the victor nations tried the highest-ranking officials of Nazi Germany and Japan.

Of the Japanese, Gen. Hideki Tojo was considered one of the chief architects and perpetrators of the Pacific war. Intensely ambitious and an avid expansionist, by 1944 Tojo had, for all practical purposes, become dictator of Japan. As his power grew, so did his titles, which at various times included prime minister, minister of home affairs, minister of war, and chief of staff of both the Army and Navy. Shortly after the surrender, Tojo shot himself in the chest even as military police arrived at his house to take him into custody.

After his recovery from the botched suicide, the general joined his fellow war criminals in Tokyo's Sugamo Prison, where he became the patient of a young Navy dentist, Lt. (jg) Jack Mallory.

In June 1945 I was a brand-new lieutenant (jg), DC, USNR, on active duty at a Navy facility in the San Francisco Bay area. In the summer of 1946, the Army found they had a shortage of dentists and the Navy a surplus. The Navy loaned something like eight hundred of their dentists to the Army, and they served in Army facilities all across the United States and overseas. I was one of a group of those loaned that shipped out of Seattle to Japan that August.

Along with another one of our group, Jack MacMahon, I was assigned to the 361st Station Hospital in Tokyo, on the bank of the Sumida River. I was the dental prosthetics officer. The general dental clinic up on the main floor took care of all the operative needs—fillings, routine extractions, and so forth. Downstairs was the prosthetic department, a single chair with a laboratory. I had three Japanese dentists— two women and one man—working for me who have remained friends of mine right up to this day by correspondence.

My friend George Foster arrived shortly. Like myself, he was a general dentist at that time but specialized in oral surgery later on. For whatever reason, George was picked to go to the Sugamo Prison two or three times a week.

Sugamo was the prison in Tokyo where a dozen or so of the high-level Japanese officials were being held and tried for war crimes. Other war-crimes trials were taking place all over the Far East. The International Military Tribunal Far East was Japan's equivalent of Germany's Nuremburg.

One night George came back from a trip to Sugamo and said to me, "Guess who was my patient today? Hideki Tojo, the prime minister. His mouth is in terrible condition and I know I will have to take out all his upper teeth, and I don't know what we're going to do with the lowers. How about coming to the prison with me and tell me what you think, because you're going to have make the dentures."

I was naturally excited to be able to see and meet one of the then world's most famous (or infamous) persons, probably second only to Adolf Hitler.

The dental operatory at Sugamo was a little room that was very rudimentary to say the least. But George was able to do the necessary fillings and extractions there on both staff and prisoners. They brought Tojo in with two or three guards. He was wearing his typical kimono and was accompanied by his dentist and attorney. It was his right to have his people there whenever a procedure involving him was going on.

Tojo didn't look at all like the man we had seen in pictures. He and Hitler were always caricatured as the epitome of evil. Tojo's caricatures always included buck teeth and a butch haircut to give him a sharp, harsh look. But he was basically bald. His nickname was the Razor; I don't know where he got that. But the man I now confronted was a rather tired, grandfatherly, innocuous-looking little old Japanese man.

George extracted all his upper teeth. He had seven lower anterior teeth left, one of which was just a carious root. These few remaining teeth were in very bad shape periodontally as well. Today we'd do some great heroics and probably save them, but the treatment at that time was to extract them.

I wondered what that dentist had been doing all those years, but you have to remember that they had few materials and all resources were going to the military. Here was a man at the very top of the government and his mouth was in a horribly deteriorated condition. You'd think he would have had access to something during that time. Obviously he hadn't had his mouth open to a dentist for years and years.

Speaking through the interpreter, I said, "Mr. Tojo, these lower teeth are very bad, and it would be very poor dentistry to make an upper denture that would hit against just six or seven lower anterior teeth." I learned later that Tojo spoke fair English but he chose not to. "The denture," I said, "would simply rock back and forth and beat your upper anterior ridge traumatically. We really need to remove those teeth and make a full lower denture to go with the upper."

He pondered my words for a moment and then said something to the interpreter, who said to me, "Mr. Tojo says those teeth will last him for six more months, and after that he won't be needing any teeth." Everyone in the room broke out in a chuckle. And pretty soon, he started laughing too. That was in November 1946. As it turned out the trial wasn't over until December of '48 so he lived for two more years.

When I took the impression of the lowers, one of the seven came out in the impression. It was an artificial crowned tooth that had a dowel post down the non-vital root canal. The remaining root was so carious around the dowel that the crown came out in the impression. I still have it.

When we made a dental prosthetic appliance for American military personnel, we left a recess in the acrylic body of the appliance and then typed name, rank, and serial number on a piece of paper, put it in the recess, and applied some clear acrylic over the top. It tied that appliance to a specific individual and could then be used for identification purposes.

Of course, the slogan Remember Pearl Harbor was certainly still ablaze in the minds and hearts of any good red-blooded American. We all thought of it. George did. I did. Many of the doctors and the administrative personnel of the hospital knew I was making this denture. "You've got a chance that nobody else has. Make this sucker chew on those words, *Remember Pearl Harbor,*" was typical of the advice I was getting from all sides.

But you just don't do things like that, in or out of the military. Even at that young age, I had enough brains to know that this would be a mistake from a professional and military ethics point of view. Here's a man on trial for his life and in the American way of justice you're not guilty until proven so. Moreover, you just don't debase somebody like that. So I refrained from the impulse.

But I figured a compromise was possible. I had been an amateur radio operator and knew the international Morse code. I could slip that in there and nobody would know it. So I took a little round burr, and inside the circumference of the denture's peripheral border I inscribed the words *Remember Pearl Harbor* in dots and dashes.

```
.-. .   - -  .  - -  -...  .  .-.
.- -  . .  .-  .-.  .-..
....  .-  .-.  -...  - - -  .-.
```

A denture by nature of its usage is never dry. In the mouth it's covered with saliva. You take it out and wash it and it's wet. And when it's wet many of the cracks and crevices and idiosyncracies of its tissue-bearing surface are indistinguishable. So what I had done was not readily seen when it was moist. But if you dried it, it stood out very plainly.

I finished the denture in mid November of '46. The only ones who knew about it were George, my other roommates, and myself. All were sworn to secrecy lest George and I find ourselves in some kind of trouble. I suppose it also would have been a humiliating thing for the officials there at the prison.

In February 1947, three Baylor University classmates of one of our roommates showed up in Tokyo for dental assignment. One of them was sent to work with us. The Tojo thing was still fresh in our minds and was a big thing for young bucks like us. So we took them out to the prison on the pretext of checking up on Tojo. We called him down to the dental clinic. These newcomers stood around while I got the denture and took it over to wash it off and let them see the Remember Pearl Harbor. And then we told them that it was really a secret and they weren't to tell anybody about it. They were very much impressed with our prank on this man of such world notoriety.

The secrecy of it all didn't last long. This is the way the story got back to me. One of the new dentists wrote the story to his parents in Texas, whereupon his father passed it on to his brother, who proceeded to retell it on his small-town radio station. And then it really hit the fan in a big way all across the country and the world. In fact, a friend of mine who was a missionary in Indochina heard it out there. When he heard that a Navy dentist had done this trick he said, "That's got to be Jack Mallory!" I guess I had a reputation as a prankster from early college years.

One afternoon a reporter from the International News Service there in Tokyo called, asking for an interview. At first I thought this was my good friend Jim Wasley, from a close-by hospital, trying to con me, but when he asked directions out to the hospital, I knew I was in trouble.

I went upstairs to my dental commanding officer, Maj. Bill Hill, and confessed the story. Major Hill was a world-wise regular Army man, and he said, "That's as funny as hell, but it could get us into trouble. You have your office tell him you're not available and you go into hiding. I'll talk to the reporter."

When the reporter showed up he talked to Major Hill, who denied everything. The reporter started getting belligerent because he knew there was more to the story, but Hill stuck to his story and the newsman left pretty angry.

Nevertheless, that night it was out over the Evening Armed Forces Tokyo Radio Station, WVTR. Major Hill called us and asked if we had heard the broadcast. We said we had. He asked if we would be able to grind it out of the denture. When we told him yes, he said, "You guys get your butts out to that prison right now and get that out!"

So on Valentine's Day night 1947, we commandeered a jeep and drove about twelve miles in a snowstorm to the prison. When we got there a Valentine's Day party was in full swing at the officers' club. We just mingled because we didn't want to be too obvious. George was waiting for a guard he knew real well to come on duty.

Sometime around eleven o'clock the young GI arrived, and George asked him to go up to Tojo's cell, get his denture, and bring it down. The guard was puzzled, but, knowing and trusting George, he disappeared and finally came back with the denture.

Down in the dental operatory, we pulled the blinds down and I got a heatless stone and, as lightly as I could, removed the offensive dots and dashes. There were some joe-dandy disks there and I tried to obliterate the marks left by the heatless stone grinding. It was all pretty crude. Then the guard took the denture back to Tojo's cell.

The next morning the story was on the front page of the *Stars and Stripes,* telling how Navy dentists—not naming names—had already gotten their revenge on Tojo by inscribing in his denture the words he would most like to forget. Right after breakfast, George was called to the telephone. It was the very tough colonel in charge of the prison. As I recall, this is how the conversation went:

"Lieutenant Foster!"

"Yes sir!"

"Have you seen the front page of *Stars and Stripes* this morning?"

"Yes sir!"

"Is there any truth in this report that Remember Pearl Harbor is inscribed in that denture?"

"No sir."

"Have you personally seen it recently?"

"Yes sir!"

"And you're really sure it's not there?"

"Yes sir!"

"Can I invite the press to come out and examine it for themselves?"

"Yes sir!"

"Thank you, Lieutenant."

And that was it. I have no idea if he ever invited the press to the prison and so the story ends very anticlimactically. Nothing more was heard. There was only speculation of what might have been our fate had we been caught with the goods.

My tour of duty in Japan ended in early summer of 1947. In late May I had an opportunity to visit the war-crimes trials. A panel of judges presided over the trials, one from each of the Allied nations—the United States, Britain, France, the Netherlands, China, and the rest. The president of the tribunal was the Australian Sir William Webb, on leave from his position as chief justice of their supreme court, or its equivalent. During my tour in Tokyo, Sir William had come to me as a dental patient and had taken a liking to George and me. And so he arranged for me and my friend Jim Wasley to sit in reporter's boxes right in the center of the courtroom. Over on the left was the prisoner's dock. In between were many tables. Up in the balcony facing me were all the Japanese people, who were free to come and watch the proceedings.

The defendants filed into their box as they had been doing for over a year and half. Tojo sat down and looked all around the room in a bored manner. I was sitting about twenty-five or thirty feet away from him. His eyes then came to rest on me and he stopped and seemed puzzled. It looked like he was thinking, "Now there's a face I don't usually see in this courtroom." It was as though he was saying to himself, "I know that guy from somewhere." He studied me for what seemed a long time and finally his eyes lit up and he broke into a big smile. Pointing a finger to his teeth, he bowed toward me in a gesture of thank you, which was nice on his part.

That was the last time I saw Tojo. The trials lasted approximately another eighteen months. When he was hanged, he was without the denture I had made him. Shortly thereafter I saw a newspaper article in the *San Francisco Chronicle,* accompanied by a photo of Mrs. Tojo kneeling before his shrine in her home. And there were his trademark big horned-rimmed glasses, and the false teeth he wouldn't be needing anymore.

DAY OF PEACE

A veteran of Saipan and Iwo Jima, PhM2c Laddie Vacek spent his war as an X-ray technician serving with the Marines. He was in Hawaii awaiting the next campaign when the war ended. Even though the shooting had ceased, sudden and ironic death had not. Excerpts from his wartime journal follow.

Last night Tokyo radio reported that it has accepted Potsdam terms. I was attending the 2000 movie at the time. Today about 1330 it was officially announced from Washington, D.C., and England, that Japan has surrendered. Official V-J Day won't occur until the actual signing of surrender terms by Japan. MacArthur is to be "boss" of Japan.

This afternoon a serious jeep accident occurred. Three patients were X-rayed here. The fourth is dead!! The deceased is 19 years of age, has gone thru four invasions, and today—the day of peace, he dies. His mother is probably rejoicing over the end of the war, not knowing that here her son lies dead.

Many are the men that are inebriated tonight. My barracks is a mad house.

I thank God with all my heart for His Goodness, Mercy and Compassion upon us in ending this war.

✚

MEN WERE STILL ARRIVING

The news of Japan's surrender on 14 August 1945 triggered a torrent of joyful emotion from San Francisco to New York City. A nation united in purpose to achieve victory had grown weary from nearly four years of war and was primed to let down its hair and celebrate. The photograph of a sailor exuberantly kissing a young nurse in Times Square has become a metaphor for the end of World War II.

But although the end had come at last, the men who had paid the price for peace in burned and mutilated bodies, and those still responsible for putting them back together, saw it all differently. Shortly after the war, one of the caregivers, HA2c Irving Feld, told the way it was at Oak Knoll Naval Hospital in California.

Word of war's end came to Oak Knoll Tuesday afternoon before the beginning of the liberty hour. At first patients received the news with a quick excitement, a short-lived reaction, universal and inevitable. Throughout the wards this fleeting excitement was followed closely by a passive observance, which in turn surrendered to almost complete indifference.

The anticlimactic announcement—long awaited and entirely expected—provoked little show of unbridled feeling. Radios that heralded the news for nearly four days were soon silenced.

Long siren blares immediately clarioned the official note throughout the hospital. The siren's prolonged sound, caused by jamming, was in itself the only humorous relief of the event. To the staff this noise seemed to stab the ears with twofold effect: a brief moment of joy and a poignant, awful reminder of still-unfulfilled obligation. The shrill whistle clearly sounded, "Relax for a minute, you have earned a respite. But do not abate your vigilance. Remember your responsibility."

The patients' reactions were epitomized most accurately by a survivor of the *St. Lo.* When he heard the news, the wounded air crewman said, with a grin completely absent of malice or cynicism, "It's swell. It's swell for them for whom this is the end." All too clearly, Oak Knoll was filled with men for whom no words or sounds could mean an ending.

Patients were generally satisfied with the unqualified terms of the truce. None had been willing to concede the Japanese their earlier condition upholding the sovereignty of the emperor. There were men like the Marine corporal who wears the Bronze Star Medal with his Purple Heart. After Guam and Iwo Jima, he and thousands of others owned a personal stake in the Pacific and wanted full measure for their paid price. All longed for absolute victory. Yet the word *victory* was seldom heard. Nor did anyone exclaim, "By God, we beat 'em!"

Men who had engaged the enemy preferred the word *peace.* These were the men who were silently thinking of lasting peace at this moment, the lasting peace of the men they had loved who had fallen beside them and the lasting peace they trusted would belong to their children. There were other thoughts of relief for the now-assured safety of comrades yet overseas.

On the crowded wards, in medical service buildings, beneath the covered walks—wherever we gathered—there was the mist of peculiar sensation. There was the feeling that to observe the end of such torturous suffering with an orgy of celebration would be akin to sinful sacrilege. A smile, set in a face that had served only as a pattern for a smile before, was the most lasting and intimate expression. But it was no more than a smile, and not laughter. True, there was a common apprehension that peace could come so cheaply and without further bloodshed. This misgiving also served to temper unrestrained joy.

An hour after the news came, most Oak Knoll patients, bedfast and ambulatory, had resumed their occupational or recreational habits. Hospital routine was soon the same as it perforce must be for months to come. Volleyball, horseshoes, reading, weaving, model building, card playing, checkers—and fixed staring—took up where they had left off. It was after chow. The recess that the news brought was barely noticeable. Without interruption nurses continued giving medication. Dressing-room Waves were still changing bandages. Hospital corpsmen were beginning the evening back rubs. There was little rearrangement in the benignly serious features of the doctors' faces.

All familiar hospital sights and functions—the operating rooms, the laboratory, physical therapy, the post office, ship service, the OD's desk—displayed their usual desultory appearance in this first important hour. Peace Day was not unlike other days at the unsettled time of closing up. Now, without an apparent transition and oblivious only to the cry of time, the hospital passed into the beginning of an era at the end of a day.

Staff chow lines were only slightly shorter by the mess halls that evening. A heavy attendance overcrowded the movies as usual.

When darkness descended on the hospital compound the scene was that of the night before, the week before, and the year before. The wards were silent. Blue-capped nurses hurried over the wooden sidewalks on their rounds. A doctor quickly left the OD's desk to visit a still-critical patient. Under starry skies a chaplain's gold cross shone luminously on a sleeve that turned a corner. White-uniformed hospital corpsmen assigned to night duty stood jesting and smoking on the administration-building porch. Without marked change they awaited their regular muster and inspection before reporting for duty.

Few patients were physically able to leave the hospital and attach themselves to the riotous mob that ravaged San Francisco's Market Street. Those who began to participate soon stopped with a sickened disinterest, fully conscious that they were witnessing the enactment of a mockery that shamed the history their agony had written.

But the blind were still the blind. In stiff bodies, nerves were not miraculously revived. Crippled limbs and arms failed to recapture motion. Burned and shell-torn faces did not heal and reshape themselves. Peace did not grow a mission leg.

And at the receiving room, men were still arriving.

GLOSSARY

Adrenalin: The trademark for preparations of epinephrine, a hormone secreted by the adrenal medulla. Epinephrine stimulates contraction of the muscular tissue of the capillaries and arteries. In its synthetic form, Adrenalin is used as a cardiac stimulant and to increase blood pressure.

Albumin: Serum albumin is the principal protein of blood plasma. When administered intravenously, albumin draws fluid from surrounding tissues and helps increase blood volume to counteract shock.

Antitoxin: The antibody formed when immunizing with a given toxin, used in treating certain infectious diseases or in immunizing against them.

Atabrine: Trade name for quinacrine hydrochloride. A bright yellow crystalline powder developed by the German chemists of I.G. Farben in the 1920s. Used during World War II as an antimalarial, it largely replaced quinine, which was in short supply because of limited access to cinchona bark.

Autoclave: An apparatus employing steam and pressure for sterilizing.

Belladonna: The dried leaves and flowering or fruiting tops of the *Atropa belladonna,* or deadly nightshade. Used to relieve pain, as a cardiac and respiratory stimulant, and for its sedative action upon the gastrointestinal tract.

Beriberi: A disease caused by thiamine (vitamin B1) deficiency. Characterized by pain in and paralysis of the extremities, and by severe emaciation or swelling of the body. In the dry variety, paralysis, muscular degeneration, and enlargement of the heart are common. Wet beriberi is marked by cardiac failure and edema, but without nervous-system involvement. Both wet and dry varieties are endemic in regions such as in Southeast Asia, where polished white rice is the staple food.

Bismuth: The salts of bismuth were once used for the treatment of inflammatory diseases of the stomach and intestine, and for syphilis.

Bleeder: Any large blood vessel cut during a surgical procedure.

Caecum: The cul-de-sac in which the large intestine begins. Also called the blind gut.

Cannula: A tube for insertion into a duct, cavity, or blood vessel.

Cauterization: The destruction of tissue with a hot iron, electric current, or caustic substance such as phenol.

Debridement: The surgical removal of foreign material and dead or contaminated tissue from or adjacent to a wound, until surrounding healthy tissue is exposed.

Dengue: An infectious, eruptive fever characterized by severe pains in the joints and muscles. It is caused by a virus and most commonly transmitted by the *Aedes aegypti* mosquito.

Digitalis: The dried and powdered leaf of *Digitalis purpurea*, or purple foxglove. Used as a stimulant to increase the force of heart contraction. The administration of this drug, called digitalization, was often the treatment of choice for patients suffering cardiac failure or insufficiency.

Dysentery: An infectious disease marked by inflammation and ulceration of the lower part of the intestines. Characterized by chronic diarrhea and severe dehydration.

Edema: A swelling caused by abnormally large amounts of fluid in the subcutaneous tissues.

Elephantiasis: A chronic filarial disease caused by the nematode *Wuchereria bancrofti* and characterized by inflammation and obstruction of the lymphatics and enormous enlargement of the legs and scrotum.

Fascia: A sheet or band of connective tissue surrounding, supporting, or binding together internal organs or parts of the body.

Gangrene: Death of large amounts of tissue due to an interruption of circulation followed by invasion of bacteria and putrefaction.

Hemoglobin: The oxygen-carrying pigment of red blood cells.

Hemostat: A small surgical clamp for constricting a blood vessel. Sometimes used as a locking plier for gripping a suture needle or surgical blade.

Hemothorax: A collection of blood in the pleural cavity.

Hernia: The protrusion of an organ or tissue through an abnormal opening of the body, especially in the abdominal region.

Leishmaniasis: An infection caused by the parasitic *Leishmania* protozoa.

Laparotomy: A surgical incision into the abdominal cavity through any point in the abdominal wall.

Ligation: The application of any substance such as catgut, cotton, silk, or wire, used to tie a vessel or strangulate a part.

Malaria: Any of a group of diseases characterized by chills, fever, and sweating. Caused by five or more species of parasitic protozoa transferred to the human bloodstream by the *Anopheles* mosquito. The protozoa occupy and destroy red blood cells.

Merthiolate: A water-soluble powder used as an antiseptic.
Morphine: An opium derivative used as a narcotic painkiller.
Nasogastric tube: A tube inserted into the nose and down the throat, through which nourishment can be administered.
Novocain: Procaine hydrochloride used as a local anesthetic.
Optic atrophy: Atrophy of the optic disk resulting from degeneration of the nerve fibers of the optic nerve.
Optic neuritis: Inflammation of the optic nerve that can lead to blindness.
Paregoric: A camphorated tincture of opium used to check diarrhea.
Pellagra: A disease caused by a deficiency of niacin in the diet. Characterized by skin changes, severe nerve dysfunction, and diarrhea.
Penicillin: The so-called miracle antibiotic of World War II. Noted for its antibiotic properties in 1928 by Sir Alexander Fleming, penicillin was first isolated from the penicillium mold in 1940. In the next several years, U.S. pharmaceutical firms began producing penicillin in quantities that made a huge impact in the treatment of Allied casualties.
Peritoneum: The strong colorless membrane that lines the abdominopelvic walls and surrounds the viscera.
Petrolatum: An ointment obtained from petroleum, used as a protective dressing. Also called petroleum jelly.
Phenol: A caustic substance used as an antimicrobial agent. Also called carbolic acid.
Pilonidal cyst: A hair-containing cyst that opens into the anus.
Plague: An acute febrile, infectious disease with a high fatality rate, caused by *Yersinia pestis*. It begins with fever and chills, quickly followed by prostration and frequently attended with delirium, headache, vomiting, and diarrhea. It is transmitted by fleas from infected rodents to man. Bubonic plague is characterized by swelling of the lymph nodes, forming buboes in the femoral, inguinal, axillary, and cervical regions. Pneumonic plague is characterized by extensive involvement of the lungs.
Plasma: The liquid part of blood as distinguished from the suspended elements, such as platelets and red blood cells. Before serum albumin and whole blood were available, plasma was commonly used as a blood-volume expander for the prevention and treatment of shock.
Pneumothorax: An accumulation of air or gas in the pleural space that can lead to a lung collapse.
Quinine: An odorless, white crystalline powder. In its pure chemical form (quinine sulfate), or the cinchona bark extract (cinchona sulfate), quinine is used as an antimalarial.
Salvarsan: A yellowish red arsenic compound once used for the treatment of syphilis, yaws, and other spirochete infections, but later replaced by penicillin.
Shock: A collapse of circulatory function caused by severe injury, blood loss, or disease, and characterized by pallor, sweating, weak pulse, and very low blood pressure.
Sodium pentothal: A commonly used anesthetic administered intravenously to induce general anesthesia.
Strangulated hernia: A hernia that is tightly constricted and likely to become gangrenous.

Sulfa drugs: A group of antibacterial compounds first introduced in 1936, commonly used to prevent or treat infection before penicillin came into general use in the mid-1940s. The wartime sulfa quintet included sulfanilamide, sulfapyridine, sulfathiazole, sulfadiazine, and sulfaguanidine. By July 1941, the Navy Medical Department had begun including sulfanilamide powder in each corpsman's medical-aid bag.

Scurvy: A disease marked by swollen and bleeding gums, weakness, and anemia. Caused by a deficiency of vitamin C in the diet.

Syrette: A single-dose, collapsible tube with an attached sterilized hypodermic needle sealed in tinfoil. During World War II, corpsmen in the field commonly used Syrettes with premeasured doses of morphine.

Tetanus: An infectious, often fatal, disease caused by the toxic effect of *Clostridium tetani*. The bacteria usually enters the body through wounds. Characterized by violent muscle spasms, rigidity resulting in trismus (lockjaw), and respiratory failure.

Traction: The act of drawing or exerting a pulling force used principally in the treatment of fractures.

Triage: The sorting and classification of casualties to determine priority of need and proper place of treatment.

Triturate: To reduce to a fine powder by grinding or rubbing.

Xerophthalmia: Dryness of the conjunctiva and cornea due to vitamin A deficiency. The condition begins with night blindness and ends with the possible destruction of the cornea.

Yaws: A systemic infectious disease caused by the spirochete *Treponema pertenue*, commonly occurring in tropical regions.

Zinc oxide and eugenol: When mixed, the powder (zinc oxide) and eugenol (oil of cloves) is used as a temporary filling material in dentistry.

BIBLIOGRAPHY

BOOKS

Bird, Tom. *American POWs of World War II.* Westport, Conn.: Praeger, 1992.
Bureau of Medicine and Surgery (BuMed). *Medical Department of the United States Navy with the Army and Marine Corps in France in World War I.* Washington, D.C.: BuMed, 1947.
Daws, Gavan. *Prisoners of the Japanese: Pows of World War II in the Pacific.* New York: William Morrow and Company, 1994.
Goodhart, Philip. *Fifty Ships That Saved the World.* Garden City, N.Y.: Doubleday and Company, 1965.
Hill, Max. *Exchange Ship.* New York: Farrar and Rinehart, 1942.
Kerr, E. Bartlett. *Surrender and Survival: The Experience of American POWs in the Pacific 1941–1945.* New York: William Morrow and Company, 1985.
Maisel, Albert Q. *Miracles of Military Medicine.* New York: Duell, Sloan and Pearce, 1943.
Miles, Milton E. *A Different Kind of War.* Taipai, Taiwan: Caves Books, Ltd., 1967.
Morison, Samuel Eliot. *History of United States Naval Operations in World War II: Leyte, June 1944–January 1945,* vol. 12. Boston: Little, Brown and Company, 1958.
———. *History of United States Naval Operations in World War II: The Rising Sun in the Pacific,* vol. 3. Boston: Little, Brown and Company. 1951.
Naval Historical Center, Navy Department. *Dictionary of American Naval Fighting Ships.* Washington, D.C.: U.S. Government Printing Office. Vol. 1, 1959; vol. 2, 1963; vol. 4, 1969; vol. 5, 1970; vol. 6, 1976.

PERIODICALS AND STUDIES

Beadle, Christine, and Stephen L. Hoffman. "History of Malaria in the United States Naval Forces at War: World War I Through the Vietnam Conflict." *Clinical Infectious Diseases* 16 (1993): 320–29.
Bruenn, Howard G. "Clinical Notes on the Illness and Death of President Franklin D. Roosevelt." *Annals of Internal Medicine* 72 (1970): 579.
Duff, Ivan F. "Medical Study of the Experiences of Submariners as Recorded in 1,471 Submarine Patrol Reports in World War II." BuMed, Washington, D.C., 1947.
Laforet, Eugene G. "Cecil Coggins and the War in the Shadows." *Journal of the American Medical Association* 243 (25 April 1980): 1653–55.
Levin, Dan. "Briefing for Iwo Beach." *Hospital Corps Quarterly* 18 (May 1945): 35–36.
Newhouser, Lloyd R. and Eugene L. Lozner. "Human Serum Albumin (Concentrated): Clinical Indications and Dosage." *U.S. Naval Medical Bulletin* 40 (April 1942): 277–79.
Woodruff, Lorande M. and Sam T. Gibson. "The Clinical Evaluation of Human Albumin." *U.S. Naval Medical Bulletin* 40 (October 1942): 791–99.

UNPUBLISHED MANUSCRIPTS

Davis, Robert G. Diary, 8 December 1941–7 September 1945. Typescript in BuMed Archives, Washington, D.C.
Kentner, Robert W. Journal, 8 December 1941–5 February 1945. Typescript in BuMed Archives, Washington, D.C.
Sartin, Lea B. "Report of Activities of the United States Naval Hospital in the Philippines from December 8, 1941, to January 30, 1945." Typescript in BuMed Archives, Washington, D.C.
"U.S. Navy Medical Department Administrative History, 1941–1945: Narrative History," vol. 2. Chapters 9–18 and chapter 17. Typescript in BuMed Archives, Washington, D.C.

SOURCES OF FIRST-PERSON ACCOUNTS

Interviews

All interviews were conducted by Jan K. Herman unless otherwise specified.

Bell, Dr. A. Milton. 18 September 1995.
Berley, Dr. Ferdinand V. Several conversations throughout 1995.
Bernatitus, Ann A. Exeter, Pa., 25 January 1994.
Bonacker, Beryl A. 25 October 1995.
Bookatz, Samuel. Washington, D.C., 10, 14, and 17 August 1984.
Bruenn, Dr. Howard G. Riverdale, N.Y., 31 January 1990.
Burwell, Dr. Walter B. 16 February 1994.
Bush, Robert E. 31 October, 1 November 1995.
Coggins, Dr. Cecil H. Conducted by Dr. Katherine Herbig, Monterey, Cal., 9, 12, and 19 August 1985 (used with permission).

Conard, Dr. Robert A. Setauket, N.Y., 9 November 1993.
Dabrowski, Stanley E. New Britain, Conn., 23 August 1994.
Danner, Dorothy Still. Baton Rouge, La., 3 and 4 December 1991.
DePalma, Dr. Anthony F. 24 May 1994.
Erickson, Ruth A. 30 March 1994.
Falk, Dr. Victor S. 22 February 1995.
Fast, Chester K. 8 February 1995.
Feduik, Frank R. Elmhurst, Pa., 26 January 1994.
Gibson, Madge Crouch. Bethesda, Md., 22 November 1995.
Gibson, Dr. Sam T. Bethesda, Md., 13 November 1995.
Groom, Dr. Dale L. 26 May 1994.
Haynes, Dr. Lewis L. Newton, Mass., 5 and 22 June 1995.
Heimlich, Dr. Henry J. Cincinnati, Ohio, 15 December 1994.
Irvin, Ernest J. Alexandria, Va., 1 and 22 February, 24 March, and 22 May 1986.
Kelley, Sara Marcum. 14 and 15 April 1994.
Lally, Grace. Conducted by Irene Matthews, Gulfport, Miss., 1961 (used with permission).
Lipes, Wheeler B. Conducted by Jan K. Herman and Dr. Robert C. Bornmann, Corpus Christi, Tex., 3 March 1993.
Mallory, Dr. Jack. 5 January 1996.
Moore, Thomas A. 30 April 1993.
Pribram, Kathryn Van Wagner. Alexandria, Va., 6 January 1995.
Ramsey, Helen Pavlovsky. 14 and 15 April 1994.
Sherman, Dr. Samuel R. 29 April 1993.
Smith, Dr. Alfred L. Richmond, Va., 16 December 1985.
Soucy, Lee B. 11 February 1995.

REPRINTS AND EXCERPTS

Bolster, Richard L. "Rice Is Life," reprinted from *Hospital Corps Quarterly* 20 (April-May-June 1947): 3–6.
DeWitt, Gill USN. "First Flight Nurse on a Pacific Battlefield," reprinted with permission from a pamphlet published by the Admiral Nimitz Foundation, Fredericksburg, Tex., 1983.
Eckstam, Dr. Eugene E. "The Tragedy of Exercise Tiger," excerpted from *Navy Medicine* 85 (May–June 1994): 5–7.
Feld, Irving. "Men Were Still Arriving," reprinted from *Hospital Corps Quarterly* 20 (July-August-September 1947): 20–21.
Fountain, Dr. Freeman P. "Nagasaki Up Close," excerpted from *Navy Medicine* 86 (September–October 1995): 28–29.
Fultz, Harold F. "Forest Fires, Lightning, and the Moon," excerpted from *Navy Medicine* 75 (July–August 1984): 9–18.
Vacek, Laddie J. "Day of Peace," condensed from journal of 14 August 1945. Manuscript in BuMed Archives.
"The Women of Bountiful," from a typescript in "Hospital Ship" file (*Bountiful*), BuMed Archives.

INDEX

Abandon ship, 20–22, 141, 152–56, 162
Admiralty Islands, 212
Admiral W. S. Benson, USS (AP-120), 185
Adrenalin, 133–34
Africa. *See* North Africa
Air attacks, Japanese, 19–23, 39–41, 135, 145–46
Air Group 5, 144
Alcohol, 23
Alfred, 1
American Red Cross. *See* Red Cross
American Revolutionary War, 1, 3
Amputations, 38, 58, 99–100, 146, 173, 178, 180
Anemia, 215
Anesthesia, 120, 125, 173, 180
Apothecaries, 3
Appendectomies, 120–28, 145
Argonne, USS (AP-4), 24
Arkansas, USS (BB-35), 195
Armed Forces Radio, 188
Army Nurse Corps, 3, 161
Arnest, Gertrude, 25

Artificial respiration, 132
Atabrine, 84, 92
Atomic bomb, 150–51, 188, 238–40
Augusta, USS (CA-31), 202
Australia, 60

Bainbridge, USS (DD-246), 13–17
Banko, Andy, 196–97
Baruch, Bernard, 216, 219
Basham, George, 185
Bataan, 36–45, 49, 52
Battle dressing station, 39, 41, 131–33, 136, 138–40
"Bayman," 3
Bell, A. Milton, 178–80
Benevolence, USS (AH-13), 174–75, 235
Beriberi, 64, 227
Berley, Ferdinand V., 8–12, 37–42, 68–73, 230–34
Bernatitus, Ann, 45, 55–60, 226 n
Biak, 164
Bilibid prison, 62–64, 66–70, 79–82, 224–25, 228

259

Bismarck, 16
Bismarck Sea, 163
"Black Tuesday," 87–90
Blewitt, Kenneth L., 92
Blood, 111, 173, 179–80, 203, 209, 211–12
Board of Navy Commissioners, 2
Boettiger, Anna Roosevelt, 213, 217–18
Bolster, Richard L., 49–50, 73–79
Bombings. *See* Air attacks, Japanese; Atomic bomb
Bonacker, Beryl A., 91–93
Bookatz, Samuel, 208, 221–23
Bookman, John, 71–73, 230, 233
Botulinus toxin, 184
Bougainville, 134–35
Bountiful, USS (AH-9), 102, 143, 170–74
Boyington, Pappy, 118, 144
Bray, James F., 67
Brisbane, 161–62, 164
Brixham, 191–92
Bronchitis, 212
Brooklyn Navy Yard, 149, 198
Brown, Emerson, 108
Brown, Wilson, 218
Bruenn, Howard, 208, 212–21
Brunson, Clyde W., 26
B-17s, 212
B-29s, 70, 93, 102, 229
Buckner, Simon B., Jr., 169
Bulmer, USS (DD-222), 9
BuMed. *See* Bureau of Medicine and Surgery
Bureau of Medicine and Surgery, 2–4, 123, 128, 189–90, 208
Burials, 12, 134, 193; at sea, 132, 148
Burlingame, Creed, 124–27
Burns, 140, 142, 146, 152, 157, 177, 179–80, 206
Burwell, Walter B., 137–43
Bush, Robert E., 114–18
Byrd, Richard E., 233
Byrnes, James F., 218

Cabanatuan, 62, 68, 80–81
Camden Naval Shipyard, 130
Camp Four (Inner Mongolia), 186–88
Camp Holcomb, 50
Camp Limay Hospital #1, 56–57
Camp O'Donnell, 62
Cañacao Naval Hospital, 45–50, 53, 55, 79
Canopus, USS (AS-9), 45–47
Cavite Navy Yard, 36–38, 42–43, 46–47, 50, 52–54, 119
Cecil J. Doyle, USS (DE-368), 156–57
C-47s, 235
Chaplains, 240, 249
Chekiang Province, 182
Chemical agents, 192
Cherbourg, 197
Chicago, USS (CA-29), 134
China, 181–88
China Strait, 162–63, 167
Chinese National Airways Corporation, 185–86
Cholera, 152
Chungking, 186
Churchill, Winston, 213, 217–18
Civil War, 2–3, 158
CNAC. *See* Chinese National Airways Corporation
Cockroaches, 48–49
Coggins, Cecil H., 28–33, 182–84
Cohn, Edwin, 209–11
Comfort, USS (AH-3), 158
Comfort, USS (AH-6), 160–70
Conard, Robert A., 130–37
Condon, Jean, 173–74
Congressional Medal of Honor, 4, 84, 114
Continental Congress, 1
Continental Navy, 1–2
Convoys, 161, 165, 169, 191, 198
Coral, 91–93
Corregidor, 36–45, 49–50
Crehan, Edward Patrick, 14
Crews, Jeremiah, 44–45
Crossing-the-line ceremony, 132
Crouch, Madge, 174, 235–37
Current, 165
Curtis, Don, 39

Dabrowski, Stanley E., 94–103, 212
Dartmouth, 191
Daub, Jack, 17
Davenport, Roy, 124–26
Daws, Gavan, 62
D-Day, 189–207
Dealey, Sam, 17
Delano, Laura, 219
Delirium, 155
Dengue, 64
Dental Corps, 3
Dental hygiene and care, 127, 137, 236, 241–46
Denver, USS (CL-58), 133
DePalma, Anthony, 176–78
Depth charges, 127
Desolation Point, 166
Destroyer Division 58, 9
Destroyer Division 62, 13
DeWitt, Gil, 104–6
Diarrhea, 90, 155, 229
Dietz, David, 221
Dinagat Islands, 165, 168
Divine guidance, 169–70
Dogfight, 171
Doolittle, James H., 40
Drinking water, 155
Drownings, 155, 193
DUKWs, 202
Duncan, Robert, 214
Dysentery, 58

Early, Steve, 215
E-boats, 191–92, 201–2
Eckstam, Eugene E., 191–94
Eden, Anthony, 218
Edsall, USS (DD-219), 9
Efate, 176
Elephantiasis, 64
Eleventh Airborne Division, 226
Empress Augusta Bay, 135
Eniwetok Atoll, 167, 174
Epinephrine, 198
Erickson, Ruth A., 25–27
Espíritu Santo, 176
Ethiopia, 5

Evening Armed Forces Tokyo Radio Station, 244
Exercise Tiger, 191–94
Explosions, 184
Explosives, 183
Eye problems, 65, 148

Falk, Victor S., 86–90
Fast, Chester K., 66–68
Feduik, Frank, 194–98
Feld, Irving, 247–49
Ferrall, William E., 120–21
Fires: forest, 164, 168–69; shipboard, 141–42, 146–47, 152
Flight nurses, 85, 104–13
Food, 8, 40, 47–49, 59, 64, 69–72, 81, 90–91, 95, 111, 231. *See also* Rice
Ford Island, 22
Forrestal, James, 117–18
Foster, George, 241–46
Fountain, Freeman P., 238–40
Fowey, Cornwall, 190, 192, 199
Fox, George, 147
Foxy 29, 192, 198, 204
Fractures, 236
Fraleigh, Claud, 57
Franklin, USS (CV-13), 129, 144–50
Fuelling, James, 147
Fuel oil, 23, 26–27, 45, 154–55, 157
Fultz, Harold F., 160–70
Furman, Robert R., 151
Fu Tso Yi, General, 186

Gallbladder colic, 219
Gangrene, 173
Gary, Donald, 147
Gas warfare, 148, 192
Geneva Accords, 160, 162, 176
Gibson, Sam, 208–11
Glassford, William A., Jr., 51
Glusman, Murray, 230, 232, 234
Gobi Desert, 186
Gonorrhea, 240
Grayback, USS (SS-208), 120
Greene, Ralph, 193
Grenades, 116

Groom, Dale L., 198–204
Guadalcanal, 86–87, 97, 133–34, 176, 194
Guam, 106–12, 149, 157, 177–78, 211, 228, 233
Guerrillas, 182, 187
Gyrocompass, 169

Hallucinations, 155
Halsey, William F., 33–34, 136
Hannigan, Robert E., 215
Harper, John, 214
Harrison, Joseph, 1
Hart, Lynn, 127
Hart, Thomas C., 51
Harukaze, 10
Haruna, 88
Hayes, Thomas, 38, 41–42, 66
Haynes, Lewis L., 13–17, 150–57
Heat problems, 133, 135
Hecla, HMS, 15
Heimlich, Henry J., 185–88
Henderson, USS (AP-1), 53, 170
Hill, Bill, 244
Hill 362, 101–2
Himes, Ethel, 170–72
Hitler, Adolph, 5
Hobcaw, 213, 216
Holdredge, Willard B., 44
Hollandia, 162–64, 166–69
Hollier, Fred, 117
Hogan, Bartholomew, 157
Homonhon, 165, 168
Hospital Corps, 3
Hospital ships, 143, 158–80
Howard, Sam, 12
Hsiao Sin-ju, Colonel, 183
Hurricanes, 16
Hypertension, 212
Hypothermia, 193
Hysteria, 155

India, 185
Indianapolis, USS (CA-35), 150–57
Inner Mongolia, 186–87
Intelligence, 29

International Military Tribunal Far East, 241–42, 245
Irvin, Ernest, 42–45, 234–35
Isabel, USS (PY-10), 12
Italy, 194
Iwo Jima, 93–110, 112–13

Jungferman, Rhea A., 173

Kamikaze, 139, 150–51, 170, 177, 232
Kelley, Sara Marcum, 205–7
Kempe, 232
Kempetai. *See* Kempe
Kendeigh, Jane, 102, 104–6
Kerama Retto, 177
Kilpatrick, MacGregor, 147
Kinkaid, Thomas C., 226 n, 227
Kirbow, Jack, 44
Kobe International Prisoner of War Hospital, 70–79, 231, 234
Koh Jin Tsuh, Colonel, 182
Kongo, 88
Kula Gulf, 136
Kurita, Takeo, 138
Kwashiorkor, 228

Lahey, Frank H., 214
Lally, Grace, 27–28
Landaal, Henry B., 199, 202–3
Latrine facilities, 80, 239
Laws, Clyde C., 174–75
Layton, Edwin T., 28
Leahy, William D., 218
Le Havre, 197
Leishmaniasis, 51
Lexington, USS (CV-2), 147
Leyte, 138, 165–68, 177, 211, 227
Liberty, 8, 240
Liberty ship, 198
Lice, 70
Lido Beach, Long Island, 192, 198
Life jackets, 141, 153–56
Lightning, 164, 168–69
Lingayen, 168, 226
Link trainer, 107
Lipes, Wheeler B., 5–8, 45–50, 120–25

Liu, Eddie, 183
Loblolly Boys, 1–3
Lockwood, Charles A., Jr., 122
Los Baños, 226–27
LST-293, 198
LST-314, 199–200
LST-338, 194–95
LST-357, 200
LST-391, 194
LST-507, 192
LST-515, 193
Luftwaffe, 197, 201
Lurline, 87
Luzon, USS (PG-47), 50–52
Lyme Bay, 191

MacArthur, Douglas, 56, 58, 213, 216 n, 217, 226, 227 n, 247
McDuffie, Basil, 88
MacInnis, Angus A., 186
McIntire, Ross T., 35, 128, 212–15, 220, 222
MacLeod, James J., 201
MacMahon, Jack, 241
McVay, Charles, 151–52
Malaria, 64, 83–84, 89
Malinta Tunnel, 39, 41, 44–45, 58
Mallory, Jack, 241–46
Manhattan Project, 150
Manila, 168, 224–28
Marine Corps, U.S., 28th Marine Regiment, 95–103
Maruyama, 230–32
MASH. *See* Mobile hospitals
Matsonia, 87
Mayfield, Irving, 29
Meat Grinder, 101
Medal of Honor. *See* Congressional Medal of Honor
Medical care: in air, 104–13; of Marine ground units, 83–103; in submarines, 119–28; in surface ships, 129–43
Mercy, USS, 143
Mercy ships. *See* Hospital ships
Merrill, Stanton, 135

Miles, Milton, 181–83
Miles, Pete, 226
Mindanao Sea, 168–69
Mindoro Strait, 168
Mines, 169, 196, 199
Mitre Rock, 164
Mobile hospitals, 182
Molotov, Vyacheslav, 218
Montgomery strap, 109
Montpelier, USS (CL-57), 130–37
Moon, The, 164–65, 168
Moore, Thomas, 120, 124–28
Morale, 71, 90, 112, 136
Morphine, 49–50, 84, 99, 109, 127, 133, 142, 153, 196, 198
Mount Suribachi, 94–100
Mussolini, Benito, 5

Nagasaki, 238–40
Nanking, 4, 53
Naval Group China, U.S., 181–86
Naval Medical School, Bethesda, Maryland, 211
Navigation, 162–65, 169
Navy Base Hospital #12, 204–5
Navy Commissioners, Board of, 2
Navy Department, 2
Navy Medical Department. *See* Bureau of Medicine and Surgery
Navy Nurse Corps, 2–3
Negros Island, 168
New Georgia, 134
New Guinea, 162–63
Newhouser, Lloyd, 211
New Zealand, 176
Nimitz, Chester W., 33, 128, 143, 149, 213, 216 n, 217
Nitro, USS (AE-2), 5–6
Nolan, James F., 151
Norfolk Naval Hospital, 3
North Africa, 190
Northern Ireland, 199
Nouméa, 137
Nurses, 25–28, 38, 53–60, 102, 167; on hospital ships, 170–75. *See also* Flight nurses; Navy Nurse Corps

Oak Knoll Naval Hospital, 222, 247–49
Oil, 23, 26–27, 45, 154–55, 157
Okinawa, 113, 130, 169, 177
Omaha Beach, 190–96, 201, 204
Osaka Red Cross Hospital, 230–34
Osborne, Weeden, 4
Overton, USS (DD-239), 13–17

Pact Doc, 182
Panay, USS (PR-5), 4–5, 50
Panic, 141
Parrott, USS (DD-218), 9–10
Paullin, James E., 214, 220
PBYs, 58
Pearl Harbor, 19–34, 175
Peleliu, 90–93, 157
Penicillin, 109, 171, 179, 187, 194, 206–7, 240
Peter Bent Brigham Hospital, 209–10
P-40s, 43–44, 52
Philadelphia Navy Yard, 131
Philippine Sea, 150
Phosphorus wounds, 110
Pidgeon, USS (AM-47), 49, 73
Pierson, Arthur H., 177
Pinkney, USS (APH-2), 176
Pittsburgh, USS (CA-72), 148
Plasma, 146, 173, 179–80, 198, 209–12
Plastic explosives, 183
Platter, George, 124–28
Plymouth, 191
Poland, 219
Polio, 215
Pottsdam Declaration, 235, 247
POWs. *See* Prisoners of War
Prettyman, Arthur, 220
Prinz Eugen, 16
Prisoners of War: American prisoners of the Japanese, 61–82, 224–37; German prisoners of the Allies, 196–97, 204; Japanese prisoners of the Allies, 30–33
Prostitution, 9–10, 240
Providence, 1
Psychiatric problems, 194
Puget Sound Navy Yard, 143

Pulsus alternans, 219
Purvis, Ann, 104–5
Purvis Bay, 136

Queen Mary, 194
Quincy, USS (CA-71), 217, 219 n

Radar, 136, 162
Radiation, 151
Ramsey, Helen Pavlovsky, 205–6
Ranger, USS (CV-4), 144
Ravdin, Isidor, 210
Raven Channel, 163, 167
Rector, Darrell Dean, 120–23
Red Beach, 165
Red Cross, 81, 193, 232–34
Red Rover, 2–3, 158
Reilly, Michael F., 217
Relief, USS, 4
Rendova, USS (CVE-114), 150
Rennell Islands, 133
Reuben James, USS (DD-245), 13–17
Rice, 74–80
Rice Paddy Navy, 182–86
Ringness, Henry R., 88–89
Rixey, USS (APH-3), 176–78
Roby, Harry, 120
Roe, USS (DD-418), 17
Roosevelt, Eleanor, 220, 222
Roosevelt, Franklin D., 13–14, 212–22
Royal Victoria Hospital, 204–5
"Ruptured Duck," 117

SACO. *See* Sino-American Cooperative Organization
Sacred Twenty, 3
St. Lo, USS, 248
Saipan, 136, 170–71
Sakamaki, Kazuo, 30–33
Salvarsan, 10
Samaritan, USS (AH-10), 102
San Bernardino Strait, 138
Sanders, Stan, 98
San Francisco Chronicle, 246
Sangley Point, 37–40, 42
Santee, USS (CVE-29), 139

Sante Fe, USS (CL-60), 147–48
Santo Thomas, 226
Schistosomiasis, 229
Seabees, 206
Seadler Harbor, 143
Seadragon, USS (SS-194), 47–48, 120
Sealion, USS (SS-195), 46–47, 123
Seasickness, 131, 161, 178–79, 195
Secret Service, 220
Serum Albumin, 101, 115, 209–12
Shanghai, 9–12
Shark, USS (SS-174), 46
Sharks, 150, 155–56
Shell shock, 207
Sherman, Samuel R., 144–50
Shmueck, John A., 153
Shock, 99, 112, 149
Shortland Islands, 135
Shoumatoff, Elizabeth, 220
Shuri Line, 113
Silversides, USS (SS-236), 120, 123–24
Sino-American Cooperative Organization, 181–86
Sisters of the Order of the Holy Cross, 2
Slapton Sands, 191
Smallpox, 239
Smith, Alfred L., 50–52, 57, 63–65, 224–25
Smith, Francis Kurt, 147
Smith, Stan, 230–32
Smoke screens, 177
SNAG 56, 205
Snow weasels, 197–98
SOC-1, 132
Sodium pentothal, 180
Solace, USS (AH-5), 4, 20, 27, 102, 158–59, 175
Soucy, Lee B., 20–25, 33–34
Spanish-American War, 3
Spearfish, USS (SS-190), 59
Sproul, Mary, 211
Spruance, Raymond, 33, 151
Stalin, Joseph, 213, 217–18
Stegall, Richard, 125
Steichen, Edward, 104
Sternberg Army Hospital, 53–55

Stettinius, Edward R., Jr., 218
Stewart, USS (DD-224), 9
Still, Dorothy, 53–55, 225–28
Stratton, Darrell A., 195
Sturtevant, USS (DD-240), 13–17
Subic Bay, 168
Submarine duty, 45–49, 119–28
Suckley, Margaret, 219
Sugamo prison, 241
Suicides, 136–37, 241
Sulfa drugs, 109, 171, 187, 206–7
Sulu Sea, 168
Sumner, Gordon, 22–24
Supplies, 97, 141, 203
Surgeon's steward, 3
Surrender, Japanese, 247–49
Suwannee, USS (CVE-27), 137–43
Syphilis, 9, 187
Szabo, George J., 203

Tacloban, 168
Taffy 1, 138
Taffy 3, 138
Tai Li, Lieutenant General, 181–84
Tarawa, 138
Tetanus, 71
Texas, USS (BB-35), 6–7, 195, 202
361st Station Hospital, 241
Tillinghast, Henry, 1
Tinian, 151
Tiny Tim heavy rockets, 146
Tojo, Hideki, 240–46
Tokyo, 230–31, 241–46
Tokyo Bay, 235
Tokyo Express, 134
Tokyo Rose, 162, 167
Torpedo attacks, 133–34, 152–54, 192–93, 199
Traveling Lizard, 17
Truman, Harry S., 118
Tryon, USS (APH-1), 176
Tsuruga Camp, 229
Tuberculosis, 64, 69–70, 236
Tufi Leads, 162–65, 167
Tung An, 182
Turkey Knob, 101

Turnbuckle, 178
28th Marine Regiment, 95–103
Typhoon, 166, 232

U-boats, 13, 16–17, 198
Ulithi Atoll, 148–49, 169
Ushijima Mitsuru, 113
Utah, USS (AG-16), 20–25, 34
Utah Beach, 190–94

Vacek, Laddie, 246–47
Van Wagner, Kathryn, 106–13, 228–29
Venereal disease. *See* Gonorrhea; Syphilis
V-J Day, 247
Voge, Richard, 47

Wainwright, Jonathan, 58, 66–67
War crimes trials. *See* International Military Tribunal Far East
"Washing Machine Charlie," 89

Wasley, Jim, 244–46
Watson, Edwin M., 218–19
Webb, William, 246
Weller, George, 120, 122–23
West Point, USS (AP-23), 60
Wheeler Point, 39–41
Wilson, Louis, 118
Woodruff, Lorande, 209–10
World War I, 3, 5
Worthington, Robert, 126
Wounds, 54, 111–12, 130, 140

X-ray, 177, 247

Yalta, 217–19
Yangtze Patrol, 4
Yokohama, 230–31, 233, 235
Yorktown, USS (CV-5), 147

Zeilin, USS (APA-3), 87
Zero (Japanese fighter), 111, 171

ABOUT THE AUTHOR

Jan K. Herman received his master's degree in history from the University of New Hampshire, where he was a Ford Foundation teaching fellow. After serving in the U.S. Air Force, he became a public affairs specialist in the Department of State and assistant to the department spokesman. Mr. Herman joined the Navy Bureau of Medicine and Surgery in 1979, becoming editor of *Navy Medicine* magazine, historian of the Navy Medical Department, and curator of the old U.S. Naval Observatory.

Mr. Herman has lectured for the Albert Einstein Planetarium of the National Air and Space Museum, the National Academy of Sciences, the Smithsonian Institution Resident Associate Program, the Explorer's Club, the Historical Society of Washington, and the Naval Historical Center. He represented the U.S. Navy at the Longitude Zero Conference commemorating the centennial of the Greenwich Meridian at the National Maritime Museum in Greenwich, England. In the summer of 1992, he represented the Navy Medical Department as guest lecturer for Project Marco Polo, the joint Navy–National Geographic Society expedition to Egypt, the Mediterranean, and Greece.

The **Naval Institute Press** is the book-publishing arm of the U.S. Naval Institute, a private, nonprofit, membership society for sea service professionals and others who share an interest in naval and maritime affairs. Established in 1873 at the U.S. Naval Academy in Annapolis, Maryland, where its offices remain today, the Naval Institute has members worldwide.

Members of the Naval Institute support the education programs of the society and receive the influential monthly magazine *Proceedings* and discounts on fine nautical prints and on ship and aircraft photos. They also have access to the transcripts of the Institute's Oral History Program and get discounted admission to any of the Institute-sponsored seminars offered around the country.

The Naval Institute also publishes *Naval History* magazine. This colorful bimonthly is filled with entertaining and thought-provoking articles, first-person reminiscences, and dramatic art and photography. Members receive a discount on *Naval History* subscriptions.

The Naval Institute's book-publishing program, begun in 1898 with basic guides to naval practices, has broadened its scope in recent years to include books of more general interest. Now the Naval Institute Press publishes about 100 titles each year, ranging from how-to books on boating and navigation to battle histories, biographies, ship and aircraft guides, and novels. Institute members receive discounts of 20 to 50 percent on the Press's nearly 600 books in print.

Full-time students are eligible for special half-price membership rates. Life memberships are also available.

For a free catalog describing Naval Institute Press books currently available, and for further information about subscribing to *Naval History* magazine or about joining the U.S. Naval Institute, please write to:

Membership Department
U.S. Naval Institute
118 Maryland Avenue
Annapolis, MD 21402-5035
Telephone: (800) 233-8764
Fax: (410) 269-7940
Web address: www.usni.org